MW01122505

THE CREATIVE THERAPIES
AND EATING DISORDERS

_160201_

THE CREATIVE THERAPIES AND EATING DISORDERS

By

STEPHANIE L. BROOKE, Ph.D., NCC

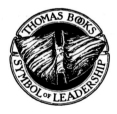

CHARLES C THOMAS • PUBLISHER, LTD.
Springfield • Illinois • U.S.A.

Published and Distributed Throughout the World by

CHARLES C THOMAS • PUBLISHER, LTD.
2600 South First Street
Springfield, Illinois 62704

©2008 by CHARLES C THOMAS • PUBLISHER, LTD.

ISBN 978-0-398-07758-7 (hard)
ISBN 978-0-398-07759-4 (paper)

Library of Congress Catalog Card Number: 2007012283

With THOMAS BOOKS *careful attention is given to all details of manufacturing and design. It is the Publisher's desire to present books that are satisfactory as to their physical qualities and artistic possibilities and appropriate for their particular use.* THOMAS BOOKS *will be true to those laws of quality that assure a good name and good will.*

Printed in the United States of America
CR-R-3

Library of Congress Cataloging-in-Publication Data

The Creative therapies and eating disorders / [edited] by Stephanie
L. Brooke.
   p. ; cm.
Included bibliographical references and index.
ISBN 978-0-398-07758-7 (hard) -- ISBN 978-0-398-07759-4 (pbk.)
1. Eating disorders--Treatment. 2. Creation (Literary, artistic, etc.)--
Therapeutic use. 3. Arts--Therapeutic use. I. Brooke, Stephanie L.
[DNLM: 1. Eating Disorders--therapy. 2. Psychotherapy--methods.
3. Sensory Art Therapies--methods. WM 175 C912 2007]

RC552.E18C73 2007
362.196'852606--dc22

                                                           2007012283

CONTRIBUTORS

I extend my deepest appreciation to the following contributors for sharing their expertise and experience about their work with eating disorders. Each of these contributors was selected on the basis of his or her experience with respect to clinical issues, diversity in theoretical orientation, or treatment modality. As you read each chapter, it is my hope you will share in my appreciation for the insights contributed by the following individuals:

Geneva Reynaga-Abiko, Psy.D.

Julia Andersen MA.,ATR-BC.

Brian L. Bethel, M.Ed., PCC, LCDC III

Donna J. Betts, Ph.D., ATR-BC

Marah Bobilin, MA, MT-BC

Michelle L. Dean, MA, ATR-BC, LPC

Claire Edwards, MA (Hons) Art Therapy

Cosmin Gheorghe, MFT

Annie Heiderscheit, Ph.D., MT-BC, FAMI, NMT

Shinta Hermanns, PG Dip, MA

Lisa D. Hinz, Ph.D., ATR

Kate Hudgins, Ph.D., TEP

Amy Jerslid, M.S.W.

Kathryn N. Klinger

Charles E. Myers, M.A., LPC, LMHC, NCC, NCSC, RPT-S

Sheila Rubin, LMFT, RDT/BCT

Priyadarshini Senroy, MA, DMT, CCC

PREFACE

The *Creative Therapies and Eating Disorders* is a comprehensive work that examines the use of art, play, music, dance/movement, drama, and spirituality to treatment issues relating to eating disturbance. The author's primary purpose is to examine treatments approaches which cover the broad spectrum of the creative art therapies. The collection of chapters is written by renowned, well-credentialed, and professional creative art therapists in the areas of art, play, music, dance/movement, and drama. In addition, some of the chapters are complimented with photographs of client art work, diagrams, and tables. The reader is provided with a snapshot of how these various creative art therapies are used to treat male and females suffering from eating disorders. This informative book will be of special interest to educators, students, and therapists as well as people struggling with eating disorders.

S.L.B.

CONTENTS

THE CREATIVE THERAPIES
AND EATING DISORDERS

And now?

Somewhere inside the stone I see my breath against the glass
At the centre behind the glass, suffocation
Hospital smells and sticky dimpled peas glued to steaming plastic trays
The walls here are thick and no one hears me
My hands, clawing, praying, hoping
My legs crimp, paralysed expression
My cries are swallowed, something inside me pulls my voice downwards
Famine
Only faint echoes, no one must hear
Shh . . .

I am cold, shivering
My stomach swells
Powdered pills and false compassion
Darkness intrudes, the path is full of shadows
I am floating
Pushing from the inside
Light, light as a feather
Trying to get out
I do not feel
Trying to be released
The silence hammers into my head
Alone, marrying my appetite
Do not speak, do not move
Craving freedom
Blackout, curtain . . .
Gingerly crawling back behind the stone
I look through the glass
Only remnants of my breath, clinging
I cease to be

Chapter 1

EATING DISORDERS ACROSS THE WORLD

Stephanie L. Brooke

Was macht mir umbricht, macht mir starker.
Nietze

Introduction

Although typically thought of as a woman's disease, eating disorders affect men and women alike as they emerge into culture and society. Research from the course of the latter half of the twentieth century indicate that eating disorders exist in many corners of the world, even those thought to be protected from such disorders (Nasser et al., 2001). Why is there an obsession with food across cultures? Why is there an epidemic of suffering among people at a moment when men and women are reaching out to find a place for themselves in society? Some view eating disorders as a inherent struggle with identity (Chernin, 1985). The purpose of this chapter will be to take a look at the research of eating disorders in countries across the world.

Widely considered a Western phenomena, eating disorders are also pervasive in Eastern cultures and appeared in their literature in the 1970s (Soh, Touyz, & Surgenor, 2006). In fact, eating disorders were thought to be rare in non–western cultures. However, as far back as the seventeenth century, eating disorders have been recognized as a problem. For instance, in Japan, the word, fushokubyo or non–eating illness was described in Kagaywa in the seventeenth and eighteenth centuries (Soh, Touyz, & Surgenor, 2006). Most of the people were women and the illness was thought to be psychological in origin.

Many cross–cultural studies will look at ethnicity in relation to the development of eating disorders. Specifically, it is thought that the more acculturated the person, the more likely he or she will develop an eating disorder (Al–Subaic, 2000; Furukawa, 2002). The results in the literature have been quite mixed on this line of thought:

3

Thus exposure to Western culture is not irrefutably associated with eating disturbances, nor with body image issues and their associated desire for slimness which are commonly appearing variables in etiological models of eating disorders. However, interpretation of the results is hampered as many cross–cultural studies only take ethnicity into account and do not quantitate the degree of acculturation into Western society or the level of retention of traditional values. (Soh, Touyz, & Surgenor, 2006, p. 57)

Culture itself is a complex term referring to language, beliefs, myths, customs and symbols associated with a culture. "The experience and exposure to the difference between two cultures, rather than a particular culture itself, is also hypothesized to contribute to the etiology of eating and body image disturbances" (Soh, Tyouyz, & Surgenor, 2006, p. 58). A class between the traditional culture and the adopted culture may cause a disruption in eating and body disturbance.

Africa

One study used a survey method to establish levels of eating disorders in Black and White female students is South Africa. Young Black females that showed high risk for developing or having an eating disorder were interviewed. Although thought to be a problem of Caucasian South Africans, the survey found that Black girls were as likely as White girls to have eating disorders. The girls ranged in age from 15–25. In some cases, this was also true of males. As opposed to self–starvation, the common disorder found among Black South Africans was bulimia nervosa. The incidence of eating disorders in young girls from other African countries was rarely reported. The authors mentioned the problems with surveys followed up by interviews. "Relying on self–report measure alone will provide an indication of eating disorder pathology, but not a eating disorder diagnosis" (LeGrange et al., 2004, p. 440). Therefore, the authors recommend a two–stage screening process – surveys followed by interviews. Out of the rapid socio–cultural change in South African, there has been a rise in eating disorders in Black youth. LeGrange and colleagues (2004) found significantly greater eating disorder pathology in Black high school students than their white or mixed race counterparts in South Africa. LeGrange and colleagues postulate several reasons for this emergence of eating disorders. First, the rapid socio–political changes in South Africa have challenged the traditional gender roles leaving Black women unprepared for the new role and thus vulnerable to developing an eating disorder. Second, with the abolition of Apartheid in 1994, there is increased exposure to the Western culture. This has caused a shift from collectivism to individualism.

Australia and Hong Kong

Sheffield and colleagues (2005) conducted a cross–cultural study to test the validity of a biopsychosocial mediation model that hypothesized a variety of biological, psychological, and social variables would have an impact on eating disturbance through the mediation of body image dissatisfaction. Hong Kong has shown a considerable rise in eating disorders. "While Chinese people have traditionally emphasized that attractiveness is based on the beauty of facial features rather than body shape, recent research has shown that young Chinese women in Hong Kong share the same ideal of slimness as Caucasian women in western societies, although relatively few engage in serious dieting" (Sheffield, Tse, & Sofronoff, 2005, p. 114). One hundred Australian females, ranging in age from 17–28, and 48 women from Hong Kong were examined. Although no significant differences were found between the groups of women in levels of body dissatisfaction and eating disturbance, different variables in the biopsychosoical model predicted their risk of developing eating disorders. The researchers found important cultural differences in aspects of dieting and body images between the two groups. For Australian women, body dissatisfaction directly influenced and mediated the effects of self–esteem. For Hong Kong women, body dissatisfaction was no longer a significant predictor of eating disturbance, while self–esteem had a direct effect on eating disturbance. "The results indicate that risk factors contributing to body dissatisfaction and eating disturbance are not the same for Australian and Hong Kong women, signifying that cultural differences appear to exist in the prediction of eating disorder symptomotology" (Sheffield, Tse, & Sofronoff, 2005, p. 120).

China

A study of 301 Chinese immigrants in New Zealand examined eating disorder symptomotology using the Eating Disorder Inventory (EDI), the Positive and Negative Perfectionism Scale (PANPS), the Multigroup Ethnic Identity Method (MEIM), and the short form of the Marlow–Crown Social Desirability Scale (MCSDS) (Chan & Owens, 2006). As measured by the EDI, negative perfectionism (e.g., drive for thinness, bulimia, and body dissatisfaction) significantly predicted more eating disorder symptoms. Positive perfectionism was associated with some psychological correlates of disordered eating through some components of acculturation and ethnic identity. "The relationship between Negative Perfectionism and disordered eating may be partly explained in the context of Chinese culture, in conjunction with the influence of Confucian heritage. The Confucian emphasis, on social norms and behaviors, should be modeled with reference to ideal types to avoid shame" (Chan & Owens, 2006, p. 60). When immigrating to another country, Chinese women may want to save face by escaping disapproval and avoiding shame, thus eating disorders may develop. There were limitations to this study. The population of New Zealand is diverse making the question of acculturation to the dominant culture complex. The authors admit that the population sample may represent more traditional Chinese values as opposed to those who were acculturated. The study did find some avenues for preventing eating disorders in an at–risk Chinese population.

Japan

"As the first non–Western nation in contemporary history to become a major industrialized economic power, Japan is central to the debate on cultural relativism in psychiatric nosologies, and the study of eating disorders in Japan contributes to the complex discussion of the impact of culture and history on the experience, diagnosis, and treatments of such disorders" (Pike & Borovoy, 2004, p. 493). The authors contribute the rise in eating disorders in Japan to increasing industrialization, urbanization, and the breakdown in traditional family forms following World War II. Pike and Borovoy (2004) used a case approach to examine the etiology of eating disorders in Japanese women. Their work analyzed the cultural factors associated with the rise of eating disorders in Japan: (1) dominant cultural expectations for young women in contemporary Japan and models of marriage, gender, and adulthood; (2) cultural dimension of society beauty ideals specifically with respect to weight and shape. Beginning in the 1970s, case reports of eating disorders in Japan emerged in the literature. Through the 1980s, documented cases began to grow, increasing twofold from the previous decade. In the 1990s, it increased fourfold. "The data from the most recent studies indicate that the number of Japanese women pursuing the thin ideal is still increasing, and such weight data may be intimately linked with increases in eating disorders as well" (Pike & Bovoroy, p. 497).

Germany and Japan

Kusano–Schwartz and von Wietersheim (2005) compared data for women with bulimia nervosa and to a healthy control group for both Germany and Japan. They used the Eating Disorder Inventory (EDI–2). Interestingly, the Japanese control group showed significantly higher values on nearly all EDI scales as compared to the German control group. Comparing the German and Japanese bulimia nervosa patients, Kusano–Schwartz and von Wietersheim (2005) found that Japanese women showed higher scores on three EDI scales compared to the German group but these results were negligible. The authors concluded that sociocultural factors, specifically, the dependence on social norms, may have contributed to the high EDI values in Japanese women. In German culture, society values independence, self–assertion, self–confidence, and individuality. Whereas in Japanese culture, attentiveness, modesty, and respect toward other people are important values. Both societies may deal differently with the value of slimness. The study did have weaknesses such as the lack of matching samples and the fact that the EDI Japanese version was not validated.

Mexico

In a non–urban area, Michoacan, Mexico, Bojorquez and Unikel (2004) found a dangerously high incidence of eating disorders among teenage girls. Using a sample of 458 girls, 27.9 percent were seriously concerned about weighing too much, 14.3 percent were dieting or fasting to lose weight, and 2.4 percent binged and vomited. This was significantly higher than a representative group of Mexico City girls. They propose that culture is a important risk factor in the development of eating disorders. "The ED/culture relationship could be better understood if we stopped using the concept of culture in its vaguest sense in favour of a more precise definition. The use of analytical tools such as concepts of ideology, gender construction and gender demonstration would allow a more useful vision of the relation between cultural values and individual practices" (Boroquez & Unikel, 2004, p. 2001).

Conclusion

"As more eating disorder cases are identified around the globe, certain identifiable risk factors (e.g., female gender) and social conditions (industrialization, democratization, and rapid social change) appear to be common denominators in setting the stage for the development of eating disorders" (Pike & Borovoy, 2004, p. 4949). Psychological, developmental, and biological individual differences interact with cultural dimensions to account for the reason why people develop eating disorders. This chapter is by no means a comprehensive view of all cultures but is meant to give a glimpse of cultural issues and eating disorders around the world.

This book will take a look at the use of the creative therapies as a possible treatment option for working with clients who are diagnosed with eating disorders. For instance, art therapy with people with eating disturbance reveals body image disturbance, depression, and obsessive compulsive features in the art work (Acharya, Wood, & Robinson, 1995). Chapters 2 through 5 cover art therapy.

Using a case approach, play therapy has been used to treat very young children with eating problems (Honjo et al., 2005). Chapter 6 covers play therapy and discusses sandtray work. Chapter 7 provides an overview of play therapy techniques with children who have been diagnosed with eating disorders.

Cognitive behavioral music therapy as been used in a women's residential treatment facility for eating disorders (Hillard, 2001). "Quite often, primary therapists reported that patients retold incidents of when music therapy assisted them through a crisis helped them challenge cognitive distortions, and gain insight" (Hillard, 2001, p. 112). Chapters 8 through 10 cover music therapy. In addition, Chapter 10 discusses the use of poetry therapy in treating eating disorders. Woodall (1983) found that poetry therapy produced significant change in anorexic patients.

Drama therapy has been used in the treatment of eating disorders. (Jacobse, 1995)

By setting less rigid boundaries, the anorexia nervous patient will extend her role repertoire. By setting clearer boundaries, the bulimia nervosa patient will learn to avoid melting into her role, the scenery or other actors. The contrasts in particular between the two patient groups, mean that the two groups have a lot to offer to and learn from each other. (Jacobse, 1995, p. 142)

Callahan (1989) used psychodrama in the treatment of bulimia. "I have found psychodrama techniques to be highly effective for many bulimic clients, in particular, helping people in their efforts to overcome blocks to emotional experience and to gain access to hidden parts of the self" (Callahan, 1989, p. 106). Chapters 11–14 cover drama therapy

"The symptoms of eating disorders serve to disconnect affect from the body, particularly as sexuality, trauma, and cultural influences contribute to conflict in the woman's developmental struggle for self–identity" (Krantz, 1999). Krantz used dance therapy to help eating disordered clients reconnect the body with feelings, to recognize meaning in behavior, and to develop psychophysical unity. Chapters 13 and 14 combine drama and movement therapy for treating eating disorders.

Chapter 15 is a unique work focusing on the use of spirituality as a creative modality for treating eating disorders. Chapter 16 covers supervision issues and the Therapeutic Spiral Model. And last, Chapter 17 discusses ethical considerations when using the creative therapies to treat people with eating disturbances.

Appendix–Terms

Acculturation–The modification of the culture of a group or individual as a result of contact with a different culture. The process by which the culture of a particular society is instilled in a human from infancy onward. http://www.answers.com/topic/acculturation

Anorexia nervosa–Anorexia nervosa is an eating disorder that occurs primarily among girls and women. It is characterized by a fear of gaining weight, self–starvation, and a distorted view of body image. The condition is usually brought on by emotional disorders that lead a person to worry excessively about the appearance of his or her body. There are generally two types of anorexia: one is characterized by strict dieting and exercising; the other type includes binging and purging. Binging is the act of eating abnormally large amounts of food in a short period of time. Purging is the use of vomiting or other methods, such as laxatives, to empty the stomach. An individual who suffers from anorexia is called anorexic. http://www.faqs.org/health/Sick–V1/Anorexia–Nervosa.html

Bulimia nervosa–Bulimia is an illness defined by food binges, or recurrent episodes of significant overeating, that are accompanied by a sense of loss of control. The affected person then uses various methods–such as vomiting or laxative abuse–to prevent weight gain. Many, but not all, people with bulimia may also suffer from anorexia nervosa, an eating disorder involving severe, chronic weight loss that proceeds to starvation. http://www.nlm.nih.gov/medlineplus/print/ency/article/000341.htm

Collectivism–Collectivism is defined as the theory and practice that makes some sort of group rather than the individual the fundamental unit of political, social, and economic concern. In theory, collectivists insist that the claims of groups, associations, or the state must normally supersede the claims of individuals. http://freedomkeys.com/collectivism.htm

Culture–(from the Latin cultural stemming from colere, meaning "to cultivate"), generally refers to patterns of human activity and the symbolic structures that give such activity significance. Different definitions of "culture" reflect different theoretical bases for understanding, or criteria for evaluating, human activity. http://uk.answers.yahoo.com/question/index?qid=2007012 2130531AASvfzM

Cultural relativism–Different cultural groups think, feel, and act differently. There are no scientific standards for considering one group as intrinsically superior or inferior to another. Studying differences in culture among groups and societies presupposes a position of cultural relativism. It does not imply normalcy for oneself, or for one's society. It, however, calls for judgment when dealing with groups or societies different from one's own. Information about the nature of cultural differences between societies, their roots, and their consequences should precede judgment and action. Negotiation is more likely to succeed when the parties concerned understand the reasons for the differences in viewpoints. http://www.tamu.edu/classes/cosc/choudhury/culture.html

Individualism—Individualism is at once an ethical–psychological concept and an ethical–political one. As an ethical–psychological concept, individualism holds that a human being should think and judge independently, respecting nothing more than the sovereignty of his or her mind; thus, it is intimately connected with the concept of autonomy. As an ethical–political concept, individualism upholds the supremacy of individual rights. http://freedomkeys.com/collectivism.htm

References

Acharya, M., Wood, M. J. M., & Robinson, P.H. (1995). What can the art of anorexic patients tell us about their internal world: A case study. *European Eating Disorders Review, 3*(4), 242–254.

Al–Subaic, A. S. (2000). Some correlates of dieting behavior in Saudi schoolgirls. *International Journal of Eating Disorders, 28*, 242–246.

Bojorquez, I., & Unikel, C. (2004). Presence of eating disorders among Mexican teenage women from semi–urban area: Its relation to a cultural hypothesis. *European Eating Disorders Review, 12*, 197–202.

Callahan, M. L. (1989). Psychodrama and the treatment of bulimia. In L. M. Hornyak & E. K. Bakers (Eds.), *Experiential therapies for eating disorders* (pp. 101–120). New York: The Guilford Press.

Chan, C. Y., & Owens, G. (2006). Perfectionism and eating disorder symptomotology in Chinese Immigrants: Mediating and moderating effects of ethnic identity and acculturation. *Psychology and Health, 21*(1), 49–63.

Chernin, K. (1985). *The hungry self.* New York: Times Books.

Furukawa, T. (2002). Weight changes and eating attitudes of Japanese adolescents under acultural stresses. *International Journal of Eating Disorders, 12*, 71–79.

Hillard, R. (2001). The use of cognitive–behavioral music therapy in the treatment of women with eating disorders. *Music Therapy Perspectives, 19*, 109–113.

Honjo, S., Sasaki, Y., Murase, S., Kaneko, H., & Namura, K. (2005). Transient eating disorder in early childhood: A case report. *Early Child Adolescent Psychiatry, 14*, 52–54.

Jacobse, A. (1995). The use of dramatherapy in the treatment of eating disorders. In D. Dokter, (Ed.), *Arts therapies and clients with eating disorders: Fragile board* (pp. 124–143). Philadelphia, PA: Jessica Kingsley Publishers.

Krantz, A. M. (1999). Growing into her body. Dance/movement therapy for women with eating disorders. *American Journal of Dance Therapy, 21*(2), 81–103.

Kusano–Schwartz, M., & von Wietersheim, J. (2005). EDI results of Japanese and German women and possible sociocultural explanations. *European Eating Disorders Review, 13*, 411–416.

LeGrange, D., Louw, J., Breen, A., & Katzman, M.A. (2004). *Culture, Medicine and Psychiatry, 28,* 439–462.
Nasser, M., Katzman, M. A., & Gordon, R. A. (2001). *Eating disorders and cultures in transition.* London: Brunner–Routeledge.
Pike, K. M., & Borovoy, A. (2004). *Culture, Medicine and Psychiatry, 28,* 493–531.
Sheffield, J. K., Tse, K. H., & Sofronoff, K. (2005). A comparison of body image dissatisfaction and eating disturbance among Australian and Hong Kong women. *European Eating Disorders Review, 13,* 112–124.
Soh, N. L., Touyz, S. W., & Surgenor, L. J. (2006). Eating and body image disturbances across cultures: A review. *European Eating Disorders Review, 14,* 54–65.
Woodall, C. (1983). *Eating disorders, body image and self–hate.* Unpublished doctoral dissertation, Rutgers State University, Newark, NJ.

Biography

Stephanie L. Brooke, Ph.D., NCC, teaches sociology and psychology online at the University of Phoenix, Excelsior College, University of Maryland, and Capella University. She also has written books on art therapy and edits books on the use of the creative therapies. In October 2006, she was the chief consultant for the first Creative Art Therapy Conference in Tokyo, Japan. Doctor Brooke continues to write and publish in her field. Further, Dr. Brooke serves on the editorial boards of PSYCCritiques and the International Journal of Teaching and Learning in Higher Education. She is Vice Chairperson for ARIA (Awareness of Rape and Incest through Art). For more information about Doctor Brooke, please visit her web site: http://www.stephanielbrooke.com.

Chapter 2

ART THERAPY APPROACHES TO WORKING WITH PEOPLE WHO HAVE EATING DISORDERS

DONNA J. BETTS

This chapter provides information about the use of art therapy with an adolescent and adult population of individuals who have eating disorders. The Canopy Cove eating disorder clinic in Tallahassee, Florida, is described, including an overview of the Recovery Model treatment approach (Reiff & Reiff, 1992). The benefits of art therapy with this patient population are discussed, and a description of art therapy approaches for individuals and groups is offered. Treatment goals are delineated in the context of recommended art interventions.

Canopy Cove Eating Disorder Treatment Center

Canopy Cove is a partial hospitalization program located in Tallahassee, Florida, that provides clients with an independent living situation (Canopy Cove, 2006a). Clients must demonstrate medical stability in order to be eligible for the program. Only eight clients are accepted at a time, which enables the staff to individualize treatment plans to meet specific needs. The patient population consists of adolescents, men, and women with anorexia nervosa, bulimia nervosa, binge eating/overeating disorders, and eating disorder not otherwise specified.

Clients live in the city of Tallahassee for the duration of their treatment, and as a part of their therapeutic experience, they reside in a one–bedroom apartment furnished by the clinic. This unique situation provides an environment that is more similar to what clients would experience when at home: They prepare all of their own meals, shop for groceries (with staff guidance), and face the daily task of dealing with food, both at the clinic during the daytime and at their apartment in the evening.

The program requires a minimum stay of 30 days. Often, a 45–60 day stay is necessary to resolve underlying issues and to stabilize the severe symptoms of an eating disorder. Each client recovers at his or her own pace, and the staff continually make recommendations for a decreasing level of treatment based on client needs. Step–down/aftercare can continue for as long as is required.

Weight Stabilization and Meals

In order to ensure continued medical stability and progress, weight stabilization is addressed on an individual basis. Meal plans are developed to make certain that each person who needs to gain weight does so in a safe and gradual manner. Canopy Cove patients meet weekly with a nutritionist, who aids them in creating a balanced meal plan. Each day the clients prepare and eat their breakfast with the staff beginning at 8:30 a.m. Staff facilitators participate in each meal and are present to guide both the meal time and the meal process session, which entails a discussion of food and feelings about the meal experience. Lunch takes place from 12:00 p.m. until 1:00 p.m., and an afternoon snack follows at 3:45 p.m. Process time takes place after meals, and clients are encouraged to discuss any successes and/or difficulties they may have experienced. In the evenings, clients are held accountable for preparing and eating their own dinner, according to their meal plan.

Medical Services

Consulting physicians and psychiatrists work closely with the Canopy Cove staff. Patients are seen as often as is needed during their treatment stay. The office visits help to ensure medical stability and provide ongoing monitoring of bone density, heart rate, blood pressure, other indicators of health, and medications. It is common practice to prescribe anti–depressant, anti–anxiety, and anti–psychotic medications to clients with eating disorders. For example, an anti–psychotic such as Geodon can facilitate reduction of obsessive thoughts related to food and body image distortions.

Daily Schedule

In the partial–hospitalization program there are 10 forty–five–minute therapy sessions most days from 8:30 a.m. until 4:30 p.m. After breakfast, group members share their individual homework exercises in the opening session. These exercises, completed the evening before, give clients the opportunity to reflect on their feelings and responses to daily events, thereby increasing their self–awareness and sense of self–efficacy. Following afternoon snack, there is a closing session that includes directed planning for the evening. Throughout the day, various mental health professionals facilitate all of the therapy sessions. The staff includes psychologists, social workers, an art therapist, a music therapist, a dietitian, a spirituality counselor, and a yoga instructor. The daily sessions are a combination of individual and group therapy, as well as weekly family therapy sessions. Equine–assisted therapy is also offered.

Therapy: The Recovery Model

Many different approaches are used in the treatment of eating disorders. Two of the most recognized are the Addiction Model (or the Twelve Step Model), and the Recovery Model (Reiff & Reiff, 1992). Canopy Cove operates under the premise that the Recovery Model is more effective than the Addiction Model in treating eating disorders. The Addiction Model stipulates that recovery from an eating disorder is not possible, and that food is an addictive substance. Many have criticized this position (Costin, 1999). Conversely, the Recovery Model maintains that a full recovery is possible, and the eating disorder is identified as a symptom of deeper, unresolved issues (Reiff & Reiff, 1992).

The Recovery Model encompasses behavioral change, personal growth, and the development of life management skills. It is not enough for a person with anorexia to put on weight: His or her distorted body image must also be corrected in order to sustain recovery (Kaslow & Eicher, 1988; Mitchell, 1980). Fundamental problems in the client's functioning must be acknowledged (Mitchell, 1980). Thus, in addition to developing a more balanced relationship with food, patients are assisted in identifying and resolving the underlying causes of their eating disorder through psychotherapy, as well as the expressive therapies.

Step–Down and Aftercare

Toward the end of a client's minimum required stay, the treatment team makes recommendations to meet the client's continued needs. This can range anywhere from an additional 15 days of treatment, to a few days a week, etc., eventually culminating in out–patient care with several sessions during each week.

This section provided an overview of the program at Canopy Cove, and a description of the Recovery Model. Information about the nutrition program, medical services, therapy, step–down and aftercare was delineated. The remainder of this chapter focuses on the benefits of art therapy in working with this population. Techniques and treatment goals employed in the art therapy program at Canopy Cove are outlined.

Art Therapy and Eating Disorders

Art therapy is an effective modality for helping people with eating disorders (Kaslow & Eicher, 1988; Matto, 1997; Mitchell, 1980; Naitove, 1986; Schaverien, 1995; Wolf, Willmuth & Watkins, 1986; Zerbe, 1993). The creative arts promote new insight and awareness for clients through the process of self–expression (Mitchell, 1980). This treatment approach also provides the individual with freedom of expression and the opportunity to develop a better understanding of his or her underlying psychological issues in a non–threatening environment. When making art, the client creates new and more positive associations with his or her True Self: in this context, "True Self" refers to the attributes of an individual's identity that contribute to a sense of wholeness and well–being. One client explained that her eating–disordered thoughts make it hard for her to be fully present, in the here–and–now, but that when she is engaged in the creative process she is more present and in touch with her True Self than at any other time of the day.

The symbolic behaviors of people with eating disorders correspond with qualities inherent in arts therapies approaches (Naitove, 1986). For example, control and perfectionism issues can be directly addressed by using art materials. Clients can gain a sense of self–efficacy when they experience mastery of the materials, or they can confront their feelings about being imperfect when a painting does not turn out exactly the way they had expected.

Art materials and food share this commonality – they are tactile, substantive products with texture (Schaverien, 1995). Sometimes this similarity manifests itself in the way clients use art materials. For instance, people with bulimia might have a looser and more excessive way of working with art media, whereas those with anorexia might have a more restrictive and selective approach (Matto, 1997). Thus, challenging clients to experiment with various art materials and to modify their way of relating with the media can assist them in confronting their maladaptive belief systems about food.

Eating disorders, particularly anorexia nervosa, are characterized by a "disturbance of delusional proportions in the body image and the body concept" (Mitchell, 1980, p. 54). The expressive arts therapies help the client to create an inner image of his or her body in a safe manner (Zerbe, 1993). Furthermore, many arts therapies techniques are conducive to the development of a trusting relationship between the client and therapist, and in turn, between the client and his or her body. Body image is multidimensional and includes affective, cognitive, perceptual, and interpersonal levels (Kaslow & Eicher, 1988). Thus, a multimodal treatment approach is ideal for helping clients cope with significant body image disturbance.

The most effective method for dealing with body image issues includes both verbal and non–verbal psychotherapy approaches (Kaslow & Eicher, 1988). Unlike verbal therapy, art has a material presence – it takes on a life of its own, whereas words simply vanish (Wolf et al., 1986). "Since a primary vehicle of communication for anorexics is their body it was thought that a model of therapy that combined both verbal and non–verbal approaches was essential in helping these individuals to develop a more realistic, positive, and integrated sense of their bodies" (p. 179). Art therapy combines verbal and non–verbal work (Rabin, 2003). A client can work on a non–verbal, sensory level using art materials and then discuss the product and the art–making process. Discussion further assists in helping the patient to operate on a cognitive/intellectual level, thereby providing closure to the session.

Art Therapy at Canopy Cove

The program at Canopy Cove includes individual and group art therapy services. As the clinic's full–time art therapist, I have developed and/or modified several techniques, which are customized to patient goals, to assist in the recovery process. The activities that I have found to be the most successful in combating an eating disorder are detailed in this section, including the following individual techniques: the Bridge Drawing technique; Separation from the Eating Disorder; Self as a Developing Seed; feelings work; and splatter painting. Group themes include: mirroring activity; boundaries/personal space project; group island mural; and termination puzzle.

Individual Projects

The Bridge Drawing. The Bridge Drawing is an art therapy assessment developed by Hays and Lyons (1981). I have found it to be a very useful tool in determining my clients' weekly progress. In my modification of the original Bridge Drawing instructions, I ask patients to "draw a picture of a bridge going from one place to another. Specifically, please draw a landscape on one side of the bridge to represent life with your eating disorder. On the other side of the bridge, please draw a landscape that represents what recovery might look like." I have administered this technique in individual and group sessions. Typically, clients will draw a bleak, dark landscape on the left side of their bridge, and a sunny, flourishing landscape on the right side. Figure 1 represents the Bridge Drawing of Lisa (pseudonym), an adult female client with anorexia.

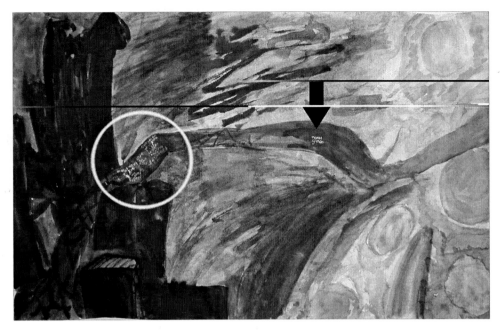

Figure 1. Bridge Drawing

In this Bridge Drawing, the left side of the page represents the eating–disordered landscape that Lisa was so accustomed to in her life. It is a dark city painted in black, purple, and blue. The right side is a bright place, where orange and yellow dominate. Once a week for 5 months, Lisa was asked to place a dot somewhere on the bridge to show where she would locate herself on that given day. Alongside the dot, she would also place the date, and an arrow to show the direction she would be traveling in. Most of her dots are placed in the same region on the beginning of the bridge to the left, indicated by the white circle. It is apparent that she spent most of her time at the clinic slowly climbing a steep slope at the start of a journey out of the eating disorder.

Upon her discharge from the clinic, Lisa was able to place a dot on the far right side of the bridge (under the black arrow) to represent the emotional progress she had made. Unfortunately, her distorted body image was still very much intact, as represented by another dot that she placed back on the left side. As clients progress in treatment, some reach a point when they feel that they are in two places on the bridge. This occurs when the client feels that he or she has made some emotional progress (e.g., increased self–awareness, positive outlook), but body image is still a problem. This usually coincides with the client's improved ability to separate from his or her eating disorder.

Separation from the Eating Disorder. Many of my clients who have had their eating disorder for several years explain that the disorder provides a false sense of safety and security, and that it becomes a way of functioning in the world – a coping mechanism. Naitove (1986) described a patient who preferred to continue with his pain rather than surrender it and have no feelings at all. This suggests a fear of emptiness without the eating disorder, as though the disorder were a friend – someone without whom the patient would feel unreal and unsafe.

Given the sense of emptiness and fear described by many clients, it is important to ensure that as treatment progresses – as the clinicians work to help the client defeat the eating disorder – the patient learns how to replace the eating disorder and associated negative behaviors with healthy, productive behaviors.

Bruch (1978) and Claude–Pierre (1997) found that people with anorexia tend to feel split, as though they have two minds. In the Recovery Model approach used at Canopy Cove, clients are taught how to separate, or differentiate, themselves from their eating disorders. In essence, this split encompasses a True Self that is lost to an overpowering entity – the eating disorder. Claude–Pierre (1997) would classify the True Self as the "Actual Mind," and the eating disorder as the "Negative Mind." No matter what label is used to identify the sense of a split self, however, the concept is the same – dualism. To achieve recovery, the eating disorder must be separated from the True Self.

The client can engage in more adaptive ways of functioning when he or she separates the eating disorder from his or her True Self. "Anorexics often benefit from therapy that aids in achieving a sense of self–autonomy and dealing with their disturbed self–concepts and self–images" (Mitchell, 1980, p. 57). Art therapy is particularly conducive to this goal.

I developed an art technique to help clients symbolize the separation/differentiation process: "Separation from the Eating Disorder." This technique is administered early in treatment, in individual or group format, and is usually completed in two to three sessions. First, the client is asked to name his or her eating disorder. Some typical examples are: "Satan," "Ed," or "It." Second, the client is asked to create a picture of the eating disorder ("ED") (Figure 2, left side); a picture of the client as his or her True Self, without the eating disorder (the "True Self" picture) (Figure 2, right side); and an environment to hold the ED and True Self once these figures are cut out (background, Figure 3).

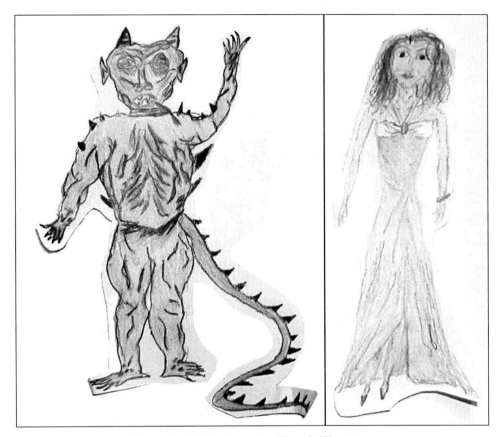

Figure 2. "ED" picture & "True Self" picture

The background is made from a piece of mural paper, cut to a size that comfortably accommodates an environment/landscape. This environment should be large enough to include the figures as well as two different shelters, one for each figure. The picture as a whole reflects the client's current reality of having to share his or her life with the eating disorder, with the ultimate goal of moving farther and farther away from the disorder until this shared environment becomes obsolete, and the True Self reigns. Once a week, clients use their Separation picture to gauge their progress, by moving the ED figure and the True Self pictures accordingly. Figure 3 shows Lisa's True Self still in the grips of her eating disorder, placed at the mouth of his treacherous cave dwelling. Lisa had this to say about her "Separation" project:

I placed my True Self in (ED's) lair, under his power/arm because I still feel stuck in his world (in terms of thoughts, body image, fear of gaining weight,

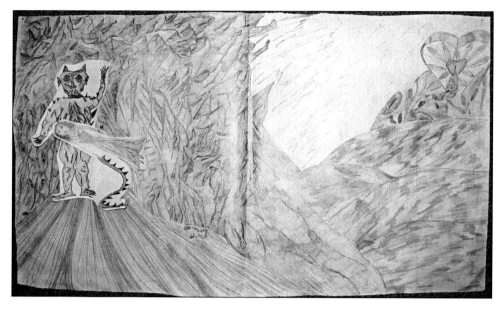

Figure 3. "Separation from the Eating Disorder"

self–acceptance, etc.). However, I can see the "Abode of the True Self" and am looking towards it. I am not at the coffin in the back–I have moved away from it, but (ED) is still threatening to steal one more year of my life (he has half of it on the cave wall) and wants to claim the rest and pin it up. There is a power struggle going on between us. The floor to the cave is very enticing and beckons me back in towards death, but I look forward to the heart and unconditional love where serenity, happiness, and health thrive–the cup of life awaits me there.

Upon termination of her five–month stay at Canopy Cove, Lisa knew she had yet to achieve recovery. Once she returned to her hometown, aftercare included regular meetings with a psychologist and a nutritionist. Clients rarely recover after one or two months of treatment, so they are encouraged to bring their "Separation" pictures home and continue to use them until they are able to conquer their eating disorder.

Self as a Developing Seed. In an individual or group session, clients are asked to "represent yourself as a developing seed." This technique helps clients to reflect on where they have been in the course of life and what their future goals encompass. A piece of paper can be divided into sections to illustrate the stages of development. This task can also be modified to use with clay. Molly (pseudonym) drew a picture of a seed buried under the ground which flourished with help from the elements. She wrote the following response to her "Seed" picture:

At first there seems to be no hope of the seed's inner being displaying itself to the world. Then the rain comes gently to wake it and encourage – it barely stirs, it just let the dream of more echo in its heart. Next the sun inspires and probes telling it of beauty and demonstrating its own strength . . . the seed responds . . . in fact it keeps struggling and daring to believe it can become like the sun and rain. After a few moons of determined liberalism the seed can now show what it once hoped it might have, and it rejoices in its new life by giving a gift of nourishment to the things around it along with protection and strength.

The content of this passage reveals the way in which eating disorders are used to deny sexual maturity and to reject adulthood (Crowl, 1980). Molly's drawing helped her to identify and address her maturity fears. In a follow–up session, she was able to portray herself as a fully grown tree, indicating her increased confidence to face the inevitability of becoming a woman, and instilling in her a sense of hope.

Feelings Work. People with eating disorders are typically unaware of their inner psychological and physiological processes, thus it is important that the therapist assist patients learn to identify and honor their needs, feelings, and impulses, and to be accountable for them (Luzzatto, 1994; Mitchell, 1980). This is essential in order for clients to develop skill in the areas where they have chosen not to function or have been denied learning (Mitchell, 1980). There are several ways in which I assist my clients to increase awareness of their inner processes. At the beginning of each session, I ask them to state a word describing how they are feeling physically, and a word to describe how they are feeling emotionally. This aids in distinguishing between bodily sensations and emotional states, which people who have eating disorders typically confuse.

We often remind our patients that "it's not about the food – it's about the feelings." As clients gain mastery of their actions through art production, their need to control eating patterns is reduced (Luzzatto, 1994). Once a client learns how to effectively confront his or her psychological issues and the related emotions, he or she can develop a more positive relationship with food.

An art intervention that I find particularly effective in identifying and acknowledging feelings is borrowed from the Diagnostic Drawing Series (Cohen, Hammer & Singer, 1988). The client is invited to "draw how you are feeling using lines, shapes and colors." By working in the abstract, deeper feelings tend to emerge. To help the client identify the feelings expressed in the abstract picture, the artwork can be discussed. Art therapist Linda Chapman's (n.d.) list of verbal prompts to talk about art provide effective follow–up for this project (Table 1).

Table 1. Ways of Looking at and Talking About Artwork

- If you could be in this picture, where would you be?
- Comment on what you actually see–colors, shapes, lines, form, etc. Avoid interpreting or making reference to possible content/meaning.
- What do you like, dislike about the image?
- Ask parts to be introduced, does the red line know the green dot?
- What does the blue circle have to say?
- Invite parts to talk to each other. What does _____ have to say to _____?
- Who is in charge, who is most vulnerable?
- Does the image have anything to say?
- Look at the image another way–upside down, sideways, from above, below.
- Any questions for the image?
- Is there anything you would like to change?
  Invite the person to change the image. Pay attention to body sensations, pains, and other physical responses when client alters the image. Physical sensations are common.
- Stick to color, line, form, shape, texture and the client's own associations and interpretations.
- Try to stay in the metaphor.
- Find closure.

These questions help the therapist uncover some of the more deep–seated feelings and issues that the eating disorder would prefer to keep hidden. It is safe to do this work in art therapy because the boundaries of a page act as a container for even the most difficult feelings, thus demonstrating to the client that it is possible to survive these feelings.

Splatter Painting. Expressive therapies are particularly applicable for this client population because eating disorders have a physical, somatic component and they cause a disturbance in the individual's body image (Canopy Cove, 2006b). Art, drama, movement, and music therapy techniques assist clients to creatively express representations of their inner self. Furthermore, these modalities assist clients in identifying feelings of bodily experience and stored memories because they may have difficultly understanding physical sensations and recollections at a conscious level.

Because many patients with eating disorders are out of touch with their bodies, movement work is very important. One art therapy approach that is effective in engaging the whole body is the splatter painting technique. It is a personal experience that can be facilitated during an individual or group session, preferably outside in an open space. The client is instructed to use washable tempera paint, large brushes, and large pieces of mural paper, to create huge paintings. Following a mild physical warm–up (arm rotations, knee bends, etc.), brushes can be dipped in paint, and clients are prompted to make use of their whole body, while standing, to throw the paint onto the paper.

People with eating disorders tend to impose a great deal of control over themselves, their families, and their environment (Crowl, 1980). "The patient feels and recognizes the body as her own, but controls it as if it were not. In this mechanistic conceptualization, the focus is internal mechanical control" (Crowl, 1980, p. 147). Bruch (1978) explained that many clients with eating disorders experience their bodies as separate from themselves, and that the hated and unmanageable body must be controlled. This need to control results in a loss of spontaneity (Crowl, 1980). Rigid, obsessive–compulsive behaviors are typical, as they serve to reduce anxiety, and this often extends into the patients' artwork. Pictures tend to be compulsively organized and decorative with "rote repetitions" and "stereotyped symbols" (p. 147). Kaslow and Eicher (1988) would explain that the kinesthetic exploration involved in the splatter painting technique helps the perfectionist client loosen up. In turn, this process decreases the client's need to control, thereby increasing trust and spontaneity. Paint cannot be easily controlled when splattered, and once a client is ready for this activity, he or she can experience the freedom inherent in letting go.

Group Projects

Mirroring Activity. This activity, borrowed from a workshop with art therapist Judy Rubin (personal communication, January 2003), involves two to three clients. Two clients sit directly across the table from one another. One client starts out as the "Leader"; the other begins as the "Mirror." Using a marker, the Leader draws a line and develops it into a scribble while the Mirror follows on his or her own piece of paper. An extra group member can be used as an observer of the process. Alternatively, as suggested by Kaslow and Eicher (1988), the therapist can serve as the Leader first and then the mirror. This provides a way to re–enact the separation–individuation process and is thereby conducive to increasing clients' sense of self–efficacy. During follow–up discussion, patients explore their feelings about being a leader vs. a follower, and talk about non–verbal communication processes. This discussion tends to heighten self–awareness and increase understanding of how one's behavior can affect others.

Kinesthetic exploration provides the opportunity to learn about our environment. It is an important part of normal development and formation of normal body image (Kolb, 1975). As with the splatter painting exercise, the kinesthetic aspect of mirroring can also facilitate improvement of body image (Kaslow & Eicher, 1988).

Boundaries/Personal Space Project. Clients' tendency to be emotionally disconnected from their bodies can be addressed with boundary work. Art is particularly conducive to this work, as paper has four edges, thereby framing the contents of the image. With this art therapy technique, each group member claims his or her own space on a large piece of mural paper, using art materials. Clients are then invited to connect to others' spaces on the page. This experience affords clients the opportunity to actually create and see their own physical space and to witness the way in which their space fits within the context of the group, thereby increasing awareness of their own limits while gaining respect for others' boundaries.

Group Island Mural (and Supplementary Questionnaire). People with eating disorders tend to isolate themselves from others. It is easier for them to engage in their dysfunctional rituals and behaviors when they are alone. Mitchell (1980) described the therapeutic goal of increasing social interaction so as to help clients decrease the tendency to withdraw and isolate themselves. To achieve this goal, the therapist can encourage the client to participate with others.

At Canopy Cove, I developed the group island mural technique to address the goal of increasing social interaction. In facilitating this intervention, begin by asking clients to imagine going on a week–long boat trip together. Have them make their own lists of items that they would take with them on this fantastic voyage–their "Personal List." Then, have them designate one member to serve as the group secretary. Instruct this individual to create a list of items that would be on the boat itself, with other clients verbally contributing to this "Boat List."

The journey: Start by telling the clients that they are on the trip, enjoying themselves, when suddenly the weather turns bad. Lightning strikes the boat. Everyone is okay, but the clients must remove half of the items from their Personal List, then as a group they must eliminate half of the items from the Boat List. After the storm, everyone wakes up on a sunny beach. Explain that the boat was shipwrecked on a deserted island. No one is harmed, but they must remove half of the items from their Personal List (again), then as a group they must also eliminate half of the items from the Boat List.

Once these tasks are complete, have the clients make a mural together. If desired, the art–making can be done in a subsequent art therapy session. Follow up on the entire process with the Island Mural Experience Post–Session Questionnaire (Table 2):

The questionnaire enables clients to reflect on their inner experience and to consider their role as a group member. When a client gains awareness of his or her ability to communicate and work with others, eating disordered behaviors are no longer needed as a way of coping with underlying problems (Mitchell, 1980). Increasing social interaction in the group setting can also address obsessional thoughts about the body and food that impede progress, by helping clients to learn more adaptive behaviors, such as using positive affirmations and healthy thoughts.

Table 2. Island Mural Experience Post–Session Questionnaire

1. On a scale from 1–10, how easy/difficult was it for you to come up with ideas for your list of personal items?
2. On a scale from 1–10, how easy/difficult was it for you to delete objects from your list of personal items?
3. On a scale from 1–10, how easy/difficult was it for you to come up with ideas for the group list of items on the boat?
4. On a scale from 1–10, to what extent did you participate in making the group list of items on the boat?
5. On a scale from 1–10, how easy/difficult was it for you to delete objects from the group list of items on the boat?
6. Please identify your role in the making of the group mural (check one):
   ☐ I took charge.
   ☐ I helped to lead the group.
   ☐ I was an equal participant.
   ☐ I kept to myself and worked more or less independently.
   ☐ I did not participate.
7. On a scale from 1–10 ("not great" vs. "great"), how do you feel about your level of participation in making the mural?
8. On a scale from 1–10 ("I made no effort" vs. "I made every effort"), to what extent did you include other group members, and encourage them to participate?
9. On a scale from 1–10 ("I did not enjoy it" vs. "I enjoyed it immensely"), overall, what was this experience like for you?
10. Finally, please write a few sentences about your level of enjoyment – why you feel this way.

Termination Puzzle. Canopy Cove clients usually develop solid relationships with each other and with the staff because they are in treatment for at least 30 days. Thus, when the time comes for a client to step down from the program, it is important to acknowledge this transition. In art therapy, I facilitate an art project that aids in the departing client's transition, the termination puzzle. First, the client who is leaving divides a piece of 18"–by–24" white poster board into the number of people who are in the group, including the therapist(s). For example, five clients and one therapist would yield a six–piece puzzle (Figure 4). The pieces should have some shape to them, and fit together. Second, the client is instructed to flip the board over and draw an oval shape, known as the circle that connects all of the puzzle pieces (and the clients who created the puzzle). Then, the person who is leaving cuts out the puzzle pieces and distributes the pieces to group members and therapist(s). Group members are asked to use the side of their piece that has a segment of the oval line in it, and to incorporate this line into their image. The image should be about the person who is leaving, for example, group members can be directed to think of what they would like to give this person, such as peace, strength, freedom, etc. Once everyone is finished embellishing their pieces, the person leaving collects these and assembles the puzzle.

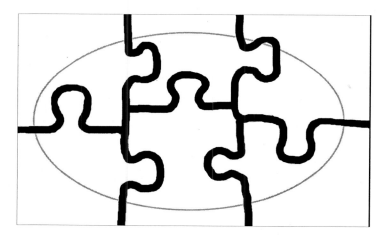

Figure 4. Termination Puzzle

The art therapy interventions described in this chapter are those that I have found to be the most successful in combating an eating disorder. I recommend that other art therapists employ these techniques, and develop additional activities that address the goals and objectives specific to this client population.

Although I employ many of the art therapy techniques that are available to help patients work on treatment goals and objectives, I also endeavor to take the clients' lead in directing the course of each session. This approach empowers clients and provides me with an opportunity to learn more about the people who have accepted me as a guide along their path to recovery. This acceptance yields a strong relationship between the patients and me, and is a vital tool in the recovery process.

References

Bruch, H. (1978). *The golden cage: The enigma of anorexia nervosa*. Cambridge, MA: Harvard University Press.

Canopy Cove. (2006a). About Canopy Cove. Retrieved July 10, 2006, from www.canopycove.com.

Canopy Cove Eating Disorder Treatment Center. (2006b). *The Recovery Model.* [handout]. Tallahassee, FL: Author.

Claude–Pierre, P. (1997). *The secret language of eating disorders.* New York: Times Books.

Cohen, B. M., Hammer, J., & Singer, S. (1988). The Diagnostic Drawing Series (DDS): A systematic approach to art therapy evaluation and research. *Arts in Psychotherapy, 15*(1), 11–21.

Costin, C. (1999). *The eating disorder sourcebook.* Lincolnwood, IL: Lowell House.

Crowl, M. A. (1980). Art therapy with patients suffering from anorexia nervosa. *Arts in Psychotherapy, 7*(2), 141–151.

Hays, R. E., & Lyons, S. J. (1981). The Bridge Drawing: A projective technique for assessment in art therapy. *Arts in Psychotherapy, 8*(3–sup–4), 207–217.

Kaslow, N. J., & Eicher, V. W. (1988). Body image therapy: A combined creative arts therapy and verbal psychotherapy approach. *Arts in Psychotherapy, 15*(3), 177–188.

Kolb, L. (1975). Disturbances of the body image. In S. Arieti (Ed.), *American handbook of psychiatry* (2nd ed., Vol. 4, pp. 749–769). New York: Basic Books.

Luzzatto, P. (1994). Anorexia nervosa and art therapy: The "double trap" of the anorexic patient. *Arts in Psychotherapy, 21*(2), 139–143.

Matto, H. C. (1997). An integrative approach to the treatment of women with eating disorders. *Arts in Psychotherapy, 24*(4), 347–354.

Mitchell, D. (1980). Anorexia nervosa. *Arts in Psychotherapy, 7*(1), 53–60.

Naitove, C. E. (1986). "Life's but a walking shadow": Treating anorexia nervosa and bulimia. *Arts in Psychotherapy, 13*(2), 107–119.

Rabin, M. (2003). *Art therapy and eating disorders: The self as significant form.* New York: Columbia University Press.

Reiff, D. W., & Reiff, K. K. L. (1992). *Eating disorders: Nutrition therapy in the recovery process.* Gaithersburg, MD: Aspen Publishers, Inc.

Schaverien, J. (1995). The picture as transactional object in the treatment of anorexia. In D. Dokter (Eds.), *Arts therapies and clients with eating disorders* (pp. 31–47). London: Jessica Kingsley Publishers.

Wolf, J. M., Willmuth, M. E., & Watkins, A. (1986). Art therapy's role in the treatment of anorexia nervosa. *American Journal of Art Therapy, 25*(2), 39–46.

Zerbe, K. J. (1993). *The body betrayed: Women, eating disorders, and treatment.* Washington, DC: American Psychiatric Press.

Biography

Donna J. Betts, PhD, ATR–BC, hails from Toronto, Canada. She received a Bachelor of Fine Arts from the Nova Scotia College of Art & Design in 1992, a Master of Arts in Art Therapy from the George Washington University in 1999, and a PhD in Art Education with a specialization in Art Therapy from the Florida State University in 2005. Dr. Betts served on the Board of Directors of the American Art Therapy Association (AATA) from 2002–2004. Dr. Betts is an adjunct professor in the art therapy department at FSU, and works as an art therapist with people who have eating disorders at Canopy Cove in Tallahassee, FL. She is the Recording Secretary and Virtual Assistant for the National Coalition of Creative Arts Therapies Associations (www.nccata.org), and serves on the Editorial Board of *The Arts in Psychotherapy* journal.

Chapter 3

BRINGING "THE WORLD" INTO THE ROOM: ART THERAPY, WOMEN AND EATING ISSUES

CLAIRE EDWARDS

Eating Issues and Art Therapy

Images of slenderness are never "just pictures" as the fashion magazines continually maintain (disingenuously) in their own defense. Not only are the artfully arranged bodies in the ads and videos and fashion spreads powerful lessons in how to see (and evaluate) bodies, but also they offer fantasies of safety, self–containment, acceptance, immunity from pain and hurt. They speak to young people not just about how to be beautiful but about how to become what the dominant culture admires, how to be cool, how to "get it together." To girls who have been abused they may speak of transcendence or armoring of too–vulnerable female flesh. For racial and ethnic groups whose bodies have been marked as foreign, earthy, and primitive, or considered unattractive by Anglo–Saxon norms, they may cast the lure of assimilation, of becoming (metaphorically speaking) "white" [Bordo (2003), pp. xxi–xxii].

"I could not talk about being big" (Butler, 1983, p. 67)

Eating issues and body image dissatisfaction present a serious health threat to girls and young women which is increasing in severity across the developed world (Bordo, 2003; Malson, 1998). This chapter describes a community based, feminist informed art therapy intervention conducted in South East Queensland, Australia. The purpose of the intervention was to explore and develop an alternative approach to the medically based treatments, sometimes incorporating art therapy, which are usually offered to women with serious eating issues. It was conducted in 2000, as part of a research Masters project.

At the clinical end of the spectrum, serious eating issues such as anorexia and bulimia are complex and difficult to treat (Wood, 1996). At the non–clinical end of the spectrum, popular women's magazines regularly feature stories about the fluctuating body sizes of various female celebrities, alongside fashion shoots and advertisements which feature rail thin models, dieting articles, and recipes (Bordo, 2003). Perhaps unsurprisingly given this environment, body image dissatisfaction and eating issues are experienced by many women who otherwise have no significant mental health issues (Brown, 1993), and who do not develop anorexia or other serious eating issues. Eating and body image issues, it would seem, are pervasive and full of contradictions for young women who are struggling to forge their own identity within a climate which gives them conflicting and unpalatable messages about how to be. Brown's concept of a "continuum of eating distress," which aims to encapsulate both clinical and non–clinical responses by women to food and body image, may help to shed light on this complex area.

Art therapists working with women with eating issues have identified a number of factors which they consider are significant in the etiology and treatment of eating issues. These include: denial (Maclagan, 1998; Mitchell, 1980); perfectionism and control (Crisp, 1980; Lawrence, 1979; Maclagan, 1998; Murphy, 1984); autonomy and identity (Bruch, 1974; Fleming, 1989; Mitchell, 1980; Robertson, 1992); enmeshment with the mother (Levens, 1987; Murphy, 1984; Welsby (1998); distorted body image (Crowl, 1980; Murphy, 1984); and concrete thinking (Levens, 1987, 1990). There is however a range of issues art therapists have failed to address (Edwards, 2005). For example, Wood (1996) has highlighted the lack of gender analysis by art therapists with regard to eating issues, which is curious considering the vast majority of individuals with serious eating issues are female. Similarly, although there are many published articles on art therapy and eating issues (Wood, 1996), and although a feminist approach to eating disorders has been suggested by *psychotherapists* such as Orbach (1998) and Kearney–Cooke (1989, 1991), relatively few art therapists have discussed a feminist approach to art therapy with this client group (Edwards, 2005).

The purpose of this chapter is to suggest that incorporating a feminist analysis of eating issues into art therapy may be beneficial to female clients who are struggling with eating issues. A feminist approach is outlined firstly in terms of theoretical foundations, and secondly in terms of practical strategies which may be implemented in art therapy interventions. A description of working as an art therapist within a feminist framework is given in the form of a case study.

Feminist Art Therapy

Theoretical Foundations

Since Orbach's (1978, 1998) groundbreaking, *Fat is a feminist issue,* was published, clients and clinicians alike have had access to an alternative perspective on the meaning and genesis of eating disorders. As art therapists, we may be particularly conscious of the impact of visual imagery on vulnerable young women, and how this affects their psychological development. I will argue that working as an art therapist with these clients needs to include a consideration of the cultural influences, such as magazine images, which put a premium on slimness, especially for young women. A feminist approach to art therapy takes account of socio–cultural influences on women, and how these influences impact on body image and eating behaviours.

In recent years, a feminist art therapy perspective has been developing (Hogan, 1997a). Whilst arguing that feminist therapy is "a philosophical approach . . . rather than a prescription of techniques" (p. 90), Joyce (1997) outlines a model for feminist art therapy, which includes the following principles:

- Awareness of issues of power, racism, and gender
- Strengths and skill–building focus
- Rejection of sex–role stereotyping
- Working with the client's goals
- Using explicit methods

Joyce (1997) argues that art therapy may offer women a more palatable alternative to traditional medical models of mental health care. In considering how feminist art therapy may differ from a more "traditional" psychoanalytically informed art therapy, we need to consider a range of factors. These include: increased awareness of socio–cultural issues; the art therapist as a positive role model; the importance of multiple perspectives; a supportive, collaborative approach; adopting the goal of the empowerment of women; and so on.

Socio–cultural Awareness

Feminist art therapists have argued for the inclusion of a socio–cultural context in their therapeutic framework (Waldman, 1999; Waller, 2006). Feminist therapists combine a therapeutic approach with a political and gender analysis – as Eichenbaum and Orbach (1983) have argued: "As feminist psychotherapists we bring in our political and personal attitudes, biases and values to the work we do. We hear what our clients say with a particular ear, no more special in its peculiarity than other therapists, but with a stated bias that sees women as the oppressed sex within patriarchy" (p. 69).

In addition, feminist *art* therapists in particular may include an analysis of the way images of women's bodies appear both within the history of art, and in the popular media. In this way, they provide clients with a critical cultural lens through which to view images in general, as well as those created in art therapy (Hogan, 1997b; Rust, 1987). These therapists enable the exploration of the links between aesthetics and cultural theory, and their impact on individual psychological development, from a feminist perspective.

Both of these areas come into play when considering a feminist approach to eating issues. Aspects of this approach include an awareness of the particular pressures girls and women face in regard to body image and weight loss, especially from the popular media. Feminist therapists aim to increase clients' awareness of these pressures. In effect they are engaged in a consciousness–raising exercise which aims to assist female clients to start to challenge some of the cultural messages they have internalized about body image and the desire to lose weight in order to gain peer approval or acceptance.

Multiple Perspectives

Making a parallel with modernist and postmodernist art, as well as drawing on feminist theory and feminist art practice, Davis Halifax (1997) suggests that feminist art therapy needs to include multiple perspectives, arguing for the consideration of gender and race, sexual orientation, and ability in therapeutic practice. Power issues (between client and therapist) need to be considered, as do the strengths and competencies of the client:

> A feminist and relational model of therapy is able to value what each participant brings to the relationship. At its best, it is capable of containing and tolerating the confusion that may arise with the admission of difference, and multiple points of view. This kind of therapy suggests that people entering a supportive, collaborative, empowered, therapeutic relationship will carry that experience with them into their world. (Davis Halifax, 1997, p. 51)

Supporting and Empowering Clients

In their description of an art therapy group for women in the community, Otway and Ellis (1987) claim that the use of art therapy offered the participants unique opportunities to meet their needs for support, space, and the expression of feelings in a safe and non–threatening environment: "Since women are expected primarily to take care of others it is often extremely difficult for them to recognized or admit need for support. Afraid too of being unable to articulate feelings and of possible stigmatization, women may be hesitant to approach somebody with whom they can talk over their fears ... art therapy can offer a gradual way of exploring feelings, since its versatility can allow communication on many different levels" (Otway & Ellis, 1987, p. 16).

Matra Robertson (1992) makes a link between feminist approaches to the treatment of eating disorders and the use of art in therapy, seeing art therapy as a break from more traditional treatment methods:

> Feminist theory on anorexia nervosa and feminist psychoanalytic theory give rise to a greater sense of optimism about treatment for women who self–starve. Crisp (1980), Mitchell (1980), and Bruch (1974) have used art in their otherwise traditional treatment of women diagnosed as anorexic. Art can provide an avenue for expression of aspects of the self that are difficult to verbalise. Women can also use painting and artwork in a non–hierarchical, subversive manner to explore the diverse realities common to all women in a patriarchy. (Robertson, 1992, p. 71)

The use of art for encouraging non–verbal expression is familiar to art therapists. Additionally, the use of art for "subversion" may be a less obvious function of art therapy. Skaife (1995) argues that "art therapy by its nature is radical. It is about empowering people ... art therapy is nearly always a subversive activity" (p. 2). The reasons given by Skaife include art therapy's emphasis on imagination and play, its messiness, and its active involvement of the client. In addition, according to Skaife, its very antithesis to the medical approach emphasizes the radical nature of art therapy.

When compared to the biomedical approach to anorexia, for example, which is often forced to impose behavioural treatment regimes on unwilling patients, art therapy may be experienced by the client as a much more palatable and less invasive form of treatment. The client may well perceive medical treatment as persecutory, abusive, invasive and judgmental, whereas art therapy (by comparison) is seen as empathic, empowering, and fundamentally benign. Art therapy in and of itself may have unique qualities which make it particularly suitable for challenging the "dominant paradigm," whether that be psychoanalysis or the medical model, and for working in a more empowering and sensitive way with female clients.

A Collaborative Approach

Art therapy may have other qualities which make it a particularly suitable treatment for women with eating issues. In their meta–analysis of therapeutic factors, and echoing Robertson (1992) and Skaife (1995), Orlinsky, Grawe and Parks (1994), found that "the quality of the patient's participation in therapy stands out as the most important determinant of outcome" (Duncan, Miller and Sparks, 2004, p. 36). Duncan and colleagues continue with the assertion that "the research indicates that therapy works if clients experience the relationship positively and are active participants" (Ibid., p. 36).

As an example, Ball and Norman (1996) employed a non–directive, psychodynamic approach, in conjunction with a feminist framework, in which the content of the group was largely determined by the participants. Their values and approach are supported by a list of recommendations for working with women with eating issues, which explains clearly how the principles of feminist therapy, as they see them, are put into practice. For example, the clients have a choice about which group they participate in, and they are provided with information about art therapy prior to the group. Other factors include: the policy of non–labelling; a non–medical, non–behavioural approach; a "non–expert" role adopted by workers; and the potential for women to self–refer.

Active participation therefore does not just refer to the use of art. It also refers to "opening out" the therapy to involve the client in a consultative process, in which they provide feedback on their experience of therapy to the therapist. By addressing the power dynamic in the therapeutic alliance, and inviting the client to have a greater role in her own treatment, (whether by use of art or by discussing the progress of therapy with the client) feminist art therapists may be able to further meet her needs.

Role of Therapist

The role of the therapist working within a feminist art therapy framework is not to present a "blank screen," as in a psychoanalytic approach, but to participate to an appropriate degree, and to provide positive role models for clients. On the blank screen approach, Paul Gibney (1995) states that "the danger of working that way is its more about keeping the therapist safe than it is about facilitating the client's process" (p. 37).

Feminist therapists have frequently commented on the therapists' role, seeing it as perhaps the most significant aspect of feminist therapy. Black and Symes (1998) stress the importance of therapists listening to clients: "A feminist approach to understanding eating disorders has arisen out of listening to women and how they understand their experience of an eating disorder . . . if practitioners are to gain any real insight or understanding about the experiences of women with eating disorders it would seem obvious that there is a need to ask women themselves" (p. 10). In an art therapy context, looking carefully at the clients' art work might be as important as listening to their voices, as art is understood to be an alternative means of communication within a therapeutic relationship.

Tolman and Debold (1994) suggest that the role of feminist therapists is to provide "example, support, critical perspectives and company of adult women" (p. 313). Waldman (1999) emphasizes the importance of the therapist as a role model in art therapy. Features of the feminist therapist role, according to Kearney–Cooke (1991) include the following approach, which: "Challenges the therapist to step out of the role of a silent expert and to struggle actively with the patient . . . it challenges therapists to be clear about who they are and how they relate to others. It encourages therapists to be aware of their own struggles with shape and weight. . . . It demands an understanding of the cultural context in which an eating disordered patient's struggle takes place, as well as the provision of a relationship where the patient can clearly experience herself as having an impact on others" (p. 316).

The goal of feminist art therapists is to be clear about therapeutic goals and purpose, and about the therapists' roles and agenda within it. In the case example given, my dual role, being that of art therapist and researcher, was different from my more familiar singular role as art therapist. As researcher, I needed to be very clear and explicit about the research project, and what this meant, as well as being clear about my attitudes towards eating issues in particular and women's issues in general. As both therapist and researcher, I needed to listen to the clients and to look carefully at their art work.

Echoing Kearney Cooke (1991), Ball and Norman (1996) recommend that therapists reflect on eating issues themselves: "It is very important for workers working with women with eating problems to examine their own feelings about food, eating and body image. How a worker feels about fatness, thinness, diets, comfort–eating, fashion, mealtimes and so forth may influence how she feels about the work with women. It will be important to know why issues arising from the work arouse feelings in the worker. These issues can be explored in a confidential worker group or through supervision" (Ball & Norman, 1996, p. 59).

Art Therapy Groups as a Preferred Approach

Group work is often the preferred approach for art therapists working with women with eating issues. The art therapy groups I describe utilize a feminist approach. I have defined art therapy groups as "feminist" if the art therapist makes a conscious effort to address their clients' specific needs as women. Otway and Ellis (1987) describe a women's art therapy group in a community setting. The group was not specifically targeted at women with eating issues. According to the authors, however, at least two of the women attending used the group to work on their issues around eating and food: "An anorexic women in the group used the painting time to explore the unconscious meanings attached to her body image and eating patterns. Through her painted images she recognised the extent to which she used her body as a metaphor for her attempts to gain control over her life" (Otway & Ellis, 1987, p. 17).

In another example from the same group, a participant, the mother of a 14–month–old child "used this time for herself to focus on her own feelings of anger and hidden longings for nurturing which she had tried to deal with through eating compulsively" (Ibid., p. 17). The authors identify one of the potential benefits of attending such a group for women with eating issues, namely increased awareness of the dynamic and conflictual relationship between the body and the self in the struggle for autonomy and self–realisation.

If we accept Brown's (1993) hypothesis that eating issues exist on a continuum, it makes sense to address eating issues in generalist as well as in targeted groups. A possible benefit of the generalist group could be the exploration of this eating issues continuum, and how this affects all the participants. The group then can be a place where eating issues can be seen as less stigmatized, and therefore less shameful. Groups can help to emphasize links between women participants, and not just highlight their differences.

Ball and Norman (1996) describe a 14–week art therapy group with women with eating issues in the community. The authors discuss the benefits of group work, such as mutual support, understanding, and development of self. In addition, according to Ball and Norman, the participants in the group were able to re–experience historical traumas, take risks, and explore new ways of relating. Further, Ball and Norman describe common features in their work with women who use food, such as the mother–daughter relationship, and food as a method of control. Art therapy was used in the group in order to provide the women with a means of non–verbal expression. This was displayed through the use of art materials in relation to some of the themes expressed in the group, which included: "The inability to take in and retain anything good; the potential for the "good" to become damaging or to be destroyed by the bad; a fear of endless and overwhelming need within the group; the desperate desire to eat which may then be replaced by guilt and self–reproach; and the need to get rid of food" (Ball & Norman, 1996, p. 56).

Summary of Feminist Art Therapy Approach

The previous section explored the theoretical foundations of a feminist approach to art therapy for women with eating issues. These included: the importance of a socio–cultural perspective; an analysis of visual images in art and popular culture; a supportive, collaborative approach; active participation of clients; the importance of role modeling; and therapists' awareness of their own body image issues. The particular benefits of group work were also discussed.

The following section describes a clinical research project I developed, which consisted of a short–term art therapy intervention for women with eating issues in a community setting. The art therapy intervention incorporated many of the strategies previously outlined, in order to provide a feminist focus. The project involved the collection of qualitative data which provided a framework for gaining feedback from the participants, in order to evaluate the intervention from the clients' (as well as the therapists') perspective.

An Alternative Model for Art Therapy

Forms of psychotherapy such as art therapy represent an alternative to the mainstream, biomedical approach to eating issues, which predominates in Australian psychiatric hospitals (McDermott et al., 2002, p. 318). Gilroy and Hanna (1998) have commented on the dominance of the medical model in Australian psychiatry, and the relative lack of influence on psychiatry of psychodynamic concepts, as compared to Britain, North America, and Europe. This biomedical dominance can result in a lack of support for methods such as art therapy (or indeed psychotherapy).

A broad goal in developing this project was to demonstrate the validity of art therapy within this climate. I found that despite the above, art therapy was generally seen in a positive light by individuals working within community based agencies. This finding is supported by Gilroy and Hanna (1998), who suggest "it could be that art therapy will be in the vanguard of the acceptance and inclusion of dynamically–based treatment approaches in Australian psychiatry" (p. 272). The more specific goal of the project was to conduct and evaluate an effective, community–based art therapy intervention for women with eating issues, which incorporated a feminist approach.

My approach, therefore, was to develop a framework for art therapy with different theoretical orientations than the "traditional" biomedical or psychoanalytic approaches. I hoped to show how art therapy can offer an alternative/complementary framework for working with eating issues, which can work alongside more established approaches. This approach represented a conscious choice to work outside of the mainstream, biomedical approach, which as we have seen, predominates in Australian hospitals, and within a feminist, community–based structure.

Practical Strategies

As previously discussed, a feminist approach involves working in a more transparently and collaboratively with clients, whilst at the same time providing them with positive female role models. It may also involve working in a structured and directive manner, using particular strategies designed to enable clients to explore their eating issues from an alternative perspective. As Waller (1993) suggests, structured, theme–centered groups are well suited to short–term "outpatient" groups. In the short–term intervention described in this case study, the facilitators played an active and directive role, both in planning and actively providing structured activities in the sessions.

Practical strategies utilized in this instance included the use of magazine collage, video, cartoons and other materials which assisted clients to understand some of the external influences on their eating behaviours. Borrowing from cognitive behavioural therapy, clients were encouraged to examine their negative thought processes, which are internalized messages they have learned through these external influences. It involved clients learning to increase their ability to be safe and to self–nurture. Some of the practical strategies utilized in this case study will be discussed in order to illustrate their consistency with a feminist approach.

Collage Using Magazine Images

Rust (1987, 1992, 1994) has written extensively on art therapy with women with eating issues and has combined a feminist approach with object relations theory. She is one of the first art therapy authors to introduce political and social factors as well as intrapsychic elements into the complex arena of art therapy practice with women with eating issues. In the following example, she describes a group for women with compulsive eating issues in which participants combined guided fantasy with collage activities. Collage using magazine images, Rust (1987) suggests, is particularly apt for women with eating issues. These women are aspiring to "recreate themselves . . . using the very material that so subtly pervades, persuades and influences women – and so provokes them" (p. 153).

It is of course arguable that the process of cutting and pasting magazine images always results in an alternative meaning from that originally intended (Weiser, 1993). However, when faced with multiple images of slender young women, and a dearth of "alternative" images of women, it is difficult to see how the dominant paradigm could be challenged or subverted using this material, without some discussion of the "meanings" inherent in the images with the women concerned.

An analysis of magazine imagery in relation to gender and body image is included in Rust's (1987) approach. She suggests that collage may be a very useful medium to use in order to examine the female stereotypes and the way these images affect women. Matto (1997) makes a similar point, arguing that collage based on magazine images can link into discussions about internalized messages which can then be examined as cognitive distortions, using an approach influenced by cognitive behavioural therapy.

Safety Issues

Establishing safety is an important consideration in the treatment of women with eating issues, many of whom may have experienced some form of sexual assault or abuse (Calam & Slade, 1994). Safety is established by Ball and Norman (1996) through the negotiation of ground rules in the first session. Rust (1994) describes one particular group, where seven out of eight participants had been abused as children. Men were identified as the abusers and the Women's Therapy Centre was seen as a safe haven. Rust describes how one woman's clay sculpture of a large cobra became, using Schaverien's (1987, 1992) term, an "embodied image" for the group:

> It (the cobra) was placed in the middle of the group, squarely facing me. When we sat down together I waited with baited breath, sensing the volcano about to erupt. The woman (who made it) described the snake as a "dick" . . . the group seemed to be enthralled, frightened and outraged; the "man" had come into the room without a doubt. They spent a good deal of time looking at this object and talking about it. So much was contained in this image. They felt as though things were being dredged up from the bottom of a pond like monsters from the deep. (pp. 55–56)

Rust describes how she experienced strong counter–transference feelings of being unable to protect these women due to the number of "intruders" who came into the room in the course of this group. This experience had a parallel for Rust (1994, p. 57) with the experience of their mothers who had been unable to protect them from sexual abuse as children. Although Rust acknowledges the impact of negative life events such as sexual abuse on women, her focus is still on the mother–daughter relationship. As in much of the art therapy literature, the role of fathers, brothers and boyfriends, and indeed, the clients' experiences of rape or sexual assault, are largely unexplored. The establishment of a safe space, which is a crucial element of the therapeutic alliance, may be of particular importance for these women, since they find the articulation of feelings so difficult, and are particularly lacking in personal power.

Cognitive Behavioural Therapy

Once art therapy is understood as being capable of incorporating other theoretical models, it may also be useful to consider cognitive behaviour therapy (CBT) as an adjunct to art therapy. Rosal (2001) suggests that the main purpose of a CBT approach is "helping a client . . . to develop an internal sense (locus) of control" (p. 223). Since control is an issue frequently identified in relation to eating issues, and given CBT's suitability with this client group (Bryant–Waugh & Lask, 1995), it would seem a useful approach for art therapists to explore further.

Rosal (2001) argues that CBT can be usefully combined with art therapy for a number of reasons. She sees art as "an inherently cognitive process" (p. 217) which involves "uncovering mental images and messages, recalling memories, making decisions, and generating solutions" (Ibid). Like Rosal (2001), Matto (1997) sees art therapy and CBT as being complementary approaches, and suggests that art therapy may help overcome some of the disadvantages of a purely CBT approach, for example by allowing the emotional expression derived from art therapy to balance out the more cognitive bias of CBT, thereby avoiding "perpetuating the intellectualisation of the disorder" (p. 348). One method Matto describes is the use of art therapy as a starting point in the session, which is then followed by an exploration of the thoughts and feelings which emerge from both the art–making process and the artwork itself. She suggests this may help with reducing anxiety in relation to difficult emotions. Matto argues that the complexity of eating issues demands an integrated approach which combines art therapy and CBT, and which incorporates both hospital based and community treatment.

Project Planning and Setting Up

The art therapy sessions described in this case study were facilitated by an art therapist (the author) and a social worker. The social worker had identified a number of individual therapy clients she perceived would benefit from participation in a group on eating issues. Both workers had a similar theoretical stance on eating issues, namely a feminist approach, as outlined in the previous section. In addition, both facilitators wished to expand their knowledge and experience in this area and were committed to the use of art therapy as the primary modality of the intervention.

A major problem the facilitators faced was the low participation level, as only two women attended the art therapy sessions, although several others had registered interest but did not turn up. Both facilitators felt ethically bound to run the group, in recognition of the courage of the women who did attend. This factor had a dramatic effect on the research project, which was originally conceived as exploring the effectiveness of a group approach. Instead, the project has been treated as a qualitative case study of two individuals, although I have only focused on one of them in this chapter.

Data Collection

In designing a feminist informed, clinically based art therapy intervention for women with eating issues, I aimed to incorporate the voices and images of the women who participated, most significantly in the use of data collection, including their art work. The data collection process included two questions designed to provide an ongoing "snapshot" of the sessions from the clients' perspective. These two questions, completed weekly after the session, asked the women to nominate the "most significant event" in the session each week, as well as the "most significant image." The first question has been used before in qualitative research into the efficacy of group psychotherapy (Bloch & Crouch, 1985; Whitely & Collins, 1987), and the second has been adapted for use in art therapy group research (Gilroy, 1995). In addition, the participants' art work formed an important part of the data collected. The images in art therapy can serve to provide some of the "nuances and richness" (Yalom, 1985, p. 3) of the clients' experience, that would be missing if questionnaires were used in isolation.

The women were also given a journal to use as a therapeutic tool, for the duration of the art therapy sessions. These were not intended as research tools, however the client, "Marie" contributed some of her journal entries as research data, and these were included in the study (McLeod, 1994). The research tools provided an effective platform for continuous feedback from the participants to the facilitators, which informed both the research and the therapeutic process itself. The premise for this is a collaborative research model, in which participants are seen as co–researchers as well as "subjects."

Case Study: Marie

This following section describes the art therapy intervention, images created and comments by one of the participants, whom I shall call "Marie." Marie, was in her early twenties when she attended the art therapy sessions. Further, Marie stated that she was anorexic when she was fifteen years old.

Marie was now overweight, although she claimed not to eat much at all, never in front of other people, and seemed mystified by her large size. She struggled with depression, dissociation, and self harming/suicidal thoughts, in addition to her eating issues. Marie had lived independently from her immediate family in the past, but was currently living with her parents. She was neither employed nor studying at the time of the group. Marie clearly had significant mental health problems as well as eating issues. She was having weekly individual counseling with the co–facilitator of the group, concurrent with her group attendance.

After the initial session, which was her first experience of art therapy, Marie identified the completed image from a round robin art activity as having "really portrayed the way I was feeling after the session." In other words, right from the outset Marie was making the connection between her artwork and her feelings. The following describes four of the images Marie created, during the course of the art therapy sessions, which illustrate how a feminist art therapy approach was utilized, and how she described them.

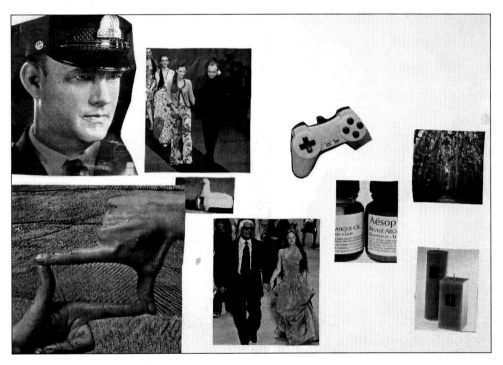

Figure 1. Powerful/powerless

Collage: Powerful/Powerless

The purpose of this task, completed in session two, was to use collage to express the contrasting themes of "powerful" and "powerless." Since it does not involve either drawing or painting, collage is often seen as a good introductory activity for clients who are not used to doing art (Makin, 2000). The women were asked to make their collage on a sheet of paper folded down the middle, to mark the division between the powerful images and the powerless ones. This task is derived from an activity described by Rust (1987).

In Marie's collage the "powerful" images on the left hand side of the picture take up more space than the "powerless" images on the right. They include: Tom Hanks in prison officer uniform from the film *The Green Mile*, as an image of male power and a picture of dirty male hands, making a frame through which we see bright green pastures. Marie related this picture to an image she had read in a poem. Other powerful images were: a colourfully dressed fashion model, walking down a catwalk with a man by her side, dressed all in black, who Marie said is "a pretty girl who can wear what she likes and doesn't care what anyone thinks"; and a duck shaped house which was again about "not caring what people think." In addition, Marie had glued a second picture of a man and a woman, similar to the first one, but in this case she placed the man on the powerful side and the woman on the powerless side. According to Marie, this was an attempt to bridge the gap between men and women, as well as a comment on gender imbalance as she saw it.

The "powerless" images for Marie included a computer game console: "when people play games, I feel powerless"; a candle, which "someone else can blow out"; a tall forest with a small person in it; and a bottle of pills, over which Marie said she felt powerless. The images themselves on the powerless side are generally smaller than on the powerful side. There was a focus on scale, as in the relative sizes of the trees and the person. Small size was indicative of powerlessness in this image, although the tiny pills, and the games console, were actually symbols of power for Marie; it's just that she felt powerless in relation to them.

There were many dualisms in this collage: the two male hands; the male and the female (twice); the two pill bottles and the two candles. This may have related to the two women in the group; her parents; herself, and a relative who had physically and emotionally abused her (given the repetition of male and female); or the two facilitators; with power being very relevant to all these possible interpretations. Marie's image of the candle was to recur in a later group (Figure 4), as an image of her eating issue.

Marie's Journal

Marie offered the following quote from her journal to describe her later reflection on this activity, particularly in relation to taking pills: "I brought up a few scary things about my eating issue today that I've never admitted to anyone, including myself. Flicking through the magazine pages the bottles seemed to call out to me. They reminded me of medicine bottles and how I sometimes take enough tablets to make myself feel sick, and to not feel hungry. To get away with not eating for longer. I feel a slight release of pressure has been lifted from me, and while I know that just admitting the issue won't make it vanish, at least I am more aware of it now. What I really need is to feel OK about me, and to not care about what anyone says or thinks. That's the difficult part."

Most Significant Image

Marie stated that the most significant image for her in this session was: "the collage on powerful/powerless because I could really think about the things in life that make me feel powerless in particular. It has left a lot of thoughts swirling through my head."

The facilitators were both surprised by the high level of self–disclosure in this second session. Marie had spoken a lot about her eating issues. This was despite the fact that the theme for the group was not specifically related to eating issues, although it reflected what we understood to be an underlying dynamic.

Drawing: "The World Seems So Unsafe"

The purpose of this session was to explore issues of identity and safety. Marie shared some memories from when she had been anorexic as a teenager, and had been regularly threatened with a syringe by her cousin's partner (whom she lived with at the time) if she did not eat. This was the physical and emotional abuse she had alluded to in the previous session. Her sister also tried to force her to eat, as did her grandmother. Her mother, who was a chef, also did not like to eat. Her father made up packed lunches, which her mother threw away. Marie's whole family, evidently, seemed to be divided between those who did not eat, and those who tried to make others eat.

As discussed in an earlier chapter, Kearney–Cooke (1989, p. 14) argues that mothers and daughters often share a negative body–image. Indeed, mothers of women with eating issues often have body image and eating issues themselves (Wooley & Kearney–Cooke, 1986). This has been noted in

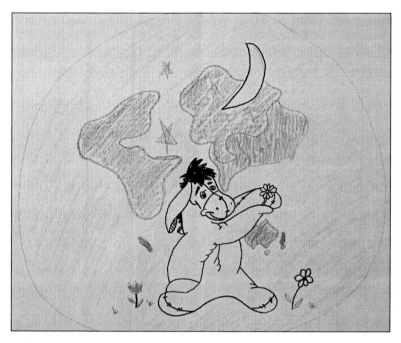

Figure 2. Self portrait as an animal in a safe and an unsafe place

my clinical practice, and Marie's family history supports that observation as well; yet, in psychodynamic interpretations the focus is often on the mother–daughter relationship being enmeshed, without specific consideration of the body image and eating issues of the mother. The phenomenon noted here may prove a more plausible explanation for their close relationship, namely the mother's identification with the daughter's issues and a resulting ambivalence about treatment.

The art therapy task was to make "a self–portrait as an animal in a safe place and an unsafe place." The participants were also asked to pick three words to describe their animal (which were in fact descriptive of themselves, as it was a self–portrait), after the images were completed. This activity is a development of an art therapy activity called a "metaphorical portrait" (Liebmann, 2004, pp. 228–229). The additional aspect is the adjunct "in a safe and an unsafe place." I added this environment element to enable further discussion about safety, and hopefully to help them start to identify the group as a relatively safe place. It also introduced the concept of a specific environmental context, which was congruent with a feminist analysis of eating issues, as previously discussed.

Marie combined her images of safe and unsafe places in one picture (Figure 2). She drew herself as a cartoon character, Eeyore (from the classic children's story *Winnie the Pooh*, by A. A. Milne), surrounded by an image of Earth, with some countries and continents depicted, the moon and stars. Marie said that Eeyore was a character she could relate to, as he is usually portrayed as miserable. Marie's Eeyore is smiling (even though he is miserable) and is holding a flower. There are two more flowers growing in the ground, one on either side of him. The three words Marie used to describe her self–portrait were "sad, lonely and fat."

Marie talked about usually feeling safe when she was alone, but still having to deal with her negative thoughts, usually about self–harming, which made her feel less safe. She said she saw the whole world as unsafe, but paradoxically felt safe at night under the stars. The image, combined with Marie's words, suggests to me a child–like ability to be "in the moment" and to forget external reality. The Eeyore figure seems to float in front of the globe, oblivious of it, lost in his own imagination. The globe appears as it would from space, with only Australia and New Zealand recognizable as countries.

Themes arising from Marie's work included, the use of cartoons, the juxtaposition of scale noted in the previous collage, and the child–like quality of her work. The image of stars was another theme for Marie, which would recur in a later image. Marie was starting to develop her own visual vocabulary to express her feelings and identity.

Most Significant Event

Marie identified the most significant event as: "the feeling I spoke about with the whole world seeming so unsafe. Everyone around me. Everything around me." Thus it was the feeling evoked in making and reflecting on her image that was most significant. This was reflected in her journal entry and in the description of the following discussion. Interestingly, her most significant *image* in this session was the image of a pig made by another client. This demonstrates the importance of asking both questions, as it enables valuable additional information to be given.

Towards the end of this session, Marie said she was feeling unsafe and wanted to take a "heap of medication" with the goal of ending up in hospital. Hospital was another place that was identified as potentially both safe and unsafe, revealing the perceived risks in getting help from the medical profession. We discussed other ways of seeking admission to hospital, which did not involve overdosing. I asked Marie to think of strategies for keeping herself "together," and she agreed to follow through on this. In my notes for this session, I wrote that "I was thrown, as usually there are some positives that come out of this activity . . . but there were none identified." This comment referred to the fact that in doing this activity, people can usually identify some positive qualities that "their" animal has. It also raises the question of my need to find positives, and perhaps my counter transference that this group was not making the women feel better, in fact they were feeling worse than before, even though we had predicted this might occur. Marie left the group feeling bad, but she did manage to "hold it all together" and stay out of hospital, which was a positive outcome for her. The opportunity for both women to express difficult emotions, and to feel them contained, was another positive outcome of the group.

Working with the Inner Critic

The purpose of this session was to explore the concept of the "inner critic." The inner critic is a term derived from CBT, and is used to describe the negative self–talk that many individuals with low self–esteem experience, in this case in relation to body image, and attitudes around eating and food. Since we were introducing a new concept, that of the inner critic, the session had a psycho–educational component, which was incorporated into the art activity.

The women were given handouts taken from *Mary Jane: Living Through Anorexia and Bulimia Nervosa* (Robinson, 1996), which illustrated the concept of the inner critic with an example from Robinson's personal experience of eating issues. The book includes cartoons by Judy Horacek, which were shown to the women as well. The use of cartoons was intended to bring humor into the discussion of an otherwise stressful and challenging topic.

Before we progressed to the art activity, we watched a brief video cartoon entitled *Gorgeous* (Cooke, 1994a). This animation illustrates the concept of the inner critic, which is personified as a "weird fairy," Deirdre, who hovers on the shoulder of Hermione, the protagonist of the video. Deirdre berates Hermione with an ongoing stream of critical comments based on the events in her day, with a particular focus on body image: this includes eating breakfast; going to the gym; buying clothes; and a consultation in the clinic of a plastic surgeon. At the end of the story, Hermione visits the art gallery (where she is applying for a job), and she converses with the images of women in the artwork about women's changing body–image represented through the history of art. The video explores the issue of the inner critic with humor, giving a graphic illustration of what many women experience daily, but are barely aware of.

After viewing the video, and discussing the concept of the inner critic, we asked the women to relate any negative messages they had received and internalized about food or body image, and to identify where these messages had come from. Eventually, Marie identified: "If you can't do something perfectly, you're a failure," which she said came from herself rather than from others. For Marie, the consequences were to drink Coke and to self-harm. She was starting to make links between her negative thoughts and her non-eating, and sometimes risky, behaviours.

Drawing: "Harpy"

The concept of the "harpy," which is derived from Greek mythology, was utilized to personify the origin of these negative thoughts. Harpies are generally depicted as obnoxious female creatures, which were sent as punishment from the Gods for some wrongdoing. In contemporary popular culture, a harpy is a woman who is very bitter and critical of others. We showed the women images of harpies and other scary mythical creatures. We then asked the women to make an image of their own inner critic, or harpy using art materials. This activity is described by Smith (1998) and it is utilized in the Brisbane agency which developed it.

Marie created a drawing of a harpy based on her hand outline, on A4 yellow card (Figure 3). She described it as a creature which sits on her shoulder and *scratches*. Marie's harpy has a cartoon-like quality, but is very different from her previous cartoon imagery. This cartoon face is like something out of a horror movie, or a Grimm's fairy tale, with bloodshot eyes, a blood-red forked tongue, and a long pointed nose. Its hair is wild and curly and it has sharp nails on its fingers, which do the scratching Marie described.

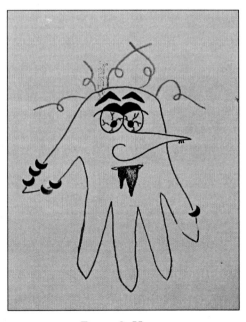

Figure 3. Harpy

Most Significant Image

Marie's most significant image after this session was "my harpy, because it is always on shoulder, scratching."

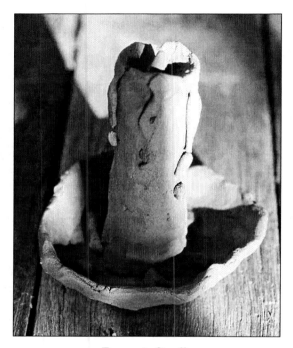

Figure 4. Candle

Claywork: Image of the Eating Issue

A documentary about a young woman with anorexia, *Bronte's Story* (26th March 2000, Channel Nine), had been shown on television in the week since we last met. This provided a good illustration of how popular culture can influence clients' perceptions of their struggles, and it sparked some discussion, with both women identifying with Bronte. Marie asked whether anorexia or bulimia was more serious. Marie stated she was "getting worse" and said she was now hardly eating at all. This was interesting in the light of the previous conversation, as Marie was not anorexic, but clearly seemed to need to demonstrate the seriousness of her eating issues. Possibly an element of competition was developing between the women at this stage.

In this session, the women were encouraged to explore their eating issue by creating an image of it. This confronting directive elicits a representation of the issue that has brought them to therapy. Marie worked in clay, which was one of a variety of media available. She sculpted a candle with wax dripping down the stem (Figure 4). Marie felt quite disturbed by it. She talked about wanting to "melt away" and someone "blowing the light out", both of which could be interpreted as metaphors for suicide or death. She had included a candle in her collage of three weeks ago, as an image that represented feeling powerless (Figure 1).

The candle with wax dripping down could also be interpreted as phallic, although this was not consciously identified by Marie. This interpretation was also suggested by the fact that Marie said she found the sensation of using the clay "disgusting," and also by her comment after the session that the most significant event that week was "just playing with the clay. Squishing and molding it with my hands." I had noticed the image of dirty (male) hands in her "powerful" collage (Figure 1), which had initially alerted me to the possibility of sexual abuse. Marie was withdrawn after making the candle, and said she felt like crying. She expressed ambivalence, saying she partly wanted to smash the candle and partly did not. Others in the room gave her permission, but she did not, neither did she cry. It seemed too hard to let go. I was relieved the candle was not destroyed – the researcher role was taking priority over the therapist here – but not just for the sake of the research. I also thought the image of the candle was a self–image in a way and Marie had already alluded to the candle being "blown out." I was unsure if it would be therapeutic for her to enact her own self–destruction. Marie was clearly making a lot of connections, but was fearful of self–disclosure in this environment. Marie's dilemma about whether to smash the candle also signified to me her ambivalence about change.

Most Significant Image

"My candle – I just want to melt away. To stop having to think anymore."

Most Significant Event

"Just 'playing' with the clay. Squishing and molding it in my hands."
Homework was given after this session, which introduced feminist concepts in relation to body image and eating, and included affirmations by Cooke (1994b).

Discussion

The purpose of this chapter has been to describe a range of strategies which were utilized in developing a feminist approach to art therapy with women with eating issues, in response to a perceived lack of feminist analysis by art therapists. The art activities outlined above are offered as examples of how a feminist approach to art therapy with women with eating issues was put into practice. The activities described represent only a small part of the intervention, which ran for ten sessions, and which included a range of strategies using art (see Appendix). The responses Marie made to the images and to her art therapy experience have been included, as a means of demonstrating the importance and relevance of collecting feedback from clients when considering the effectiveness of art therapy. From the participants' feedback, it is possible to make the following assertions in relation to the *most significant image* question:

- The process of art–making was at times as significant as the finished image.
- The image resonated with thoughts and feelings.
- The image resonated with the self.
- Participants related strongly at times to another person's artwork.
- The image increased awareness of self and others.

The following *most significant events* were identified:

- The art–making itself.
- Self–disclosure or catharsis.
- Self–understanding or insight.
- Interpersonal learning.

Women with eating issues are often seen as challenging clients who are difficult to treat (Wood, 1996). By working alongside these clients within a feminist framework, we can maximize the beneficial effects of an art therapy intervention. It may then be possible to start developing the trust, understanding and support through which positive change is able to occur.

Appendix: Weekly Schedule for Eating Issues Group

The following is the original outline of the art therapy sessions.*

Week One: Introductory Session 1. This session will look at our expectations, and thoughts about how we would like to be treated in order to feel

*In the event, the activities for Weeks Seven, Eight and Nine were modified to meet the needs of the participants, who found the idea of the Family Portrait and the Body Outline drawing in particular very confronting. In Week Seven the topic was a session review, and we discussed the rationale for changing the schedule. In Weeks Eight and Nine we focused on self–care. The women made a three–dimensional Egg–Capsule to protect "the fragile parts of themselves," and a Self–Care Poster collage to remind them to take care of themselves.

safe and comfortable. We will play some introductory and interactive "games" using drawing materials.

Week Two: Introductory Session 2. This session will involve collage activities using photos cut from magazines, and we will also have the opportunity to "play" with other art media. Again the session will be introductory, and the focus will be on "getting to know each other."

Week Three: Representation of Self using drawing activity. In this session we will be using drawing to look at ourselves in relation to our environment; in particular, where we feel safe, and where we feel uncertain. The activity will generate some ideas about our strengths, and strategies for building on them.

Week Four: Understanding negative beliefs, and challenging them. This session will explore messages we may have received about ourselves, including our body–image, from families, friends and the media. We will use collage and card to make a "harpy," which is a representation of our "inner critic," in order to externalize this voice and begin to challenge it.

Week Five: Representation of Eating Issue in a visual form. We will make an image which represents our eating issue. This can be abstract, symbolic or representational. It could be about a single incident, a feeling, a relationship, or an overall statement. Clay, paints, and dry media will be available. This activity will help us start to explore how the eating issue may be serving a particular purpose in our lives at this moment in time.

Week Six: Treasure Map. This activity identifies our wants and needs, and invites us to make a visual statement about these, as a preliminary to making sure these wants and needs are met. A photo of ourselves is needed for this collage activity.

Week Seven: Family Portrait. This activity explores our "family of origin" and helps us to look at the helpful and unhelpful dynamics we may still be enacting in our current lives. We will have a choice of either clay or collage to represent our families.

Week Eight: Body Outline drawing. We will be making a life–size drawing of ourselves using any media. We can use the body outline to represent our physical body, or our emotions, our history, in fact any aspects of ourselves, using a variety of media.

Week Nine: Closure Session 1, "Life Map." This will involve a group drawing or painting to represent, where we have come from, where we are now, and where we are heading. This can be abstract, symbolic or representational. (Alternatively, the group could decide on its own preferred theme).

Week Ten: Closure Session 2, "Group Gifts". What was gained, what was difficult, giving symbolic 'gifts' to other group members. We will review the series of groups and give feedback to the facilitators. We will explore ways to celebrate endings.

Format of Each Session

The sessions will run for two hours. Each session will start with a brief "check–in" activity (15 mins.). This will generally be followed by the main art activity (30 mins.). The second hour of the group will be a time for sharing and processing the images (artwork), and other issues arising from the session (55 mins.). There will be a brief "finishing activity" at the close of each group (5 mins.). These times are approximate only, and can be changed if necessary, to suit the needs of individuals and/or the group.

Appendix–Terms

Continuum of eating distress–This term, coined by Brown (1993), aims to encapsulate both clinical and non–clinical responses by women to food and body image. Instead of seeing women with serious eating issues as being very different from the general female population, the continuum of eating distress stresses the similarities between these clinically ill women and their "healthy" sisters. All women, Brown argues, are preoccupied with weight, dieting and body image; it is merely the severity of that preoccupation which varies. This gives us a different framework, or "lens," through which to view eating issues and causes us to consider the effect of pervasive cultural influences which help to create this phenomenon (Bordo, 2003; Edwards, 2005).

Subversion–This aspect of art therapy, identified by Skaife (1995) refers to its' potential to challenge the status quo of medical treatment and to encourage personal empowerment on the part of the client, rather than passive acceptance.

References

Ball, J. & Norman, A.M. (1996) Without the group I'd still be eating half the Co–op. *Groupwork, 9*(1), pp. 48–61.

Black, C., & Symes, J. (1998). Group work with women with eating disorders. Brisbane: Isis–Centre for Women's Action on Eating Issues.

Bloch, S. & Crouch, E. (1985). *Therapeutic factors in group psychotherapy.* Oxford: Oxford Medical Publications.

Bordo, S. (2003). *Unbearable weight: Feminism, Western culture and the body* (2nd ed.). Los Angeles: University of California.

Bronte's Story, Television documentary directed by Bibb, S., broadcast on 26th March 2000, Channel Nine, Australia.

Brown, C. (1993). The continuum; Anorexia, bulimia and weight preoccupation. In C. Brown & K. Jasper (Eds.), *Consuming passions: Feminist approaches to eating disorders* (pp. 53–68). Toronto: Second Story.

Bruch, H. (1974). *Eating disorders: Obesity, anorexia and the person within* (2nd ed.). London: Routledge.

Bryant–Waugh, R., and Lask, B. (1995) Eating disorders–an overview. *Journal of Family Therapy, 17*, 13–30.

Butler, S. (1983) Openings. In J. H. Robbins and R. J. Siegel (Eds.) *Women changing therapy* (pp. 103–111). New York: Harrington Park.

Calam, R., & Slade, P. (1994) Eating patterns and unwanted sexual experiences. In B. Dolan and I. Gitzinger (Eds.), *Why women: Gender issues and eating disorders.* London: Athlone.

Cooke, K. (1994a). *Real gorgeous: The truth about body and beauty.* St. Leonards, NSW: Allen and Unwin.

Cooke, K. (Writer). (1994b). *Gorgeous* [Video]. S. Connolly (Producer). Australia: Film Australia.

Crisp, A. H. (1980). *Anorexia nervosa: Let me be.* London: Academic.

Crowl, M. (1980) Art therapy with patients suffering from anorexia nervosa. *The Arts in Psychotherapy, 7*, 141–151.

Davis Halifax, N.V. (1997) Feminist art psychotherapy: Contributions from feminist theory and contemporary art practice. *American Journal of Art Therapy, 36*, 49–55.

Duncan, B., Miller, S., & Sparks, J. (2004). *The heroic client: A revolutionary way to improve client effectiveness through client–directed, outcome informed therapy.* San–Francisco: Jossey–Bass.

Edwards, C. (2005). *"I just want to melt away": "Treatment" of women with eating issues: A critical feminist informed view of art therapy and the exploration of an alternative approach.* Master's (Hons) thesis, University of Western Sydney, Australia.

Eichenbaum, L., & Orbach, S. (1983). *Understanding women: A feminist psychoanalytic view.* New York: Basic.

Fleming, L. (1989). Art therapy and anorexia: Experiencing the authentic self. In L. M. Hornyak and E. K. Baker (Eds.), *Experiential therapies for eating disorders* (pp. 279–304). New York: Guilford.

Gibney, P. (1995). Dr. Paul Gibney talks with Psychotherapy in Australia. *Psychotherapy in Australia, 1*(3) 36–40.

Gilroy, A. (1995) Changes in art therapy groups. In A. Gilroy & C. Lee (Eds.), *Art and music: Therapy and research* (pp. 66–81). London: Routledge.

Gilroy, A. & Hanna, M. (1998). Conflict and culture in art therapy: An Australian perspective. In A. R. Hiscox & A. C. Calisch (Eds.), *Tapestry of cultural issues in art therapy* (pp. 249–275). London and Bristol, PA: Jessica Kingsley Publisher.

Hogan, S. (1997a). *Feminist approaches to art therapy.* London: Routledge.

Hogan, S. (1997b). Problems of identity. In *Feminist approaches to art therapy* (pp. 21–48). London: Routledge.

Kearney–Cooke, A. (1989) Reclaiming the body: Using guided imagery in the treatment of body image disturbances among bulimic women. In L. M. Hornyak & E. K. Baker (Eds.), *Experiential therapies for eating disorders* (pp. 11–33). New York: Guilford.

Kearney–Cooke, A. (1991). The role of the therapist in the treatment of eating disorders: A feminist psychodynamic approach. In C. L. Johnson (Ed.),

Psychodynamic treatment of anorexia nervosa and bulimia (pp. 295–318). New York and London: Guilford.

Lawrence, M. (1979) The control paradox. *Women's studies international quarterly, 2,* (93–101).

Liebmann, M. (2004). *Art therapy for groups* (2nd ed.). London: Brunner Routledge.

Levens, M. (1987). Art therapy with eating disordered patients. *Inscape,* Summer, 2–7.

Levens, M. (1990). Borderline aspects in eating disorders: Art therapy's contribution. *Group analysis, 23*(3), 277–284.

Maclagan, D. (1998) Anorexia: The struggle with incarnation and the negative sublime. In D. Sandle (Ed.), *Development and diversity: New applications in art therapy* (pp. 78–91). London and New York: Free Association.

Makin, S. (2000). *More than just a meal: The art of eating disorders.* London and Philadelphia: Jessica Kingsley Publishers.

Malson, H. (1998). *The thin woman: Feminism, post–structuralism and the social pathology of anorexia nervosa.* London: Routledge.

Matto, H. (1997). An integrative approach to the treatment of women with eating disorders. *The arts in psychotherapy, 24*(4), 347–354.

McDermott, B., Harris, C., & Gibbon, P. (2002). Individual psychotherapy for children and adolescents with an eating disorder: From historical precedent to evidence based practice. *Child and Adolescent Psychiatric Clinical Journal of North America, 11,* 311–329.

McLeod, J. (1994). Systematic inquiry into individual cases. In *Doing counseling research* (pp. 103–120). London: Sage.

Mitchell, D. (1980). Anorexia nervosa. *The Arts in Psychotherapy, 7,* 53–60.

Murphy, J. (1984). The use of art therapy in the treatment of anorexia nervosa. In T. Dalley (Ed.), *Art as therapy* (pp. 96–109). London: Tavistock.

Orbach, S. (1978: 1998). *Fat is a feminist issue and its sequel* (2nd ed.). London: Arrow.

Orlinsky, D., Grawe, K., & Parks, B. (1994). Processes and outcome in psychotherapy–noch einmal. In A. E. Bergin and S. Garfield (Eds.)., *Handbook of psychotherapy and behavior change* (4th ed.). (pp. 270–378). Hoboken, NJ: John Wiley and Sons, Inc.

Otway, O., and Ellis, M. L. (1987) Painting their way out of the blues. *Community care,* 16–17.

Robertson, M. (1992). *Starving in the silences: An exploration of anorexia nervosa.* Sydney: Allen and Unwin.

Robinson, S. (1996). *Mary Jane: Living through anorexia and bulimia nervosa.* Sydney: Random House.

Rosal, M. (2001). Cognitive behavioural art therapy. In J. A. Rubin (Ed.), *Approaches to art therapy: Theory and technique* (2nd ed., pp. 210–225). London and New York: Brunner Routledge.

Rust, M. (1987) Images and eating problems. In M. Lawrence (Ed.), *Fed up and hungry: Women, oppression and food* (pp. 145–155). London: The Women's Press Ltd.

Rust, M. (1992). Art therapy in the treatment of women with eating disorders. In D. Waller & A. Gilroy (Eds.), *Art therapy: A handbook* (pp. 155–172). Buckingham: Open University.

Rust, M. (1994). Bringing "the man" into the room: Art therapy group work with women with compulsive eating problems In. D. Dokter (Ed.), *Fragile board: Arts therapies with clients with eating disorders* (pp. 48–59). London/Bristol, PA: Jessica Kingsley Publishers.

Schaverien, J. (1987). The scapegoat and the talisman: Transference in art therapy. In T. Dalley & C. Case, J. Schaverien, F. Weir, D. Halliday, P. Nowell Hall & D. Waller (Eds.), *Images of art therapy.* London: Tavistock.

Schaverien, J. (1992). *The revealing image.* London/New York: Tavistock/Routledge.

Skaife, S. (1995) The dialectics of art therapy. *Inscape, 1*(1), 2–7.

Tolman, D. & Debold, E. (1994). Conflicts of body and image: Female adolescents, desire and the nobody body. In P. Fallon, M. Katzman & S. Wooley (Eds.), *Feminist perspectives on eating disorders* (pp. 301–317). New York: Guilford.

Waldman, J. (1999) Breaking the mould: A woman's psychosocial and artistic journey with clay. *Inscape, 4*(1), 10–19.

Waller, D. (1993). *Group interactive art therapy: Its use in training and treatment.* London and New York: Tavistock Routledge.

Waller, D. (2006). Art therapy for children: How it leads to change. *Clinical Child Psychology and Psychiatry, 11*(2), 271–282.

Weiser, J. (1993). *Phototherapy techniques: Exploring the secrets of personal snapshots and family albums.* San Francisco: Jossey Bass.

Welsby, C. (1998) A part of the whole: Art therapy in a girls' comprehensive school. *Inscape, 3*(1), 33–40.

Whitely, S., & Collis, M. (1987). Therapeutic factors in group psychotherapy applied to the therapeutic community. *The International Journal of Therapeutic Communities, 8*(1),21–32.

Wood, M. (1996). Art therapy and eating disorders: Theory and practice in Britain. *Inscape, 1*(1), 13–19.

Wooley, S., & Kearney–Cooke, A. (1986). Intensive treatment of bulimia and body image disturbance. In K. D. Brownell and J. P. Foreyt (Eds.), *Handbook of eating disorders: Physiology, psychology and treatment of obesity, anorexia and bulimia* (pp. 476–502).

Yalom, I. (1985). *The theory and practice of group psychotherapy* (2nd ed.) New York: Basic.

Biography

Claire Edwards is currently the Program Coordinator for the Masters of Mental Health (Art Therapy) at the University of Queensland, Brisbane, Australia. She also works part–time as an art therapist at the Mater Children's Hospital in the Child and Adolescent Mental Health Service in South Brisbane. She trained in art therapy at Goldsmiths College, University of London, and completed her research Masters (Hons) at the University of Western Sydney, in which she explored a feminist art therapy approach to women with eating issues.

Chapter 4

PRESERVING THE SELF: TREATING EATING DISORDERED INDIVIDUALS WHO SELF–INJURE WITH ART THERAPY

MICHELLE L. DEAN

I feel like I am a big, open, scar. Open and bleeding. Everything is bleeding. My insides wanting to come out – to release the power it has over me. I don't feel like there is an end to this – and therefore I should try and produce an – end. An end where I have the control and power. I want to cut myself, I want to feel the warmth of the blood, the comfort of the blood. Sometimes, like now, that feels like the only comfort. I have to know that I have expressed how truly bad I feel. So, if I hurt myself, I would feel better and we could all move on.

– by a woman who has bulimia nervosa and self injures

Introduction

The symbolic expression of pain, suffering, and trauma as expressed in the patient's account in the opening of this chapter, was sublimated into a positive outcome through the use of the art therapy modality. After this young woman, a twenty–year–old bulimic and self–injurer, wrote these words about herself, a transformative process occurred, as she engaged in making an image about how she felt. During this process, her intense negative feelings that demanded action melted into greater articulation of underlying emotions and discussion of the contributing factors that led to her acute suffering. This woman who began her eating disordered and self–injurious behaviors when she was a eight escalated as she reached adolescence and her young adulthood. With several hospitalizations during her teenaged years, marked by ritualistically measuring her vomit and cutting her arms to the point that the skin on her forearms no longer resembled skin but a tough leathery surface. Her silenced childhood, full of sexual exploitation and abusive parenting, continued as she tried to tell her story to deaf ears as an ado-

56

lescent. After "failing out" of traditional talk therapy due to her non–responsiveness and "non–communicative" way of relating to others, she was referred to the author's art therapy services and began to put the piece of her life together. We worked together individually utilizing the art therapy modality, in weekly and at times twice a week sessions for six years. Finding a voice that no longer had to scream with bodily symptoms was a huge step for this young woman and the art was the portal to her inner emotional terrain.

Most eating disordered and self–injurious behaviors begin in adolescence (ANAD, 2005; Walsh, & Rosen, 1988) and many of the origins that predispose one to self–destructive behaviors in adolescence and adulthood, lie in early childhood and are pre–verbal in nature (Feldman, 2002; van der Kolk, Perry & Herman, 1991). Some of the contributing factors, which are explored in this chapter, include early childhood ruptures, trauma, and underlying personality disorders. Research and clinical observation supports the use of a "modified psychotherapy," such as art psychotherapy, to improve verbalization and symbolic expression, which is often, impaired due to damaging early childhood experiences (Bruch, 1973, 1978; Dean, 2005; Makin, 2000; Milia, 2000; Perry & Herman, 1991; van der Kolk). Theory and treatment utilizing art based interventions for eating disordered individuals who self–injure are provided through a review of current literature and the use of case examples, thus illuminating the significance of attachment ruptures and early childhood traumas, as they relate to later direct and indirect self–injurious symptom formation. While these disorders affect both men and women the author will be referring to the population in this chapter in the feminine.

Eating Disordered and Self–injurious Behaviors

Individuals who manifest eating disordered symptoms are as a group, the most lethal and self–damaging psychiatric illness currently listed in the *DSM–IV–TR* (ANAD, 2005), while the mortality rate for women with Anorexia Nervosa, ages 15–24, is twelve times the general population and it is estimated that 20 percent of women with Anorexia Nervosa will prematurely die from complications related to the eating disordered symptoms, including suicide and heart problems (The Renfrew Center Foundation, 2003). While only one percent of the general population engages in self–harm as described by Favazza (1998), it is reported as many of 50–61 percent of self–injurers have, or at one time had, a significant eating disorder (Conterio & Lader, 1998; Favazza, 1987) and as many as 32 percent of eating disordered patients self–harm (Solano et al., 2005). Knowledge has increased about the complex issues that lead to the manifestation of the spectrum of eating disordered behaviors and the direct and in–direct harm caused by such symptoms. Yet, little attention has been given to the significant subgroup of this population who also directly self–injure, through a form of self–mutilation, with few exceptions (Eberly, 2005; Farberow, 1980; Levitt & Sasone, 2002; Levitt, Sansone & Cohn, 2004; Solano et al., 2005; Vanderlinden & Vandereycken, 1997).

Most individuals who engage in eating disordered and self–injurious behaviors do not intend to commit suicide. Menninger (1938) described self–injury as a "focal suicide" in perhaps the first psychological writings on the subject, in his book *Man against himself.* Literature and clinical experience indicates that the act of self–destructive behavior serves to help preserve the psychic functioning of the individual, restoring them to an "alive" or a self–affirming state (Favazza, 1987; Menninger, 1938; Milia, 2000; Simpson, 1980; Walsh & Rosen, 1988). There are numerous accounts as to why one self–harms or engages in eating disordered behaviors. Each of the explanations include an underlying desire to symbolically act out or give voice to an internal experience that may be difficult to articulate or even identify. Some of the explanations include wanting to feel in control, or feel alive when the they feel numb or "cut off" from affective experiences. Others may be symptomatic in order to stop internal discomfort by subjugating the pain to a tangible place on the body. Schwartz and Gay (1996) described the "adaptive functions" of eating disordered symptoms, which also seem applicable to the many of the motives, albeit at times unconscious, for self–injurious acts (p. 95). These adaptive functions are listed in Table 1.

Psychotherapy approaches used to manage of self–injurious behaviors (SIB) among individuals with eating disorders (ED) are quite varied and empirical data is minimal (Levitt, Sansone, & Cohn, 2004); however, it is agreed that a modified psychotherapy, such as art therapy, is recommended for both SIB and the ED populations in order to improve verbalization and symbolic expression, thus bridging the internal states of feeling with external actions (Bruch, 1973, 1978; Makin, 2000; van der Kolk, Milia, 2000; Perry & Herman, 1991). Through art therapy based interventions, a bridging of internal emotional states to external action may mitigate and contain destructive desires to regulate affect through the symptoms associated with SIB and ED, in a constructive and socially acceptable way. By using artwork, a variety of issues may be addressed in this population.

Mitigating urges to self–harm and building self–esteem are elements that may be addressed with art–based interventions. Sanson, Levitt and Sansone (2004) describe specific strategies for managing self–harm and eating disordered behavior that includes cognitive and interpersonal restructuring, dynamic intervention, family therapy, behavioral modification, sublimation, contracting, group therapy, and crisis intervention plans, all of which may be adapted and incorporated to an art psychotherapy modality. Due to the

Table 1. Adaptive Function of Eating Disorder Symptoms

Comfort/Nurturance
Numbing
Distraction
Sedation
Energizer
Attention – Cry for help
Rebellion
Discharge of anger
Identity & self–esteem
Maintain happiness
Control & happiness
Predictability & structure
Establishment of psychological space
Reenactment of abuse (Repetition/compulsion)
Self–punishment or punishment of the body
Containment of fragmentation
Dissociation form intrusive thoughts, feelings, images
Cleanse or purify the self
Attempt to disappear (Anorexia)
Create a large body for protection
Create a small body for protection
Avoidance of intimacy
Release of tension built up from hyper vigilance
Symptoms prove "I am bad" instead of blaming abusers

Source: Schwartz & Gay, 1996, p. 95.

pre–verbal nature of the psychic injuries many of these individuals have endured, descriptions of the benefits utilizing a non–verbal and experiential, therapeutic, modality such as art therapy with clients to assist processing traumas, relationship conflicts, affect regulation, and thus decreasing direct and in–direct self–harm. Although SIB does manifest in populations such as the chronically mentally ill, such as individuals with thought and organic disorders, the mentally retarded and the institutionalized, this chapter focuses on SIB in individuals who meet eating disorder criteria in the *DSM–IV–TR.*

Between 7 and 24 million women and one million men in the United States have an eating disorder while 70 million people worldwide struggle with eating disorders (ANAD, 2005; The Renfrew Center Foundation, 2003). One–third of eating disordered clients also have a significant Axis II diagnosis, with those individuals who manifest bulimia nervosa, self–injury, and alcohol abuse had a 95 percent likelihood to also have a personality disorder, borderline personality disorder being the most common (Brownell & Fairburn, 1995; Levitt, Sansone & Cohn, 2004). This subgroup may be disproportionate diagnosed with borderline personality disorder due to the fact that the only diagnosis in the *DSM–IV–TR* that addressed self–injuring behavior is borderline personality disorder (APA, 2000a, pp. 292–293).

Self–injury may be viewed in this population in two categories, indirect and direct self–harm. Indirect self–harm may be seen in the numerous medical consequences inflicted by eating disordered behaviors (i.e., tears in the esophagus, dental, throat and stomach problems, heart and kidney functioning impairments, injuries related to loss of consciousness, falling, broken bones, and other symptoms related to starvation and dehydration). The most common form of direct self–harm as described by Fazazza (1987, 2000) is the moderate/superficial type (i.e., cutting, burning, hair pulling, piercing, tattooing and scarification). Moderate/superficial self–harm behaviors can be further divided into two subgroups: compulsive and impulsive. Impulsive SIB is characterized by two subgroups: episodic and repetitive (Eberly, 2005; Favazza & Simeon, 1995). "Compulsive self–injurious behavior is usually habitual, repetitive, and 'automatic'" (Levitt, Sansone & Cohn, 2004, p. 32). Compulsive self–injurious behavior usually has ego–dystonic overtones, despite preventing or reducing anxiety and distress" (Levitt, Sansone & Cohn, 2004, p. 32) and is closely related to obsessive–compulsive disorder (Eberly, 2005). Compulsive behaviors include "severe nail biting, hair pulling and purging behaviors such as self–induced vomiting, laxative, and diuretic abuse" (Levitt, Sansone & Cohn, 2004, p. 34).

Impulsive behaviors are not always manifested with conscious intent and are associated with a building of tension followed, an attempt to resist followed by a relief after engaging in the destructive act, such as suicide attempts, skin cutting and burning (Levitt, Sansone & Cohn, 2004). Impulsive/episodic behaviors are usually sparked by an emotional trigger and can escalate into a pattern of habitual self–injury, with individuals unable to identify themselves as "self–injurious" (Eberly, 2005). Additionally, impulsive/repetitive self–injurious behaviors differ in the rumination of about self–injury, even when not engaging in such behavior and typically individuals who engage in the repetitive behaviors, self–identify as a self–injurer (Eberly, 2005). These behaviors can be seen in individuals with an eating disorder who ruminate about restricting, purging, and bingeing.

Predisposition for Self–Harm and Eating Disordered Behaviors: Attachment Ruptures

Infancy is the time in which a child is completely dependent on her mother or primary caretaker, for safety, nurturance, and comfort (the author will be referring to primary caregiver as mother in this chapter; however, it is important to note that this person could be of either gender and not necessarily biologically related, as in an adoptive parent or relative who assumes primary care–taking responsibility of the child). Everything the infant comes to know and understand is processed through the senses: touch, taste, smell, sight, and sound. In no other place of the body, are the five senses so concentrated as in and near the mouth. She is completely dependent on the mother for her needs without other effective means to communicate desires, distress or need, except though body movements such as grimacing, crying, and other somatic defenses. Hence, Freud (1970) named this developmental period the Oral Stage, due to the infant's increased acquisitions of knowledge through the orifice of the mouth. In addition to receiving nourishment through the mouth, it can also be seen as a place of comfort, suckling long after the hunger quest has been fulfilled. A baby also mouths objects as a way to come to understand form and boundaries of self and other, or environment, experimenting with hard and soft objects. Through this receptive sensing, experimenting and play, an understanding of self and other takes place. The interaction between mother and infant is essential in the formation of a positive introject, which helps the child feels secure, trusting of her world, good about herself, emotionally and physically, able to soothe and tolerate painful affect. Through this process, an introject of mother is internalized and is later able to soothe the self in a constructive means. Though enough positive experiences, a child will emerge for this time feeling secure, nurtured, and comforted. Thus, leaving a foundation on which other experiences are to follow.

The child, in the first 18 months of life, is particularly vulnerable to attunement ruptures due to her lack of verbal communication and mobility. A secure parent–child attunement with minimal disruption leaves the child secure to venture out into her world and confident. Feldman (2002) states, "An interior symbolic world is constructed through experiences of optimal connection and separation; the baby is able to functionally to take care of himself in increasing increments . . . [and] the baby's capacity for connection also plays an important role in symbolic development" (p. 401). Personality development is one in which the child feels confident and aware of one's own and other's boundaries and separateness. In parent–child relationships in which the child receives insufficient and inaccurate feedback, she may develop poor interceptive awareness, a distorted perception of self, and a pervasive sense of ineffectiveness (Feldman, 2002). In parent–child relationships where the attachment process has had significant ruptures or trauma(s), the formation of a personality disorder may occur, particularity, borderline personality (BPD).

Early Childhood Trauma

Although there is some ambiguity about the direct relationships between SIB, ED, and trauma, current literature illuminates a correlation between childhood sexual trauma and eating disorders (Herman & van der Kolk, 1987; van der Kolk et al., 1991). Research indicates the younger the patients are when abused or neglected or in some cases, had multiple surgeries, the more likely they are to engage in self–injurious behaviors and other such destructive acts, such as eating disorders (Herman & van der Kolk, 1987; van der Kolk, 1991). "The earlier the abuse, the more self directed the aggression. Abuse during early childhood and latency was strongly correlated with suicide attempts, self–mutilation, and other self–injurious behaviors. In contrast, abuse in adolescence was significantly associated with anorexia nervosa and with increased risk taking" (van der Kolk, 1996, p. 190). Sexual abuse appears to increase the likelihood of SIB in ED patients, as many as 60–80 percent of clients with eating disorders report an underlying history of sexual abuse (Eberly, 2005; Schwartz, & Cohn, 1996; Ticen, 1987). Sexual abuse may be more predictive of bulimic rather than anorexic symptoms and is often related to the severity of symptoms (Kendler et al, 2000; Schwartz & Cohn, 1996; Wonderlich, Brewerton, Jocic, Dansky & Abbott, 1997). Thus, the more severe the abuse may indicate more severe symptoms later in life.

A personality disorder, specifically BPD, is often linked to childhood trauma and may seen as a contributing factor to SIB and the resistance to treatment in ED patients. BPD is the only diagnosis listed in the *DSM–IV–TR* that lists self–injurious behaviors as a criterion and is often given as an Axis II diagnosis for women who engage in SIB and have an eating disorder. Research demonstrated that patients with BPD had the most severe abuse histories, compared to other psychiatric populations with as many as half of BPD patients studied had physical and sexual abuse starting before the age of six (Herman & van der Kolk, 1987). It has also been demonstrated that "1.) self–mutilators had more severe character pathology than diagnostically matched nonmutilators and 2.) there was a significant correlation between SIB and impulsivity, chronic anger, and somatic anxiety. . ." (Simeon et al., 1992, p. 225). Although, Favazza (1996) advocates that SIB should be listed with its own diagnostic criteria in the DSM, separate from personality disorders, there are shared characteristics that appear to link the SIB population with BPD under its current classification system. Those characteristics include: early abuse histories, high levels of dissociative defenses, highly chaotic family environments, lack of sufficient parental support, extensive psychological stressors, and severe mood disorders (Eberly, 2005; Levitt, Sansone & Cohn, 2004).

Children who internalize trauma often develop spit off introjects and parallel schemes that coexist and follow them into adulthood (van der Kolk, 1996). These internalized schemes include: "High levels of competence and interpersonal sensitivity existing side by side with self–hatred, lack of self care, and interpersonal cruelty" (van der Kolk, 1996, p. 196). For many, there is an inability to trust others and their environment. Believing that bad things are destined to reoccur, she feels that her agency is ineffective and that there is a loss control. While others may believe that it is their responsibility to make things right through rigid controls of affect, body functions or controlling others and this early developmental trauma makes the complexity of treating this population more visible.

Another area in which trauma impairs individuals is in their ability to put feelings into words (alexithymia and somatization) and to symbolize (Milia, 2000; van der Kolk, 1996, p 185). Trauma may result in a "speechless terror," due to an increase in perfusion in the right hemisphere associated with emotional states and autonomic arousal and a decrease of oxygen utilization in the area's of the brain responsible for generating words to attach to internal experience during exposure to traumatic stimuli areas in the brain that make verbal cognition of emotional and internal experiences possible (van der Kolk, 1996). "For traumatized patients, action replaces symbolic representations. The capacity to use symbolization for soothing anxieties and delaying gratification of urges is quite weak. Instead impulsive actions to end or alter states of anxiety are used" (Milia, 2000, p. 76). Further, "Prone to action, and deficient in words, these patients can often express their internal states more articulately in physical movements or pictures than in words. Utilizing drawings . . . may help them develop a language that is essential for effective communication and for symbolic transformation that can occur in psychotherapy" (van der Kolk, 1996, p. 195).

Treatment

It is recommended a variety of techniques and interventions be utilized to assist with the continuums of SIB and ED behaviors. However, first, it is imperative to establish a base line physical health, so a medical evaluation is necessary. A comprehensive medical exam, including blood and urine screenings, such as complete blood count (CBC), liver and thyroid functions and electrolyte balance, as well as gynecological exams for women, is needed to rule out underlying medical conditions which may be causing eating disturbances, which include, but are not limited to, diseases of the thyroid, digestive, metabolic, and hormone systems (APA, 2000b). For malnourished and severely symptomatic patients, it is recommended additional blood studies be administered which include calcium, magnesium, and phosphorous levels as well as electrocardiograms and for patients underweight more than six months, a bone density examination, also known as a dual–energy X–ray absorptiomerty (DEXA) scan, given to rule out Osteopenia or osteoporosis (APA, 2000b). Due to low body weight, as seen in Anorexia Nervosa, laboratory imbalances or other changes may require inpatient hospitalization to stabilize and the re–nourish the individual before psychotherapeutic work may effective. Research indicates, only when body weight is within 90–95 percent of normal range can counseling and medication make a lasting impact and a patient's relapse rate is 50 percent if released while her weight is still below 85 percent of ideal body weight (The Renfrew Foundation, 2003).

Art Therapy and the SIB and ED patient

The approaches to art–based interventions with this population, when seen from the view of psychological theories, may best remain eclectic. Theory, which seeks to describe phenomena, is useful in that it provides a framework for understanding. However, art is a direct manifestation of psychic functioning and hence reflects the full range of human experiences that are the subject of the diverse theoretical viewpoints. Hence, in clinical practice one is led to theoretical structures through the artwork and symptomtology of the patient rather than the other way around. The author's approach is to be consistent in listening to the image and the symptoms as a symbolic manifestation of underlying issues first, and then applying such theoretical constructs as are made relevant through that approach. Some theoretical thoughts in relationship to eating disorders and self–injury are highlighted in this next section.

Destroying one Gestalt in favor of another has long been a definition of creativity thus also paralleling the process for multiple opportunities for regression in the service of the ego (Freud, 1993). The art process "recognize(s) the place of destructive activity within the creative process" (Milia, 2000, p. 177). It is through this destruction that a new form emerges. It is this idiosyncratic destruction of flesh that the individual hopes to restore them to a sate of "aliveness." Art therapy meets the "injured," pre–verbal, and child–part of the client in a contained supportive therapeutic environment. The complex work of providing a safe therapeutic alliance in which inner psychic work may take place is about creating a new experience of safety and trust, fortifying self worth, creating supportive interpersonal connectiveness, and increasing personal agency within the client. This process may include several techniques ranging from sublimation, cognitive/behavior and interpersonal restructuring, crisis intervention, group and family therapy, and contracting (Levitt, Sansone, & Cohn, 2004). Although some short–term cognitive behavioral techniques are helpful in reducing "faulty" thought processes, it is this author's belief that more profound effects occur in individuals over a longer period of time in which a multi–faceted intervention is utilized where trust is built within a supportive holding environment and interpersonal relatedness is essential in order to fortify inner supports.

The art materials and the art therapy process are inherently full of reflections of symbolic parallels between the self, nourishment, comfort, and boundaries. Patients respond to the newness of materials as if providing a gift or nourishment as found in food. The thickness of drawing paper acts a reminder of the many layers of pulp that make up each page, mimicking flesh. This building and recreating boundaries is illustrated in the delicate application of hundreds of "reparative" layers of tissue paper and decoupage, a thin glue. This is a popular technique among patients with eating disorders, which utilizes the repetitive process of covering over, and building thickness and character, layer upon layer. Acts of doing and undoing, erasures and crossing out, do not simply annihilate one symbolically but instead turn into a creative restorative process. This process was illustrated, Figure 1, by a young woman in her early twenties, who depicted how she felt and what she hoped to feel and or wanted in her life. The image on the left side of the page was created by repetitive pushing and pulling at the surface of the drawing paper until it wore away, leaving a hole. Frustrated by the hole, she then attempted to "fix" the surface through the delicate application of several layers of light blue tissue paper. Her handprint just below the torn area gives additional credence that this is where she both places and identifies herself, a nebulous unformed hole, in the delicate process of healing. On the right side of the paper was what she hoped for in her life. This incorporated figure resembles a helpless fetus, without feet and confined arms and hands, wrapped in numerous protective layers, the inner layer a cobalt blue and the outer most, represented by flames. These flames appear symbolic of warmth or hearth she longed for, as well as a fiery protection to keep others at a distance and to prevent "being burned."

"Pushed and pulled" are often words used to describe this population by clinicians, as interpersonal boundaries are stretched and recoiled in the therapy process, defining both physical and psychic boundaries. These behaviors are akin to the infant exploring her mother's breast, trying to grasp where she begins and the other ends, or the experimenting toddler who tests her parents' limits to find out how much of a behavior is enough and what type of reaction may be elicited, while needing empathic consistency. Pushing and pulling paint with hands or brushes recreates a similar dynamic to the child who mouths an object to explore all of its external properties in relationship to its own internal world. There is as much learning about the external object as the internal facets of the mouth. The world of experimentation and trial and error is the realm of art. Artists, of any experience, struggle with materials and materials may be pushed to their creative limits as a means of bridging the internal state to the external. This push and pull in art media mirrors the clients learning about the external manifestation of internal terrain.

"The skin boundary of the body provides containment, protection, and definition of the self. Likewise, artworks can provides containment, protec-

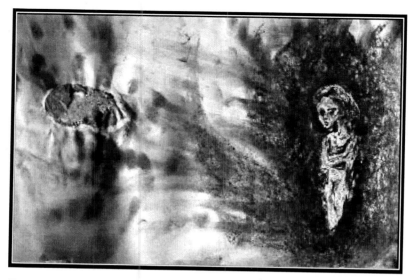

Figure 1. "Boundary Rupture." 12" x 18", pastel chalk and tissue paper on paper. *Ripping the surface of the paper and attempting to repair with layers of tissue paper underlay.*

tion, and definition" (Milia, 2000, p. 172). The artwork assists the patient in the externalizing and objectifying thoughts and feelings in a controlled manner, thus increasing feelings of power and self–awareness (Milia, 2000; Wadeson, 1980). Paint with high viscosity, or substance, such as acrylic and tempera or gouache, mimic milk and blood, filming over to form a thin skin able to be punctured and reworked. This "skin" becomes more solid but ideally remains flexible over time. Much like moving the client from a rigid or brittle posture, to one of flexibility and decreased defensiveness.

The art materials may be used in a self–stimulation, masturbatory, or soothing manner in which manipulation and mastery may be explored in socially appropriate ways. Through repetitive positive experiences of soothing oneself in creative ways increases self–esteem, self–agency and lessens the likelihood of seeking soothing or stimulating behaviors, which may be destructive. The acquisition of these skills enables clients to negotiate intolerable feelings, prolonging and ideally mitigating impulsive action. It is important to note that substitute actions toward self (i.e., snapping rubber bands, drawing on self with markers, and breaking eggs on arms) gives the message that intense, undesirable feelings require a hostile action toward self. The author believes these feelings are best sublimated in artwork and not enacted on the person.

The transitional object symbolizes "the breast, or the object of the first relationship" (Winnicott, 1971, p. 9). Art, as a transitional object, serves the purpose of suspending or minimizing anxiety caused by a separation from the positive caretaker or therapist thus creating a bridge both within the patient (internal and external realities) and between the patient and the therapist, in times of stress and anxiety. Using sculpting materials in therapy, this object may be depicted as a grounding stone, animal, or other form, which allows the person to connect in created in a "potential space." This potential space, described by Winnicott (1971), is related to the patient's inner worlds and with the actual, or external, reality. The transitional object, created in the therapy session is imbued with symbolization of the patient's internal state and hopefully as well as the positive influence of the therapist's presence, thus "creating a containing, holding environment" (Silverman, 1991, p. 100).

Graphic Indicators of SIB and ED Behaviors

Although there is no one single indicator in the artwork for eating disordered and self–injurious behaviors, clusters of these elements may be used to gain insight into functioning levels, defenses, and symptom formations. Behaviors manifested as graphic indicators phenomenologically seen in artwork of anorexic patients include: rigid and retentive affect, isolation of affect, restrictive use of space, controlled and small marks, defenses may include depersonalization, intellectualization denial as seen in "pleasing pictures" and sometimes cognitive impairments due to malnutrition which appear as temporary or permanent organic indicators (Dean, 2005, 2006b; Lubbers, 1991; Matto, 1997; Mitchell, 1980). The bulimic patients behaviors in artwork may have impulsiveness, compulsiveness, boundary issues such as difficulty creating, undoing or reinforcing forms, compartmentalization of affect as well as themes of purging such as doing and undoing. The themes of doing and undoing are especially poignant for the client who self–injurers. Commonalities among clients who demonstrate eating disordered, self–injurious behaviors, previous trauma, and borderline personality are mirrored in the manifestations of the artwork (Levens, 1987). Most striking are the slashing and cutting of body parts or objects in forms. This can also be seen in the "X–ing" out of forms or the use of crosses similar to double or single railroad tracks. There may also be much attention to the depiction of eyes such as in blacken or closed eyes with a sense of unconsciousness or depersonalization. Floating dismembered eyes and the use of wedges, as described by Spring (1993, 2005), are often seen in the artwork of trauma survivors also is commonly seen in this population.

Themes in ED and SIB patients' artwork include, the depiction of weapons and fire. Many times the weapons are turned onto the self or the symbolic portrayal of self in the artwork. The line quality may be very active and agitated thus, displacing affect and leading to a disintegration of form or reality especially as it applies to images of the body and or body boundaries. There is often use of concrete separators between people, such as walls and boxes, or empty space may be used to define oneself or a separation between people. As with the art of a patient with borderline personality disorder there is often a preferred use of black and red and there may be themes of food and blood in the artwork (Gerber & Jacobson, 1982). A very regressed patient may create an image with his or her own blood. Although never encouraged as a part of a therapeutic process, a client may bring such an image created at home to session. The author does not process such an image with the patient in order to minimize secondary gain or glorification from such destructive actions. Themes of death or coffins may manifest in the art. These images may be helpful in assessing suicidal ideation as well as discussing the desire to "kill off" negative introjects. A funeral scene may shed great insight into the patient's desire to feel connected, loved, and desired. By drawing her funeral, she may give voice to what seems like a desire to die but actually is the need to know that others care about her (Dean, 2006a). This image also may be used to identify supports in her life that perhaps are not adequately being utilized. There are many shared features in the artwork of patients with eating disorders, SIB, previous trauma, and BPD as seen in Table 2. The information in Table 2 is based on observation as well as findings in current literature about each of the populations (Brooke, 1997; Cohen–Liebman, 1995; Dean, 2005, 2006a, 2006b; Earley, 1999b; Gerber & Jacobson, 1982; Lubbers, 1991; Malchiodi, 1990; Milia, 2000; Spring, 1993, 2005; Ticen, 1987). By no means is it a complete listing nor does it imply that each indicator will apply a definitive diagnosis, or that all indicators are found in those meeting specific DSM criteria but instead it is provided to give the clinician insight into possible clusters of indicators and to the level of functioning and defenses employed.

Table 2. Graphic Indicators in Artwork

ED	SIB	TRAUMA	BPD
AN Faint hesitant line quality Small or exaggerated Tentative boundaries or omission of boundaries Restrictive/rigid line quality Omission or exaggeration of body parts	Active line quality Slashes Railroad track marks "XX" as depiction of ambivalence Doing & undoing Weapons toward self Themes of blood & fire Dehumanized & non human self representa-	Isolation, barriers Role reversal Encapsulation Compartmentalization Doing & undoing – erasures Omission of body parts Fragmented and disorganized body parts	Remains dependent when blaming others Ego centric Themes of blood & food More regressed with structure Vertical relationships Merger of human relationships – fusion or merged images

Continued on next page

Table 2.—*Continued*

Isolation, isolation of affect Intellectualization & rationalization as seen by the use of words Incorporation (i.e., circles within circles or other forms within forms) Flowers & other "pleasing picture" themes Occasionally, cognitive impairments due to malnutrition Holes in body or form, typically in mid–section Oral & anal themes BN Agitation Exaggeration of boundaries thick dark lines or multiple lines to define boundaries or form Impulsive & compulsive behaviors Compartmentalization of affect Doing & undoing – erasures Holes in body or form, typically in mid–section Omission or exaggeration of body parts Flowers with pointed petals Oral & anal themes	tions (i.e., use of fairies & other fantasy figures) Attention to eyes – blackened or closed – sense of unconsciousness Use of black & red Empty space use – to define self or separation between people Body form boundaries Concrete separation between people (i.e., boxes, walls) Themes of death, coffins Incorporation (i.e., circles within circles or other forms within forms) Incorporation (i.e., circles within circles or other forms within forms) Ungrounded, floating or disconnected images	Emphasis on upper part of body while ignoring lower parts Separation of trunk Exaggeration or minimalization of sexual features Seductiveness or avoidance of sexualization Lack of mouth or large circular mouth Protruding tongues Disembodied, highly stylized or tearful eyes Transparencies Compartmentalization Use of complementary colors Use of black & red Represents self as small Sexual themes Broken hearts Hearts with holes Floating, ungrounded images Wedges Omissions Dead trees, absence of leaves, slanted trees Clown images Presence of phallic–like objects	Body form boundaries Concrete separation between people (i.e., boxes, walls) "XX" as depiction of ambivalence Empty space use – to define self or separation between people Splitting – good & bad on opposite sides Use of black & red Multiple human ideals (i.e., angels & devils) Dehumanized & non human self representations Attention to eyes – blackened or closed – sense of unconsciousness Death or coffin themes Weapon, fire, blood Active line quality Displacement of affect Disintegration of form or reality Splitting – keeps interjects separate, lack of ability to integrate ambivalence Projective identification – denies negative attributes in self, projects ambivalence onto others Premature idealization – all good objects rarely disappoints

Eating Disorder Indicators: (Dean, 2005, 2006a 2006b; Earley, 1999b; Lubbers, 1991; Ticen, 1987).
Self–Injurious Behaviors Indicators: (Dean, 2005; 2006a, 2006b; Milia, 2000).
Borderline Personality Disorder Indicators: (Gerber & Jacobson, 1982).
Trauma & Sexual Abuse Indicators: (Brooke, 1997; Cohen–Liebman, 1995; Malchiodi, 1990; Spring, 1993, 2005).

Case Example

Bonnie began her therapeutic relationship with the author when she was a young 14–year–old girl while she was hospitalized in an inpatient eating disordered treatment facility. During those sessions, she was seen primarily within the context of group art therapy, where she was shy and timid, often refusing to speak for long periods of time. While in art therapy; however, the images she created were filled with much rage, and demonstrated affective lability. Her artwork also had symbols of trauma, such as sexual themes, isolation, barriers, encapsulation, broken hearts and hearts with holes, floating images, disembodied eyes, illustrated in Figures 2 through 6. Her inner intensity was often unable to be contained within the confines of the page and the images demonstrated of themes of death, consumption, entrapment, self–stimulation (i.e., masturbation), self–directed violence, and rage. When asked for associations to her artwork, she would shrug her shoulders in puzzlement as if the imagery and affect originated outside of her. As with so many patients with this symptom profile, she demonstrated a disconnection between her thoughts and feelings. Her depersonalization, compartmentalization, and lack of verbal articulation were evident when she tried to describe an internal emotional experience.

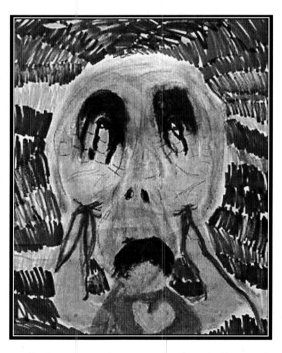

Figure 2. "Self Portrait," 12 x 18, marker, pencil, oil & chalk pastels. *A depersonalized representation of self with cut arms, truncated body and compartmentalized affect radiating from body into environment.*

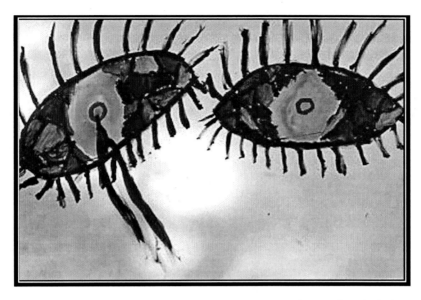

Figure 3. "Floating Eyes," 12 × 18, acrylic paint on paper. *Floating disembodied eyes demonstrating compartmentalization in the whites as well as hollow pupils. Tears flowing from pupil instead of tear ducts.*

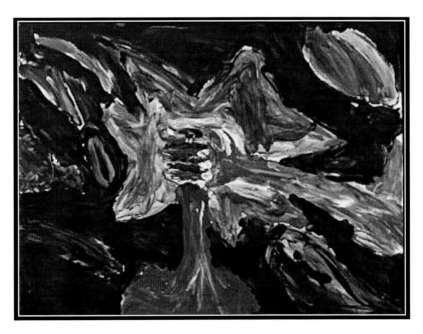

Figure 4. "My pain," 12 × 16, tempera & acrylic paint on canvas board. *A painting of how she felt on this day. Symbolic masturbation imagery apparent with much turmoil and fragmentation of affect in background.*

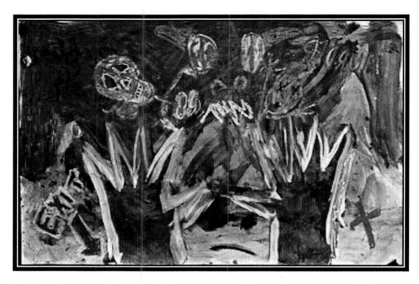

Figure 5. "Murderous exit," 12 × 18 tempera & oil pastels on paper. *A frantic attempt to visually describe her terror, murderous rage, and underlying urges to kill off painful internal introjects coupled with labile suicidal ideation.*

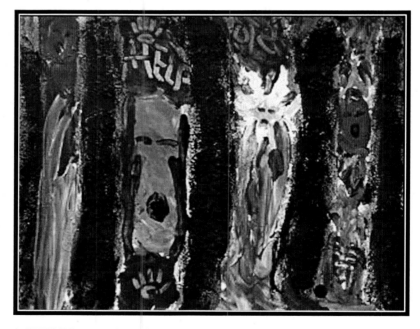

Figure 6. "HELP," 12 × 16 acrylic & paint medium on canvas board. *Images of screaming people representing aspects of self (may also be seen as a visual recapitulation of family system as there were three siblings and two parents, three people, three fingers, three fuchsia color blacks and five bars) and hands are entrapped in a prison–like container created with thick black textured paint medium.*

During the next three years, she was hospitalized three times for severe ED behaviors (bingeing, purging and restricting), and SIB (cutting and burning) and labile suicidal ideation. When she was referred to the author's private practice, she had been placed in an alternative school for children with behavioral problems, but had not been to school for over 9 months (the length of her last hospitalization) and the author no longer worked for the inpatient facility where she first meet Bonnie. Bonnie's outpatient work began when she was 17 and she attended sessions weekly, sometimes two or three times a week, until she was 21 years old. During this time, her treatment team included a psychiatrist for medication management and a physician for medical evaluation and laboratory checks on a regular basis. She refused to work with nutritionist, stating she knew as much or more than a nutritionist regarding what she was supposed to be eating. The therapy work included interpersonal, insight oriented art psychotherapy, cognitive reprocessing, behavioral interventions, and at times, crisis intervention.

Bonnie was a bright motivated young woman who possessed insight to the many contributing factors to her situation. Some of the contributing factors included an alcoholic father and an untreated bipolar mother. The mother left the patient and her older siblings when she was three and she returned for visits with her children sporadically throughout the patient's childhood. The father remarried within a year. The stepmother and her son, who was eight years older than the patient, were verbally and emotionally abusive to her and her sisters via severe criticism, belittlement, and threats of abandonment. There was suspected but unfounded sexual abuse by a relative. The "absent" father was oblivious to the abuse until the marriage failed five years later, in much rage and turmoil. The father subsequently received treatment for his alcoholism and became very involved in a support network. He was able to make great strides in his own recovery and was committed to mending his relationships with his children. By the time the father had stabilized his life, Bonnie's eating disordered symptoms and cutting behaviors were well entrenched and were escalating.

Much of the therapeutic work involved self–esteem building, the creation of positive introjects, and the realization and constructive use of power and control within relationships. Through a slow and sometimes laborious process of building self–esteem through successful mastery within an art therapy context, and positive relational mirroring, Bonnie was able to carry these skills into many spheres of her life. Places that contained much success for Bonnie included, successfully completing the of requirements of high school, discussing conflicts within the family with her father in family sessions and at home, and managing to tolerate painful affects through alternative and more constructive means other than using her ED and SIB symptoms. Bonnie was able to see that there were many ways of being in relationship to what seemed like intolerable affects (often related to separations and perceived abandonment). Further, she was able to sublimate her feelings in her art and was able to generate alternative solutions to problems which initially seemed insurmountable.

Working the Relationship

Often practicing alternative coping skills requires a conflict or stressor. Bonnie had many opportunities to practice her coping skills with her first significant boyfriend, for their relationship was tumultuous. Bonnie's boyfriend was enrolled in a nearby school for troubled youth. He struggled with drug addiction and lived in a chaotic home environment, a noteworthy parallel to Bonnie's early relationship with her father. Bonnie engaged in her first sexual activity with this young man after much discussion and deliberation in therapy. She often felt he set up hopeful but unrealistic expectations for her. They would use their symptoms to both motivate the other to not engage in their own symptoms (i.e., "If you don't use, I won't use either") and later when this did not work, they would punish each other by engaging in their symptoms (i.e., "I'll show you how much you hurt me, I'll cut my self"). Bonnie felt both liberated by the sexual relationship and also at times repulsed. He would attempt to coerce her into sex and when she was unreceptive would masturbate in front of her hoping to persuade her to join him. Toward the end of their relationship when the demise was evident, Bonnie created Figure 7, "The Jerk Off." This nearly monochrome brown image was created at home and brought to therapy for discussion. She depicted her boyfriend masturbating, smoking a cigarette, with a large red X across his featureless head. The isolation of affect is apparent in the red X over the featureless face and in the pinkness of the painted penis. Her apparent rage and hurt are evident in this image as well as the depersonalization and disconnect between the figure and the artist or audience/viewer. There are no facial features to engage or identify with only the indecipherable writing on his shirt and the action of discharge. The indecipherable writing may be reflective of her alexithymia, in that she wanted to express something but could not find the words to do so. Many of the same feelings that had been symbolically portrayed about her in earlier images had been transferred and displaced to the boyfriend (connection b/w denied or covered over thoughts and sexual action—reminiscent of previous masturbatory themes in artwork, Figure 4, in which she describes her emotional pain). The depersonalization, self-stimulation and the annihilation or undoing in this image can bee seen as both an

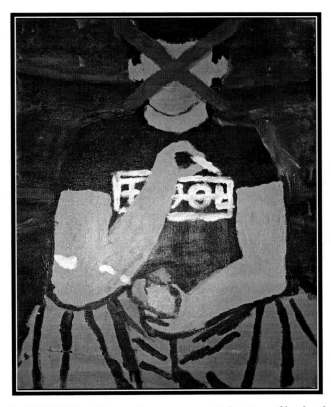

Figure 7. "The Jerk Off," 20 x 24, acrylic on canvas. *A depiction of her lost love, her boyfriend and her displaced feelings of depersonalization and annihilation for herself, anger and disappointment.*

objective sense of self and also about her feelings toward her boyfriend as they ended their relationship.

Many of the art therapy tasks Bonnie engaged in during our sessions included recognition of underlying emotional distress. This was done through free drawings, mandalas, emotional landscapes or identifying her feelings. Allowing the art to mirror her internal reality she was able to place feeling words to her previously action–oriented but verbally silent emotional terrain. Both in sessions and as homework, Bonnie was able to sublimate harmful urges into her artwork. Her artwork consisted of a multitude of two– and three–dimensional media. Over time, a broader more intricate emotional vocabulary developed as well as her ability to place behavioral "stops" in order to ward off self–injurious and eating disordered behaviors. Her artwork transformed from visual purges to symbolic representations with more content of her current experiences and immediate self.

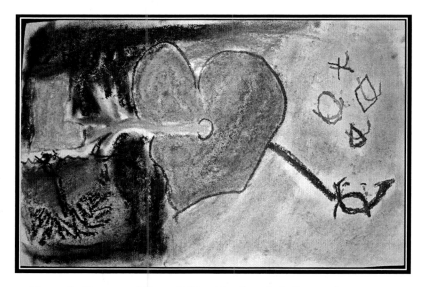

Figure 8. "Damaged Heart," 12 x 18, oil and chalk pastels on paper.

This transition continues to be visible in "Damaged Heart," Figure 8. This image created after the break up with her boyfriend depicted her feelings about relationships and her concerns of feeling "used and abused" in the past and her uncertainty about her future relationships. The compartmentalization continues to exist in the background however, the edges of the color blocks of black, pink, yellow and turquoise, begin to soften. Hearts and bodies with a hole in the middle is a motif often seen in artwork of clients who have eating disorders (Dean, 2005; Earley, 1999a, 1999b). In this image, the arrow undertakes a transformation as it emerges on the other side of the heart. Entering on the left as yellow and exiting on the right as red, on a different course, and without a point. The arrow connects to her ambivalent face, which has both a smile and a tearful frown. After she created Figure 4, our discussion included how being in relationship with others changes, which we are for the better and sometimes for the worse. The opportunity to have intimate relationships allows us to learn more about ourselves and to activate places within us that may not otherwise be awakened on our own.

Bonnie completed Figure 9 as a depiction of what she felt graduation day would be like as a way to pre–plan the day's events and to visualize the situation, thus reducing her anxiety. This day held much significance for her and her family. Just three years prior in the midst of her numerous hospitalizations, it was uncertain as to whether she would survive. In addition to the significant milestone, this day was also laden with much anxiety as she was voted by her peers and teachers as to address the graduation assembly about

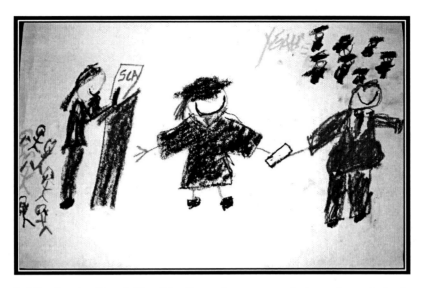

Figure 9. "Graduation Day," 12 × 18, oil pastel on paper. *A picture drawn before her graduation ceremony to help visualize this day and decrease her anxiety about addressing the assembly.*

her experience at the school and her future goals for herself and her wishes for her classmates. Her artwork although still slightly impulsive is much better organized, with less painful affect, and contains fewer trauma symptoms that were apparent in previous images.

Bonnie terminated treatment shortly after graduating high school and moved across the country to work in a five–month wilderness program. She called sporadically while away and once she returned came for "maintaince" appointments, coming only a few times in periods of stress or transition such as, finding a new job, a new relationship, and when her parents relocated to another part of the country. Bonnie continued to call on Mother's Day for several years after terminating therapy, a telling example of her transference. She reported doing well and has successful remission of both her eating disordered and self–injurious behaviors. At the time of this writing, Bonnie, has been in a serious relationship for almost two years, has secured a stable, skilled job, and is contemplating returning to school to pursue a college degree.

Implications and Recommendations

As incidents of eating disordered and self–injurious behaviors continue to grow at staggering rates, increased awareness and understanding for the complex dynamics that contribute to this cluster of symptomatic behaviors are necessary as well as awareness about effective treatment options including art–based modalities (Favazza, 1987; van der Kolk, 1996; Walsh & Rosen, 1988). Art based interventions may be utilized as a means of forming a bridge between internal emotional states and their externalization, mitigating, sublimating, and containing the destructive impulses and directing them towards more adaptive outlets as seen in the case example of Bonnie.

Further research is needed to clarify the relationship between childhood abuse, attachment ruptures, and later development of problems direct and indirect self–harm as manifested in the eating disorder population. It would also be worthy to establish the connection between the non–verbal aspects of the art psychotherapy modality and its effectiveness with direct and indirect self–harm and eating disordered behaviors. It is recommended, that along with drug and alcohol awareness and programs that are provided in many schools, that there be greater efforts to increase awareness and treatment options for individuals with eating disordered and self–injurious behaviors since most of these behaviors begin in adolescence and the mortality rate for Anorexia Nervosa is twelve times higher than the death rate of all causes of death for females ages 15–24 (ANAD, 2005). Thus, it is the author's recommendation and hope that by providing timely treatment options, which include a modified form of individual psychotherapy, such as art psychotherapy, support groups, and other services provided by trained and experienced professionals this would decrease the morality rate as well as lessen the suffering associated with these symptoms and their underlying causes amongst individuals who have self–injurious and eating disordered behaviors. This recommendation is further supported by the research that has shown that early intervention and treatment yields the most favorable prognosis for individuals who have eating disorders (Brownell & Fairburn, 1995; The Renfrew Center, 2003). This becomes particularly significant when considering, in the eating disorder population, long–term follow–up studies show a 40 percent full recovery rate, 30 percent improve and 30 percent remain chronic (Kaplan & Sadock, 1990).

Conclusion

The symbolic manifestation of eating disordered and self–injurious behaviors are often an attempt to regulate affect through the externalization of emotions. Art psychotherapy therapy interventions are relevant to bridging the symbolic language of internal and external terrain of this population, giving the pre–verbal psychic injuries a voice. Art psychotherapy interventions may be utilized to improve verbalization and symbolic expression, which is often, impaired due to damaging early childhood experiences (Bruch, 1973; 1978; Dean, 2005, 2006a, 2006b; Makin, 2000; Milia, 2000; van der Kolk, Perry & Herman, 1991). By utilizing the art–based tools, both the clinician and the patient are able to address in these multi–faceted, and challenging behaviors.

REFERENCES

American Psychiatric Association. (2000a). *Diagnostic and statistical manual of mental disorders* (4th–TR ed.). Washington D.C.: Author.

American Psychiatric Association. (2000b). Practice guideline for the treatment of patients with eating disorders (revision). *American Journal of Psychiatry, 157* 1. (January supplement), 1. Washington D.C.: Author.

Anorexia Nervosa and Associated Disorders (ANAD). (2005, February). *Facts about eating disorders.* Published 2000 [on–line], available: http://www. ANAD.org

Brooke, S. (1997). *Art therapy with sexual abuse survivors.* Springfield, Illinois: Charles C Thomas, Publisher.

Brownell, K., & Fairburn, C. (1995). *Eating disorders and obesity: A comprehensive handbook.* New York: Guildford Press.

Bruch, H. (1973). *Eating disorders: Obesity, anorexia nervosa and the person within.* New York: Harper Collins.

Bruch, H. (1978). *The golden cage: The enigma of anorexia nervosa.* New York: Harper Collins.

Cohen–Liebman, M. S. (1995). Drawings as judiciary aids in child sexual abuse litigation: A composite list of indicators. *The Arts in Psychotherapy Journal, 22,* 5, 475 – 483.

Conterio, K. & Lader, W. (1998). *Bodily harm: The breakthrough treatment program for self–injurers.* New York: Hyperion.

Dean, M. L. (2005, October). Treating clients with self–injurious behaviors with art therapy. *Professional continuing education training seminar,* Glenside, PA, USA.

Dean, M. L. (2006a). Creative Destruction: Art based interventions with eating disordered clients who self–injure. *The 16th Renfrew Center Conference,* Philadelphia, PA: The Renfrew Center.

Dean, M. L. (2006b). Preserving the Self: Art Psychotherapy applications with eating disordered clients who self–injure. *The American Art Therapy Association Conference,* New Orleans, LA: The American Art Therapy Association.

Earley, M. L. (1999a). Art therapy: Body image, media & art. *The American Art Therapy Association Conference,* Orlando, FLA: The American Art Therapy Association.

Earley, M. L. (1999b). Art therapy with eating disordered clients. *The Renfrew Center Conference,* Philadelphia, PA: The Renfrew Center.

Eberly, M. (2005). Understanding self–injurious behavior in eating disorders, *The Remuda Review, 4*(3), 26–30.

Farberow, N. (Ed). (1980). *The many faces of suicide: Indirect self–destructive behavior.* New York: McGraw–Hill Book Company.

Favazza, A.R. (2000). Self mutilation. *The Renfrew Center Conference,* Philadelphia, PA.: The Renfrew Center.

Favazza, A. R. (1998). The coming of age of self–mutilation. *The Journal of Nervous and Mental Disease, 186*(5), 259–268.

Favazza, A. R. (1987). *Bodies under siege: Self mutilation in culture and psychiatry.* Baltimore: The Johns Hopkins Press.

Favazza, A. R. & Simeon, D. (1995). Self mutilation (pp. 185–200). In E. Hollander & D. Stein (Eds.), *Impulsively and aggression.* Sussex, England: John Wiley & Sons.

Feldman, B. (2002). The lost of infancy: Symbolization, analytic process and the growth of the self. *Journal of Analytical Psychology, 47,* 399–408.

Freud, A. (1993). *Ego and the mechanisms of defense.* CN: International Universities Press, Inc.

Freud, S. (1970). Beyond the pleasure principle. In J. Stracheey, (Ed.), *The standard edition of the complete psychological works of Sigmund Freud* (Vol. XVIII). London: Hogarth.

Gerber, N. & Jacobson, M. (1982). *Identifying Borderline Characteristics in Graphic Patterns.* Unpublished paper. Philadelphia, PA. Presented at Friends Hospital CAT conference.

Herman, J. L. & van der Kolk, B. A. (1987). Traumatic antecedents of borderline personality disorder (pp. 111–126). In B. A. van der Kolk (Ed.), *Psychological trauma.* Washington, DC: American Psychiatric Press.

Kendler, K. S., Bulik, C. M. Silberg, J. Hettema, J. M., Myers, J. & Prescott, C. A. (2000). Childhood abuse and adult psychiatric and substance disorders in women: Epidemiological and co–twin control analysis. *Archives of General Psychiatry, 57,* 953–959.

Levens, M. (1987). Art therapy with eating disordered patients. *Inscape.* Summer, 2–7.

Levitt, J. L., & Sansone, L.A. (2002). Self–harm behaviors among those with eating disorders: An overview. *Eating Disorders: The Journal of Treatment and Prevention, 10,* 193–203.

Levitt J. L., Sansone R. A., & Cohn L. (2004). *Self–harm and eating disorders: Dynamics, assessment and treatment.* New York: Brunner–Routledge.

Lubbers, D. (1991). Treatment of women with eating disorders (pp. 49–82). In H. Landgarten & D. Lubbers (Eds.), *Adult art psychotherapy: Issues and applications.* New York: Brunner/Mazel.

Malchiodi, C. (1990). *Breaking the silence: Art therapy with children from violent homes.* New York: Brunner/Mazel.

Makin, S. (2000). *More than just a meal: The art of eating disorders.* London: Jessica Kingsley Publishers.

Matto, H. (1997). An integrative approach to the treatment of women with eating disorders. *The Arts in Psychotherapy, 24*(4), 347–354.

Menninger, K. A. (1938). *Man against himself.* New York: Harcourt, Brace & World, Inc.

Milia, D. (2000). *Self–mutilation and art therapy: Violent creation.* London: Jessica Kingsley Publishers.

Schwartz, M. F. & Cohn, L. (Eds.). (1996). *Sexual abuse and eating disorders: A clinical overview.* New York: Brunner/Mazel.

Schwartz, M. & Gay, P. (1996). Physical and sexual abuse and neglected and eating disorder symptoms (pp. 91–107). In M. F. Schwartz & L. Cohn (Eds.). (1996). *Sexual abuse and eating disorders: A clinical overview.* New York: Brunner/Mazel.

Sanson, R. A., Levitt J. L., & Sansone, L. A. (2004). An overview of psychotherapy strategies for the management of self harm behavior (pp. 121–133). In J. L. Levitt,

R. A. Sansone, & L. Cohn (Eds.), *Self–harm and eating disorders: Dynamics, assessment and treatment.* New York: Brunner–Routledge.

Silverman, D. (1991). Art psychotherapy: Approach to borderline adults. In H. Landgarten & D. Lubbers (Eds.), *Adult art psychotherapy: Issues and applications* (pp. 83–110). New York: Brunner/Mazel.

Simeon, D., Stanley, B., Frances, A., Mann, J., Winchel, R., & Stanley, M. (1992). *American Journal of Psychiatry, 142*(2), 221 – 226.

Solano, R., Fernandez–Aranda, F., Aitken, A., Lopez, C. & Vallejo, J. (2005). Self–injurious behavior in people with eating disorders. *European Eating Disorders Review, 13,* 3–10.

Simpson, M. A. (1980). Self–mutilation as indirect self–destructive behavior: Nothing to get so cut up about . . . (pp. 257–283). In N. Farberow (Ed.), *The many faces of suicide: Indirect self–destructive behavior.* New York: McGraw–Hill Book Company.

Spring, D. (2005). Thirty year study links neuroscience, specific trauma, PTSD, image conversion and language translation. *Art Therapy: Journal of the American Art Therapy Association 21*(4), 200–209.

Spring, D. (1993). *Shattered: Phenomenological language of sexual trauma.* Chicago: Magnolia Street Press.

The Renfrew Center Foundation for Eating Disorders, "Eating disorders 101 guide: A summary of issues, statistics and resources." Published September 2002, revised October 2003, "http://www.renfrew.org".

Ticen, S. (1987). Feed me . . . Cleanse me. . . . Sexual trauma projected in the art of bulimics. *Art Therapy: Journal of the American Art Therapy Association, 7*(1), 17–21.

Van der Kolk, B. M., Perry, C., & Herman, J. L. (1991). Childhood origins of self–destruction. *American Journal of Psychiatry, 148,* 1665–1671.

Van der Kolk, B. M., (1996). The complexity of adaptation to trauma: Self–regulation, stimulus discrimination, and characterological development (pp. 182–213). In B. M. van der Kolk, A. C. McFarlane, & L. Weisaeth (Eds.), *Psychological trauma: The effects of overwhelming experience on mind, body, and society.* New York: Guilford Press.

Van der Kolk, B. M., McFarlane, A. C. & Weisaeth, L. (Eds.). (1996). *Psychological trauma: The effects of overwhelming experience on mind, body, and society.* New York: Guilford Press.

Vanderlinden, J., & Vandereycken, W. (1997). *Trauma, dissociation and impulse control in eating disorders.* Philadelphia, PA: Brunner/Mazel.

Wadeson, H. (1980). *Art psychotherapy.* New York: John Wiley & Sons.

Walsh, B., & Rosen, P. (1988). *Self–mutilation: Theory, research, and treatment.* New York: Guilford Press.

Winnicott, D. W. (1971). *Playing and reality.* London: Tavistock Publications.

Wonderlich, S. A., Brewerton, T. D., Jocic, Z., Dansky, B. S., & Abbott, D. W. (1997). Relationship of childhood sexual abuse and eating disorders. *Journal of the American Academy of Child and Adolescent Psychiatry, 36,* 1107–1115.

Biography

Michelle L. Dean, MA, ATR–BC, LPC is a registered, board–certified art psychotherapist and Licensed Professional Counselor. She works in private practice and has been an Adjunct Professor at Arcadia University in Glenside, Pennsylvania since 1997. She is a supervisor for graduate students, ATR candidates, and mental health clinicians wanting to further their knowledge about art therapy and the therapeutic uses of art, eating disorders, and other related topics. Ms. Dean's work history includes over a decade of eating disorder experience at nationally recognized eating disordered programs. Ms. Dean has presented extensively on the therapeutic benefits of art, the use of art therapy with eating disordered clients and self–injurious behaviors. She has been invited to speak on the radio, television, at schools, colleges and numerous local and national conferences. Ms. Dean is the author of the children's book, *Taking weight problems to school* (JayJo Press, 2005). Please see her website: http://web.mac.com/michelleldean.mac/iWeb/Site/Welcome.html.

Chapter 5

THE BODY OUTLINE DRAWING TECHNIQUE: CLINICAL CONSIDERATIONS FOR EATING DISORDERED TRAUMA SURVIVORS

JULIA ANDERSEN

Introduction

Professionals involved in the treatment of clients with trauma histories deepen their knowledge when they consider the relationship between trauma, eating disorders, and body image. It has been suggested that therapies should be modified for patients with a history of traumatic abuse (Brown & Pope, 1996) due to the complexity of the issues involved including the client's physical and medical condition, the psychological impact of the trauma, and it's significant impact on the client's body image. This chapter will explore this impact, describe the use of a well–known art therapy technique known as the body outline or body tracing, to treat body image disturbances that develop as a result, and will recommend specific clinical strategies to effectively use this technique without further traumatizing the survivor in treatment for an eating disorder. Trained clinicians utilize a "stage–oriented" approach to treating the eating disordered client with a history of sexual or physical trauma (Courtois, 1999), in favor of a graduated exposure to body image treatment (Rosen, 1997). The early stages focus on crisis stabilization and establishing realistic clinical goals based on the completion of thorough assessments. The middle stages are both educational and behavioral, focusing on identifying traumatic factors while teaching coping strategies, such as stress–reduction techniques and grounding skills to use while completing regular, therapeutic meals. The later stages address underlying fears and conflicts while assisting the client to establish a motivation to change. The stage–oriented approach to treatment allows the trauma survivor to build trust in the therapeutic relationship.

The Eating Disordered Trauma Survivor

Recent literature links eating disorders and body image disturbances with a history of physical or sexual trauma (Fallon & Wonderlich, 1997; Treuer, Koperdak, Rozsa & Furedi, 2005) in as high as 75 percent of clients seeking treatment, with greater evidence linking physical abuse as a predictor in the development of eating disorders. The presence of body image distortions as measured by the Body Attitude Test (Tury & Szabo, 2000) used to determine pathological body image attitudes, indicates that various forms of abuse are associated with severe body image distortions. The most common eating disorders; anorexia, bulimia and binge–eating or compulsive over–eating, share relevant diagnostic criteria including; body dysmorphia, body image distortion, and body dissatisfaction (APA, 1994). All three eating disorders list: intense body rejection, body dissatisfaction, fear of weight gain, and obsessive thoughts regarding body shape and appearance. Clinical theorists hypothesize that bulimic symptoms, including bingeing and purging, may be the client's effort to regulate the intense affect experienced as a result of past trauma and childhood abuse, and have the highest clinical association with sexual abuse (Vanderlinden & Vandereycken, 1997). The client with anorexia may starve the body to avoid sexual development, and in this way, attempts to control maturation and interpersonal relationships (Johnson, Sansone, & Chewing, 1992). The client with compulsive over–eating may use food as a self–soothing mechanism to numb feelings and memories associated with abuse, and intentionally gain weight to a size where sexual features are covered and the body shape is unattractive. This client may successfully avoid or push away intimate relationships that bring up fears associated with trust, rejection, and abandonment due to repressed feelings associated with the original abuse.

When treating all three eating disorders of various body sizes, physical condition or attractiveness, the therapist must be aware of her own attitudes regarding body shape, in addition to expected countertransference reactions usually associated with the treatment of trauma clients (Andersen, 2000; Winn, 1994) The western–based cultural bias against having a large body size cannot be overlooked, and deserves further exploration beyond the focus of this chapter. A more complete understanding of relationship between trauma, eating disorders and body image can be explored by understanding body image concepts and development.

Body Image

Body image is the picture we have in our minds of the size, shape and form of our bodies (Slade, 1994). The "picture," in our minds, develops over time from birth and evolves throughout a person's lifetime. The infant develops awareness of the body through touch, and the experience of the mother or care–provider holding it. With close visual contact, the infant mirrors the mother's face and expressions (Mahler et al., 1975), providing a basis for its own feeling expression. Kohut (1971) describes the importance of physical touch to establish boundaries and body awareness. When the infant is given a consistent source of nurturing, secure attachments are developed and a cohesive image of the body is formed by 18 months of age. In contrast, maternal/child neglect or enmeshment creates boundary confusion (Krueger, 1989). If, for example, the mother is unable to respond to the child's natural feeding schedule or cries of hunger, feeding her only when the mother is hungry, the child will become dependant on the mother's signal for food rather than trusting her own body cues for hunger. During the first two years, the child is particularly vulnerable to these and other unnatural, disruptions in development. Confusion in body cues of hunger and fullness cause disturbances and weakness in the developing body image. Parents and care–providers have the greatest influence in the development of the child's positive body image and establishment of safe boundaries. Events that compromise the establishment of trust between the child and parents, permanently alter the child's ability to trust others and themselves. Abuse and neglect may not be visible outside the body; however, pre–verbal and non–verbal experiences are internalized and become the basis of a negative body image. All events that have ever happened to the child are stored in the body as visual or kinesthetic memory. According to one theory (Anzieu, 1989), visual and sensory experiences of early infant/child trauma and neglect are absorbed and stored as layers which surround the body like an envelope. This "envelope" continually records and responds to external stimuli and becomes the basis for the body boundary and subsequent body image, or "skin ego."

This theory suggests that early body trauma becomes the fabric of the developing ego, and internal self–concept. It is extremely important to consider this theory when treating the client with body image disturbances. Specific body areas may hold tension, shame or rage associated with the trauma. Later in development, when cognition emerges, the attitudes, perceptions and judgments regarding the body become fixed. If the abuse and body disturbance has remained undetected by others until the beginning of puberty, the stress associated with fears of sexuality and body change become too overwhelming for the weakened, negative body image and often initiate an eating disorder. Anorexia develops as an adaptive function of the ego (Johnson, Sansone, & Chewing, 1992) to avoid or manipulate body development, and the intense fears of separation and abandonment that maturation requires, In addition, natural or expected body changes which occur throughout the client's lifespan including, pregnancy and menopause in women, or the aging process can produce a similar, negative reaction in the trauma survivor. These body changes represent another loss of control and account for a recent trend in late onset eating disorders. The stress of coping with these changes may uncover repressed memories of abuse or neglect from childhood, especially if insecure attachments and weak boundaries are part of the individuals self–concept.

Trauma survivors reject the body, expressing intensely negative feelings towards it, due the experience of powerlessness, guilt, and shame associated with the abuse. When a negative body image is formed, it becomes a powerful reinforcer in the maintenance of an eating disorder (Kearney–Cooke & Streigel–Moore, 1997). Trauma survivors with eating disorders have displaced shame directly onto their bodies, and in sexual trauma cases, may fear further body violation and contamination by rejecting food (Ticen, 1987). The drive to control food in attempts to control the shape and appearance of the body through weight loss, exercise, or purging is established. The attitude that it is more acceptable to fear food, fat, and weight gain than it is to face the intolerable fear of sexual development or body change is developed. The associated meanings and feelings become the basis for the body image distortion.

It is extremely important to the recovery process that professionals involved in the treatment of trauma survivors with body image disturbances attempt to prevent shame–inducing experiences by carefully considering each intervention used in therapy. The body outline drawing or body tracing has the potential to strengthen the clients body boundary, as well as to uncover dynamic conflicts and fears held inside the body, however special considerations are necessary. When used as part of a structured art therapy group designed to support the patient's body image treatment plan, which incorporates the stage–oriented process, conflicts can be safely explored with minimal fears of additional trauma.

Art Therapy

The value of art therapy with trauma survivors has been established by some of the most prominent clinicians in the field. Evidence–based case studies (Brooke, 1995; Cohen & Cox, 1995; Gerity, 1997, Goodwin & Attias, 1999; Malchiodi, 1990; Prugh & Quirk, 1998; Spring, 1993; Ticen, 1987) report the value of the art process to safely communicate non–verbal material which transcends space and time, builds self–esteem, and describes dissociative states. Art therapy allows access to pre–verbal, non–verbal, and sensory material (Fallon & Wonderlich, 1998), externalizing the client's internal experience into a concrete form, creating a "window" (Cohen & Cox, 1995) into their world. The art–making is a safe container for the eating disordered trauma patient to express feelings, as witnessed by the trained therapist (Hornyak & Baker, 1989) and as a reparative intervention for a fragmented body image as a result of childhood trauma, towards a healthy, cohesive self (Gerity, 1997).

Art therapy is used as a clinical adjunct to traditional verbal therapies in eating disordered programs to assist the patient's behavior plan of eating meals while learning appropriate means of tolerating and expressing feelings. In addition, the drawing process is used in the assessment and treatment of a distorted body image. The management of anxiety and tension plays a significant role in integrating the feeling/emotional body with the intellect (Kearney–Cooke & Streigel–Moore, 1998). Eating disordered patients have low tolerance for anxiety and tension due to the inability to self–soothe which was not learned during childhood or disrupted as a result of physical or sexual trauma. Art expression can improve the client's regulation of body tension. Instead of relying on restricting, bingeing, purging or other means of self–injury to cope with tension and stress, the client can create artwork to channel destructive impulses (Andersen, 2004). Art therapy with the eating disordered trauma survivor can strengthen body boundaries and allow exploration of the symbolic self (Levens, 1994; Luzzatto, 1995; Waller, 1993), be used as a body–mapping process to increase body awareness and identify feelings held inside the body (Rice, Hardenbergh & Hornyak, 1989; Totentobier, 1995). It can assist therapists with grounding techniques to reduce dissociation in clients with active post traumatic symptoms (Cox, Rankin & Barnes, 1993) and most effectively as an assessment tool to treat body image distortions (Andersen, 2000b).

The Body Outline Drawing Technique

The *body outline* or *body tracing* has been used by art therapists in structured group settings to enhance body image (Schneider, Ostroff & Lebow, 1990), cope with altered body image in pediatric medical settings (Cameron, Juszczak & Wallace, 1984), in dance therapy groups with eating disordered clients (Totenbier, 1989) to improve body awareness and empathy, and to challenge cognitive distortions in perceptions of body size as part of a body image treatment program for eating disordered patients (Andersen, 1998; Andersen, 2000b). The use of this simple traced line becomes a body boundary, creating a visible container for the self and a powerful art therapy tool to temporarily hold intense, negative emotions from within the body. Anzieu's (1989) "skin ego" theory lends itself to the body tracing, allowing the client to view both inner and outer layers of the self. The drawing of the body provides a format for the eating disordered patient to safely discuss the body image treatment plan, including goals that are realistic for the hospital stay. Most art therapy techniques do not involve the whole body; however, this one focuses directly on the body capturing a two–dimensional image of the client's body shape with one drawn pencil line. Additional directives can be used throughout the entire treatment to enhance the outline, locate physical and emotional areas, and explore dynamic conflicts. Whether the therapist is addressing the degree of body distortion, or fears related to the body changing, this art therapy technique has the potential to both support the client's defenses and to challenge the presence of a body image distortion.

Therapists who question the appropriateness of using the body tracing technique with eating disordered patients, have valid concerns because of the high incidence of sexual trauma. Therapists fear that the client's experience of being traced, and of viewing the body drawing, will add to feelings of vulnerability, flooding the client with intense emotion. These fears create a false message to the client that potential reactions to the body, and feelings associated with the body, are too difficult for both client and therapist to manage. Rather the message should be on the timing and purpose of the intervention. The trained art therapist will consider each case, including issues of intimacy, space, touch, and boundaries, before introducing the body tracing as an option in therapy. Assessing the client's physical and emotional safety should always be a priority. When this has been established, and the art therapist and patient have agreed on a plan, the value of this intervention is remarkably successful.

The Body Outline Drawing Technique: Directions for Use

The client is first asked to draw a life–sized image of themselves directly on a large sheet of rolled white drawing paper which has been taped to the wall, as if they were standing in front of a mirror. The client is in comfortable, street clothing which can be held smooth to reduce wrinkle patterns during the tracing It is important that the client remain standing while drawing to facilitate a connection to the ground and build empowerment. In contrast, if the paper is placed on the floor, the client would be in a passive position which can induce feelings of powerlessness and recall victimization.

When the client drawing is completed, the therapist then asks the client to stand directly in front of the paper, facing forward, with arms and hands placed on the paper. After checking on the client's emotional state, the art therapist begins to trace the body, beginning at the top of the head and continuing to the neck, shoulders and arms, allowing the pencil to meet the edge of the client's body at a right angle. This is all done at a quick pace, to reduce the client's anxiety level. It is the pencil that touches the body, not the therapist. Physical touch should be minimized. After completing the leg line, the therapist should then check in with the client, asking if she is comfortable with the process while it is happening. The inside leg is only traced up to the knee to avoid close proximity to the client's pelvis and torso. The inner thigh line is completed by the therapist freehand after the client steps away from the wall. Another option is for the client to trace the upper leg herself while standing upright against the wall. Reassurance is needed so that at anytime the tracing can be paused to process material that may arise, and resume tracing when it is safe to do so. The choice to continue allows the client a measure of control.

At this point, the tracing becomes an interactive process between the client and therapist, as well as between the client's inner state of mind and her outer physical sensations of touch. It is a process of being seen, and connecting mind to body. If a client is unprepared for the experience or becomes flooded with negative thoughts and messages, the therapist can provide reassurance that these responses can be addressed through journaling and artwork. In the event of a post traumatic flashback or abreaction, the therapist must remain calm and use grounding strategies including deep breathing and focal points to assist the patient in re–gaining emotional safety. Even the experienced therapist with a well–planned session may be unable to prevent a dissociative or negative reaction. Although the client may have agreed to the proceed with the body tracing directive, a flashback indicates a fragile emotional state. The therapist should then re–evaluate body image goals with the client, and only resume treatment in the days or weeks that follow a dissociative event, if and when body tolerance has improved.

As soon as the tracing is completed, the client is asked to step away from the paper and view the drawings. It is important for the client to express first impressions by either journaling directly on the paper or verbalizing with the therapist. The client can react by seeing a difference between their drawing and the traced line recognizing the distortion, or she could challenge the accuracy of the tracing and deny the presence of a body distortion. Either way, the traced line is a closed shape and a concrete symbol of wholeness which has the potential to restore the connection between body and mind, and reduce fragmentation of feelings. It is a visible container for the externalization process seen in most art therapy products. It can also symbolize the shape and form of a close family member. If this member is also an abuser, the image of the body on the paper may quickly produce an identification with the abuser and cause an immediate negative reaction. Areas on the drawing and the client's body, which remind her of others can be processed in subsequent sessions. Exploring these significant factors under-lying the eating disorder and body image, can unlock doors to healing and understanding the client's illness. The results of this intervention can be com-municated to the client's clinical team to further the treatment process.

Group Therapy vs. Individual Session

The group therapy format is ideal for introducing the body tracing tech-nique to eating disordered trauma survivors for the following reasons. It can reduce social isolation and increase support between members, challenge distorted thoughts and perceptions using peer feedback, and validate intense emotional states in a safe, secure environment. Often patients in treatment will remark on the similarities between themselves and others. The group is a place like no other where irrational thoughts about the body can be open-ly discussed. Members who are further along in treatment will encourage others to "be patient" and tolerate the body changes or mirror thoughts back to a patient who is unable to make progress. Discussions about the meaning of "FAT" and fears that family or others will reject them if they were to gain weight are common, as well as disclosure of traumatic events–rape and abuse. The therapist presence in the group is extremely important (Winn, 1994). She must adhere to a classic neutral expression, and refrain from speaking directly about the body shapes seen on the wall, or make glances toward the client's body. These may be misinterpreted as judgments or eval-uations of body shape. Because the focus of the group is on the body image, the client is more vulnerable than in other groups, especially if memories of the abuse have recently surfaced and can easily be projected onto the body. One thoughtless comment could potentially sabotage the concentration and focus of the entire group. It is extremely important that the therapist herself have supervised, clinical training in trauma, educational background in art therapy, and knowledge of body image concepts to effectively use the group process. These guidelines will foster an emotionally safe experience for all members.

Conclusion

The body outline drawing process is a powerful experience for the eating disordered trauma survivor. Although it can produce remarkable results, with concrete evidence of a body image distortion and will provide a point of reference for the trauma survivor to process underlying conflicts, it should only be used by trained therapists with knowledge of body image concepts and trauma issues. Because the tracing is created directly from the body, the client is at risk for emotional flooding with body–related memories. The timing and planning for the intervention is extremely important and should only be considered when emotional safety and body tolerance have been established. With these considerations in place, the art therapist can provide a unique opportunity for the eating disordered trauma survivor to make considerable progress in one session that may typically take several months or years to achieve. The prepared therapist will gain deeper knowledge of the client when taking steps to successfully treat one of the most challenging and complex populations in the field.

Appendix A–Terms

Anorexia–A refusal to maintain body weight at or above a minimally normal weight for age and height. Intense fear of gaining weight or becoming fat, even though underweight. Absence of at least three consecutive menstrual cycles.

Bulimia–The presence of recurrent episodes of binge–eating, or consuming unusually large amounts of food within a two–hour period. A lack of control over eating during the episode. Recurrent compensatory behavior in order to prevent weight gain, such as self–induced vomiting, misuse of laxatives, diuretics, enemas or excessive exercise. Overevaluation of body shape and size.

Binge–eating–Recurrent episodes of binge–eating, eating more rapidly than normal, eating until uncomfortably full, and eating alone, at least 2 days per week for six months. Feeing marked distress after eating, disgust with oneself and guilty.

Compulsive over–eating–Repeated patterns of emotional eating.

Body image–The image of the body in the mind's eye, based on thoughts, perceptions, emotions and interpersonal experiences.

Body boundary–a psychological term to describe the physical and emotional space between self and others. Healthy boundaries are flexible and establish the self, while protecting and restoring the self image.

Body distortion–an inaccurate perception of body shape and size caused by multiple physical and psychological factors.

Body dissatisfaction–intense rejection of the body shape, size, and physical appearance, regardless of weight loss or gain.

Body dysmorphia–obsessive thinking or delusions regarding a part or the entire appearance of the body.

Body tracing–a continuous line traced around the circumference of the body to distinguish the body shape.

Body outline drawing–the development of the body tracing during subsequent art therapy sessions to assist body image treatment and self expression.

Enmeshment–a psychological term to describe a disturbance in boundaries between two persons, with one or both persons remaining dependent on the other to meet emotional needs.

Appendix B–Clinical Guidelines for Using the Body Outline Technique

1. The client must demonstrate a degree of trust with the therapist and have discussed the benefits and challenges of using the body tracing in therapy.
2. The client must demonstrate the ability to tolerate feelings about their body, without current safety issues, prior to the art therapy session.
3. The therapist must monitor the client's affect and metal state before, during and after the completed body tracing.
4. The therapist must have knowledge of body image concepts and art therapy process, have completed trauma training, and have regular clinical supervision.
5. The therapist should have group therapy training with leadership skills which foster empathy among members, and support body image recovery goals.
6. The therapist must provide follow up to the client, and attending psychiatrist, as to the effectiveness of completing the body tracing, making recommendations for continued treatment.

References

American Psychiatric Association (APA). (1994). *Diagnostic and statistical manual of mental disorders* (4th Ed.). Washington DC. Author.

Andersen. J. (1998). Tree drawings, body outlines and body image. *Proceedings of the American Art Therapy Annual Conference.* Milwaukee, Wisconsin.

Andersen, J. (2000a). Body transitions: Art therapy with eating disordered patients. *Proceedings of the American Art Therapy Annual Conference.* St. Louis, Missouri.

Andersen, J. (2000b). The body outline drawing technique: Clinical considerations for art therapy groups. *Proceedings of the American Art Therapy Association Annual Conference.* St. Louis, MO.

Andersen, J. (2004). From cutting to creating: Art therapy with clients who self–injure. *Proceedings of the American Art Therapy Association Annual Conference.* Chicago, Illinois.

Anzieu, D. (1989). *The skin ego.* New Haven, CT: Yale University Press.

Brown, L. & Pope, K.S. (1996). Recorded memories of abuse. Washington D.C: American Psychological Association.

Brooke, S. (1995). Art therapy: An approach to working with sexual abuse survivors. *The Arts in Psychotherapy, 22* (5), 447–466.

Cameron, C., Juszczak, J. & Wallace, N. (1984). Using creative arts to help children cope with altered body image.

Cohen, B. & Cox, C. (1995). *Telling without talking: Art as a window into the world of multiple personality disorder.* New York: W.W. Norton & Company.

Courtois, C. (1999). *Recollections of sexual abuse: Treatment principles and guidelines.* New York: W.W. Norton & Co.

Cox, Barnes & Rankin, (1993). *Managing traumatic stress through art. Drawing from the center.* Baltimore: Sidran Press.

Fallon, P. & Wonderlich, S. (1997). Sexual abuse and other forms of trauma. In D. Garner and P. Garfinkel (Eds.), *Handbook of treatment for eating disorders.* New York: The Guilford Press.

Fleming, M. (1995). The picture as a transitional object in the treatment of anorexia. In D. Doctor (Ed.), *Arts therapies in clients with eating disorders: Fragile board.* London: Jessica Kingsley.

Gerity, L. (1997). The reparative qualities of art therapy: Dissociative identity disorder and body image development. *Dissertation abstracts international section A: Humanities and social sciences, 58* (1–A), 63.

Goodwin, J. & Attias, R. (1999). *Splintered reflections: Images of the body in trauma.* Basic Books: New York.

Horynak, L, & Baker, E. (1989). *Experiential therapies for eating disorders.* New York: The Guilford Press.

Levens, M. (1987). Art therapy and eating disordered patients. *Inscape*, Summer, pp. 2–7.

Luzzatto, P. (1995). Art therapy and anorexia: The mental double trap of the anorexic patient. The use of art therapy to facilitate psychic change. In D. Doktor (Ed.), *Arts therapies and clients with eating disorders: Fragile board.* London: Jessica Kingsley Publishers.

Johnson, C., Sansone, R. & Chewing, M. (1992). Good reasons why young women would develop anorexia nervosa: The adaptive context. *Pediatric Annals, 21,* 731–737.

Kearney–Cooke, A., & Streigel–Moore, R. (1997). The etiology and treatment of body image disturbance. In D. Garner & P. Garfinkel (Eds.), H*andbook of treatment for eating disorders.* New York: The Guilford Press.

Kohut, H. (1971). *The analysis of the self.* New York: International Universities Press.

Krueger, D. (1989). *Body self, psychological self: A developmental and clinical integration of disorders of the self.* New York. Brunner–Mazel.

Mahler, M. S., Pine, F., & Bergman, A. (1975). *The psychological birth of the human infant.* New York : Basic Books.

Malchiodi, C. (1990). *Breaking the silence: Art therapy with children from violent homes.* New York: Brunner–Mazel.

Prugh, P., & Quirk, D. (2002). Healing the mind, mending the body: An expressive arts journey towards wholeness. *Proceedings of the American Art Therapy Annual Conference.* Washington D.C.

Rosen, J. (1997). Cognitive–behavioral body image therapy. In P. Garfinkle & D. Garner (Eds.), *Handbook of treatment for eating disorders.* New York: Guilford Press.

Schneider, S., Ostroff, S. & Legow, N. (1990). Enhancement of body–image: A structured art therapy group with adolescents. *Art Therapy*, Fall, 134–137.

Slade, P. D. (1994). What is body image? *Behavior, Research and Therapy, 32*(8): 497–502.

Spring, D. (1993). Artistic symbolic language in the treatment of multiple personality disorder. In E. S. Kluft (Ed.), *Expressive and functional therapies in the treatment of multiple personality disorder* (pp. 85–100). Springfield, IL: Charles C Thomas.

Rice, J., Hardenbergh, M., Hornyak, L.(1989). Disturbed body image in anorexia nervosa: Dance/movement therapy interventions. In L. Hornyak & E. Baker (Eds.), *Experiential therapies for eating disorders.* New York: The Guilford Press.

Totenbier, S. (1995). A new way of working with body image in therapy, incorporating dance/movement therapy methodology. In D. Doktor (Ed.), *Arts therapies and clients with eating disorders: Fragile board.* London: Jessica Kingsley Publishers.

Totenbier, S. (1989). In L.Hornyak & E. Baker (Eds.), *Experiential therapies for eating disorders.* New York: The Guilford Press.

Treuer, T., Koperdak, M., Rozsa, S. & Furedi, J. (2005). The impact of physical and sexual abuse on body image in eating disorders. *European Eating Disorder Review, 13*: 106–111.

Ticen, S. (1987). Feed me . . . cleanse me. . . . Sexual trauma projected in the art of bulimics. *American Journal of Art Therapy, 7* (I): 17–21.

Tury, F., & Szabo, P. (2000). Disorders of eating behavior: Anorexia and bulimia nervosa. "Psychiatry on the turn of the millennium" series. Budapest: Medicina Publishing.

Vanderlinden, J, & Vandereycken, W. (1997). *Trauma, dissociation and impulse dyscontrol in eating disorders.* Pennsylvania: Brunner–Mazel, Inc.

Waller, D. (1993). *Group interactive art therapy. It's use in training and treatment.* London: Routledge.

Winn, L. (1994). Experiential training for staff working with eating disorders. In D. Doktor (Ed.), *Arts therapies and clients with eating disorders: Fragile board.* London: Jessica Kingsley Publishers.

Biography

Julia Andersen MA., ATR–BC is an Expressive Therapy Coordinator and senior art therapist for The Center for Eating Disorders at Sheppard Pratt Hospital, located in Baltimore, Maryland. She has presented nationally on the subject of art therapy treatment with eating disorders, body image, and self injury. Julia is a site supervisor for the George Washington University Art Therapy Training Program.

Chapter 6

CREATING NEW WORLDS: USING SANDTRAY THERAPY WITH EATING DISORDERS

CHARLES E. MYERS AND KATHRYN N. KLINGER

Eating Disorders

A young woman is so obsessed with food and weight she misses her friend's birthday dinner. A college male wrestler spends five hours in the gym and forces vomiting to make his weight class. A sexually abused teenage girl eats compulsively to make herself physically undesirable by others. A hard–working mom worries about her image, labeling food as good or bad, as her seven–year–old daughter watches intently. Eating disorders affect everyone, men and woman, children and adults, the sufferers and their loved ones alike.

The issue of disordered eating is a well publicized topic in today's society. Various types of eating disorders and eating disordered behavior affect approximately four to five million people in the United States (Levine & Smolak, 2006). While the percentage of males diagnosed with either Anorexia Nervosa or Bulimia Nervosa is slight, it is estimated that between 40 percent and 50 percent of individuals diagnosed with Binge Eating Disorder are men (Levine & Smolak, 2006). Furthermore, in the past, the majority of individuals suffering from eating disorders were in their teens and twenties, but in recent years, women of all ages have begun to suffer from these disorders (Maine & Kelly, 2005).

Definitions of Eating Disorders

Anorexia Nervosa

The *DSM–IV–TR* (2000) defines Anorexia Nervosa as "a refusal to maintain body weight" which results in the individual maintaining a body weight of less than 85 percent the expected weight along with an intense fear of gaining weight. Anorexia Nervosa is also characterized by a distorted view of one's body and the loss of three or more consecutive menstrual cycles.

Bulimia Nervosa

Bulimia Nervosa is defined by "recurrent episodes" of binge eating followed by an inappropriate compensatory behavior in order to prevent weight gain which occur at least twice a week for three months. In addition, the individual's evaluation of self is unduly influenced by body shape or weight *DSM–IV–TR* (APA, 2000).

Eating Disorder Not Otherwise Specified/ Binge Eating Disorder

The *DSM–IV–TR* (2000) also makes mention of Binge Eating Disorder, characterized by recurrent episodes of binge eating occurring at least twice a week for six months without the use of inappropriate compensatory behavior. A diagnosis of Eating Disorder Not Otherwise Specified is provided for individuals presenting with eating disordered behavior that do not fit the full criteria for either Anorexia or Bulimia Nervosa.

Causes and Symptoms

Eating disorders are a complex phenomenon with numerous etiological factors that potentially contribute to their development (Ogden, 2003). These factors include genetics, society, family characteristics, and significant life events (Ogden, 2003). Research has shown that eating disorders run in families; the incidence of female sufferers of anorexia nervosa within families is ten times higher than in the general population. Evidence also shows an increased likelihood of developing bulimia nervosa among relatives of individuals diagnosed with bulimia nervosa (Ogden, 2003).

Eating disorders have also been viewed as an attempt to integrate opposing messages within society regarding the role of women (Maine & Kelly, 2005; Ogden, 2003). In today's society, women are faced with the demands of family and career and it has been suggested that eating disordered symptoms are an attempt to reconcile these opposing forces as women try to form their identities in light of changing social and cultural roles and expectations (Maine & Kelly, 2005; Ogden, 2003).

There are several common environmental factors present in families with an individual that suffers from an eating disorder (Maine & Kelly, 2005; Ogden, 2003). These include boundary problems, control, and conflict avoidance (Minuchin et al., 1978). Each person's experience of these conditions is unique and may manifest in different ways.

Minuchin and colleagues (1978) put forth the theory that four characteristics describe families with an eating disordered daughter or son. These are overinvolvement, overprotectiveness, rigidity, and lack of conflict resolution. In an overinvolved family, the boundaries defining autonomy are too weak to allow for appropriate individualization of members. The individual gets lost in the family system (Minuchin et al., 1978). When children grow up in families with highly enmeshed patterns of family functioning, they may make illness their identity, because they are unable to develop an autonomous self (Evans & Street, 1995; Minuchin et al., 1978). These rigid, rejecting, and chaotic patterns of functioning are often traumatic to children. This may cause individuals, believing the world is unsafe and people are unreliable, to approach interpersonal situations in a fearful and incompetent manner (Minuchin et al., 1978).

Many eating disordered individuals grow up in families with parents, specifically mothers, who are overprotective and controlling (Pole et al., 1988; Strober & Humphrey, 1987). Overprotected children may attempt to strictly control their bodies when they have little control over anything else (White, 1992). For example, in a case study of a young boy with anorexia, he stated that his goal in his eating disorder was to teach his overly controlling mother he could not be controlled (Koplow, 1993).

In addition, childhood sexual abuse has been widely recognized as a common precursor to the development of an eating disorder (Levine & Smolak, 2006; Maine & Kelly, 2005; Ogden, 2003; Zerbe, 1993). While it is difficult to determine the exact percentage of eating disordered individuals that have suffered childhood sexual abuse, estimates rate between 13 and 58 percent (Ogden, 2003).

While many factors contribute to the potential development of eating disorders, one common theme is the need for and attempt to gain some sense of control (Ogden, 2003). Eating disorder symptoms have long been characterized by an attempt on the part of the individual to gain control over uncontrollable parts of his or her life. In this way, symptoms of eating disorders have been viewed as a concrete, symbolic representation of other thoughts and feelings within the individual (Johnston, 1996; Zerbe, 1993).

Characteristics of Eating Disorders

Individuals suffering from eating disorders share many common characteristics. People that have grown up in a family environment of overinvolvement and control learn to ignore their own bodily signals of hunger and satiety, and become confused about their ownership of feelings and needs. This weak sense of self may lead the individual to build his or her identity based on those of others (Stolz, 1985). These individuals doubt their own perceptions and feel overly responsible for those around them. They often become caretakers early on and thus have difficulty gaining a sense of independence (Maine & Kelly, 2005). It is also common for these individuals to lack the skills necessary for regulating emotions and feelings. Due to this inability to effectively regulate emotion, individuals suffering from eating disorders may not be able to identify or experience their emotions. Without being able to verbalize and attend to emotions, they become overwhelming and frightening (Maine & Kelly, 2005). These individuals commonly exhibit perfectionistic tendencies, holding themselves to extreme standards and viewing life in black and white terms. These individuals struggle to believe that they will ever really be good enough and often loathe themselves for their imperfections and needs (Maine & Kelly, 2005). While they are highly intelligent, capable, and creative individuals, they commonly view themselves as worthless and incompetent (Johnston, 1996).

In addition, research shows that more than 50 percent of individuals with eating disorders struggle with alexithymia, which is a difficulty in verbalizing feelings and fantasies. This difficulty in verbalizing may cause the individual to use a body oriented, concrete activity in order to communicate inner distress (Zerbe, 1993). Eating disorder symptoms have been proposed to replace and represent verbal language in communication (Ogden, 2003). In addition, eating disorders are a way for individuals to self soothe and numb out difficult feelings (Maine & Kelly, 2005). For example, vomiting may provide a physical release of pent up emotions and stress. Eating disorders eventually allow sufferers to ignore all aspects of life other than those involving food and weight. This allows individuals to focus on something tangible and distance themselves from their pain (Johnston, 1996).

Sandtray Introduction

In a beautiful castle, a princess sings with the birds. On a battlefield, soldiers form ranks and take aim. On a snow–covered slope, children sleigh ride. Fenced away, a lone child watches the other children play. In a forest cathedral, a bride and groom make their vows of marriage. In a dark pit, a young woman is entrapped by a giant spider web. The scenes in a sandtray, called a sandworld, can be beautiful and uplifting, depressing and terrifying, even all at the same time. Sandtray is a therapeutic approach by which clients express abstract, and often traumatic, thoughts, feelings, and experiences through a concrete and physical medium. "Sandtray therapy is an expressive and projective mode of psychotherapy involving and unfolding of intra– and inter–personal issues through the use of sandtray materials as a nonverbal medium of communication, led by the client(s) and facilitated by a trained therapist" (Homeyer & Sweeney, 1998, p. 6).

Sandtray therapy effectively combines elements of play therapy, art therapy, and drama therapy, with its own unique tactile dimension (Carey, 1990). The properties of sand can be grounding for a client, both symbolically and realistically. This grounding enables a client to illustrate unconscious conflicts and materials through emerging sand scenes or sandworlds. Sandworlds are expressions of the client's experiential world and a projection of one's feelings and attitudes toward one's external world (Cockle, 1993). Sandtray therapy is a holistic process, bringing together many opposites. Through the creation of sandworlds, a client can express distress and coping, difficulties and strengths, destruction and reconstruction, concurrently releasing unacknowledged feelings and activating one's inner resources (Hunter, 1998). Sandtray therapy allows clients to express all of this through play and creation within the sandtray (Grubbs, 1994).

History

The story of sandtray therapy began with a caring father who would sit upon the floor with his two sons, playing with miniature soldiers, perhaps an early example of filial therapy. The father was the famous science fiction author H.G. Wells. Wells wrote of his experiences with his sons with great animation in his book *Floor Games* (1911/1975). In the 1920s, inspired by Wells' book, British pediatrician, Margaret Lowenfield developed the therapeutic approach known as sandplay. Lowenfield utilized sandtrays and miniatures in her counseling and shared this technique with the world in her book, *Play in Childhood* (1935/1967). Through her work with children in the 1950s, Swiss Jungian analyst, Frau Dora Kalff (2003) would have arguably the greatest impact on the development of sandtray therapy, formulating theoretical principles and training many therapists worldwide (Allan & Berry, 1987). In recent history, many therapists have contributed to the development of sandtray work. A short list of those therapists include John Allan (Allan & Berry, 1987), Lois Carey (1991), Gisela De Domenico (1999), Linda Homeyer and Daniel Sweeney (1998), and Theresa Kestly (2001).

Sandtray Defined

Sandtray therapy consists of a medium, a process, and a product. The sandtray is the medium, sandplay is the process, and the sandworld is the finished product (Allan & Berry, 1987). The medium of sandtray includes the tray, sand, miniatures, and when possible, water. There is much debate regarding the appropriate size and shape of the tray. A review of the literature shows most sandtray therapists prefer to use rectangular trays approximately 30 inches long, 20 inches wide, and 3 inches deep. This size tray is large enough to provide clients space to build their sandworld yet is small enough to allow them to take in their entire world at a single glance (Homeyer & Sweeney, 1998). Although the first author prefers this tray size in most of his work, it has been his experience that the use of different size and shape trays can be very effective in different settings. For example, a therapist may choose to use a smaller tray when space is limited or utilizing a travel sandtray kit, or the therapist may select a larger tray when doing group or couple work. The dimensions of the sandtray set limits that are both physical and symbolic (Carey, 1991), providing the client a safe space in which to work. The boundaries of the sandtray provide containment for the client's full expression of whatever one needs to put forth (Grubbs, 1994). Sandtrays are typically painted blue inside; this provides clients the simulation of sky and water if they desire. Sandtrays are normally set at waist height; this permits the client to work on the tray from a standing or sitting position with comfort.

The next component in sandtray therapy is the sand. "Sand is the basic medium for this engrossing and effective treatment modality. It is a basic elemental compound, one of the most simple and common on earth" (Homeyer & Sweeney, 1998, p. 21). Clients often feel drawn to sand. Just the feel of the sand helps to ground, center, and/or regress clients to the place they need to heal (Boik & Goodwin, 2000). In addition, sand provides clients with tactile experience and kinesthetic involvement that leads them to a concentrated focus or meditative space that allows their inner protected self to emerge (Carey, 1990). Before they are aware of it, clients are moving their hands through the sand, creating tunnels, and shaping mountains, runways, and riverbeds (Allan & Berry, 1987). There are many types of sand color and texture available. The most commonly used sand is white sand. However, there are other options, some of the most common being soft red desert sand, coarse black volcanic sand, and quicksand. Each of these types of sands can foster clients to exploring different emotions and experiences. Therapists may elect to make water, another basic elemental compound, available for client use. Water gives the sand a different texture and look, and makes it more malleable. The use of sand and water can transport clients to those areas of human experiences that need to be healed and integrated (Boik & Goodwin, 2000).

The final component of the sandtray medium is the miniatures. The language of sandtray therapy is symbolic (Carey, 1991). Clients use symbols (miniatures) to represent experiences, objects, and relationships in their lives, current, past, and future. Often clients will routinely select and use particular miniatures to represent certain people or aspects of their lives. The common usage of these symbols then develops into a shared language between the client and the sandtray therapist (Boik & Goodwin, 2000). When miniatures are added to the sandtray, whole worlds appear, dramas unfold, and client absorption into the process is total (Allan & Berry, 1987).

It is crucial for the sandtray therapist to provide clients with selected miniatures to enable them to express themselves and their experiences through the sandtray process. Therapists need be attuned to their collection, providing clients with a range of expressive opportunities. Collections should also be large enough as not to be constricting for client expression while not being so large as to be emotionally flooding (Homeyer & Sweeney, 1998). While there is no standard collection of miniatures, many sandtray therapists agree on use of certain symbolic categories. Common categories include:

- People—Ordinary, fantasy, mythological, and magical; diverse races and cultures, occupations and recreation; fighting, warring, and enslaved; death figures; religious and spiritual people and objects.
- Animals—Wild animals of the land, sea, and air; domestic; extinct, mythological and fantasy; animal habitats; bones, shells, and feathers.
- Plant Life—Natural and artificial; complete life cycle.
- Minerals—Rocks; natural and artificial gems; marbles and beads.
- Environments—Habitats of various cultures and areas; fences and bridges.
- Transportation—Land, water, and air; emergency and military vehicles.
- Miscellaneous—Planetary and earth symbols; objects that reflect and illuminate; addiction and medical symbols, aromatic objects; communication objects, containers; food; construction materials.

Sandtray Process

"There are myriads of techniques used and advocated in the mental health profession. Hurting people, however, are not healed through technique. People experience emotional healing when they encounter someone and when they encounter self. It is an inner process, a relational process, and a heart process" (Homeyer and Sweeney, 1998, pp. 18–19).

Sandtray therapy involves the development and evolution of a dynamic, interpersonal relationship between the client and the therapist (Homeyer &

Sweeney, 1998). The therapist acts as a facilitator of the process, rather than as a director. The therapist facilitates the process through providing the client with a "free and protected space" (Kalff, 2003) and empathy and trust (Bradway & McCoard, 1997). Through this facilitation, clients feel free and safe to explore emotions, thoughts, and experiences normally too threatening to face. The therapist facilitation provides clients the opportunity to fully express and explore self. This self–expression and self–exploration are crucial to the counseling process and the foundation of sandtray therapy (Homeyer & Sweeney, 1998). Clients will experience healing through a growing sense of self–control, empowerment, and safety.

Sandtray therapy commonly consists of two stages. First is the building stage, the construction of a sandworld by the client (Goss & Campbell, 2004). The process of sandtray begins with the therapist inviting the client to create a picture, or sandworld, in the sandtray. The client may choose to simply mold or shape the sand or to add and arrange miniatures as desired (Grubbs, 1994). The primary role of the therapist in sandtray therapy is to act as witness to the client's process in silent honor (Carey, 1991). It is validating for a client to have someone whom is trusted and respected to witness the expression of thoughts, feelings, and experiences (Boik & Goodwin, 2000). The process of creating a sandworld makes the client's inner world and conflict visible, allowing therapeutic growth and healing (Allan & Berry, 1987). The therapist trusts the client to direct the process and to move toward self–healing (Boik & Goodwin, 2000).

During the creation stage, clients have the freedom to express themselves in the ways they desire, with no direction or intrusion from the therapist (Grubbs, 1994). Most therapists refrain from making any verbal interaction with the client, as comments about what the client is doing may be disruptive to the process and should be avoided (Bradway, 1979). It is important for the therapist to trust that each client will do what is necessary to do at that moment in time (Boik & Goodwin, 2000). The therapist takes mental note of how the client creates the sandworld, such as the order of creation and any rearrangement of symbols, as well as the client's affect and intensity through the process. The therapist may bring this information back during the second stage of the sandtray session.

The second stage of sandtray therapy occurs after the creation of the client's world. This stage can be done verbally or in quiet contemplation. It is important to consider the client's needs in this decision. If the client is comfortably able to engage in verbal communication, the therapist facilitates the client in processing the completed sandtray (Goss & Campbell, 2004). The therapist invites the client to share or talk about the sandworld the client created. This allows the client to clarify personal meanings and to integrate new feelings and insights that may have emerged through the creation of the sandworld (Goss & Campbell, 2004). The therapist uses the client's metaphors and assists the client in enlarging the meaning of the experience. The therapist may include observations of the client during the creating stage to increase the client's understanding and self–awareness.

It is important to leave the sandworld intact until after the client has left the session. By leaving the sandworld intact, the therapist honors the client and the experience. For the client to deconstruct the sandworld is analogous to minimizing the client's thoughts, feelings, and experiences of life. Before the therapist dissembles the sandworld, the therapist documents the session through taking pictures of the sandtray and recording the story (Homeyer & Sweeney, 1998; Miller & Boe, 1990). The therapist uses this documentation to record the client's progress through therapy.

Sandtray and Trauma

Interpersonal trauma occurs when an individual experiences an event or endures conditions in which the individual's ability to integrate the emotional experience is overwhelmed (Pearlman & Saakvitne, 1995). There are many events and conditions that are generally accepted as being traumatic. However, what is considered traumatic by an individual is based on and defined by the individual's own experience or perception of the event or condition. Interpersonal trauma overwhelms an individual's healthy coping skills, causing the individual to find alternate, and often unhealthy, means to cope with the trauma. Individuals experiencing interpersonal trauma often feel out of control, helpless, and confused, and experience a loss of trust, self esteem, identity, and the ability to feel. Each person's experience is unique.

Traumatized individuals may attempt to contain their inner turmoil, being either unwilling or unable to express their pain experiences verbally. These individuals may also experience arrestment in normal development, and an inability to achieve resolution of life events and inner struggles (Wu, 2003). In an attempt to live with the overwhelming nature of their trauma, traumatized individuals frequently deny their feelings, thoughts, and experiences. Through denying their unwanted traumatic experiences, individuals shift this material, unresolved, to their unconscious.

Sandtray therapy creates a bridge, enabling an individual to bring the unconscious into theconscious through concrete expression (Boik & Goodwin, 2000). The sandtray acts as a container for the individual's unconscious material, allowing the individual to express experiences metaphorically and still keep a safe distance from them (Miller & Boe, 1990). The process of sandtray provides a language that is active, safe, and silent yet resonant (Hunter, 1998). Through sandtray, individuals are able to express symbolically, through scenes and images, their inner worlds, own true experiences in concrete form, and activate their natural healing processes (Dundas, 1992; Wu, 1993).

Homeyer and Sweeney (1998) developed a comprehensive list of rationale for sandtray therapy (pp. 11–18):

- Sandtray therapy gives expression to nonverbalized expression.
- Self–directed sandtray therapy process allows clients to be fully themselves.
- Sandtray therapy has a unique kinesthetic quality.
- Sandtray therapy serves to create a therapeutic distance for clients.
- The therapeutic distance that Sandtray therapy provides creates a safe place for abreaction to occur.
- Sandtray therapy is a truly inclusive experience.
- Sandtray therapy naturally provides boundaries and limits, which promote safety for the client.
- Sandtray therapy provides a unique setting for the emergence of therapeutic metaphor.
- The most powerful metaphors in therapy are those that are generated by the clients themselves.
- Sandtray therapy is effective in overcoming client resistance.
- Sandtray therapy, because of its non–threatening and engaging qualities, can captivate and draw in the involuntary client.
- Sandtray therapy provides a needed and effective communication medium for the client with poor verbal skills.
- Sandtray therapy cuts through verbalization used as a defense.
- Sandtray therapy creates a place for the client to experience control.
- The challenge of transference may be effectively addressed through sandtray therapy.
- Deeper intrapsychic issues may be accessed more thoroughly and more rapidly through sandtray therapy.

Sandtray and Eating Disorders

Sandtray therapy has been effectively used with a diverse range of diagnostic categories, including eating disorders (Carey, 1990). Sandtray provides clients a less threatening therapeutic approach than traditional talk therapies. It allows the individuals to soften their defenses and reduce resistance, opening an avenue to express their innermost thoughts, feelings, and experiences (Boik & Goodwin, 2000). Through the process of sandtray therapy, clients will experience healing through a growing sense of self–control, empowerment, and safety (Homeyer & Sweeney, 1998). Sandtray is a process that promotes client safety and control, enabling one to address, acknowledge, and accept emotionally charged issues. Self–discovery is a vital component of the sandtray therapy process (Hunter, 1998). Through this self–discovery or self–awareness, clients are able to integrate, and filter through, the opposing messages they receive from their environment and reconcile it their own true experiences.

Additionally, sandtray therapy provides clients with a safe, nonjudgmental, and unconditionally supportive environment (Wu, 2003). Within this calming environment, the client becomes more creative, confident, and expressive. Sandtray empowers the client, providing the opportunity to take control of one's reality (Boik & Goodwin, 2000). Sandtray therapy combines the acceptance and non–judgmental attitude of person–centered therapy, the holistic interaction of mind, body, and imagination, and the innate healing ability of all humans (Hunter, 1998).

Case Example

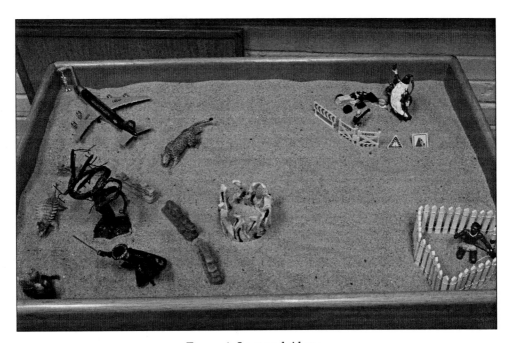

Figure 1. Lost and Alone.

A twenty–three–year–old woman expressed her perception of her family and her world at the age of 15. The woman identified herself as two figures within the tray. First, as the fairy bound in the lower left corner surrounded and under attack by a variety of threats within an inescapable wall. Second, as the wizard in the upper right corner, she choose a baby (her mother) half buried in the sand looking to her daughter (the woman) to rescue her from her own pain. The soldier in front of them represents the woman's anger toward her mother for not being there when she needed her. The small mother figure with child behind them represented the type of relationship the woman wanted with her mother. The woman used the signs to represent her feeling that in the situation her mother had created, nothing good could result. In the lower right corner is her father isolating himself from his family's pain, unavailable to help to her. The woman placed the fire extinguisher next to her father for she believed her father had the ability to help both her and her mother if he would have chosen to engage. In the upper left corner, the airplane represented the woman's desire to escape her own and her family's pain. The gallows represented the depth of her desire.

Conclusion

Sandtray therapy is a creative arts based approach to working with a variety of clients and presenting problems. Within the sandtray environment, the therapeutic healing process occurs naturally, enabling clients to freely express or re–live experiences and emotions without judgment, interruption, or criticism (Wu, 2003). Clients arrange and/or symbolically transform objects in ways that foster and promote therapeutically positive changes in their lives (Tennessen & Strand, 1998).

Individuals with eating disorders commonly feel they have little control over their lives and thus take control over something they can, food. Sandtray therapy allows clients to have total control of the action of the therapy and, consequently, to experience a sense of their own power. Individuals with eating disorders typically experience incongruent lives, trying to fit an image projected on to them from friends, family, and society. Sandtray provide clients the opportunity for self–exploration and self–expression, increasing their self–awareness and acceptance. Individuals with eating disorders may have experienced traumatic events such as sexual abuse, often lack words to describe emotionally charged experiences, or may oververbalize to avoid feelings. Sandtray therapy allows clients to express overwhelming experiences and feelings symbolically in a caring relationship, promoting healing. Sandtray therapy offers a viable and effective treatment for individuals with eating disorders.

References

Allan, J., & Berry, P. (1987). Sandplay. Special issue: Counseling with expressive arts. *Elementary School Guidance and Counseling, 21*(4), 300–306.

American Psychiatric Association. (2000). *Diagnostic and statistical manual of mental disorders* (4th ed.). Washington, DC: Author.

Boik, B. L., & Goodwin, E. A. (2000). *Sandplay therapy: A step–by–step manual for psychotherapists of diverse orientations.* New York: W. W. Norton & Company.

Bradway, K. (1979). Sandplay in psychotherapy. *Art Psychotherapy, 6*(2), 85–93.

Bradway, K., & McCoard, B. (1997). *Sandplay–Silent workshop of the psyche.* New York: Brunner–Routledge.

Carey, L. (1991). Family sandplay therapy. *Arts in Psychotherapy, 18,* 231–239.

Carey, L. (1990). Sandplay therapy with a troubled child. *Arts in Psychotherapy, 17*(3), 197–209.

Cockle, S. (1993). Sandplay: A comparative study. *International Journal of Play Therapy, 2*(2), 1–17.

De Domenico, G. S. (1999). Group sandtray–worldplay: New dimension in sandplay therapy In D. S. Sweeney & L. E. Homeyer (Eds.), *The handbook of group play therapy: How to do it, how it works, whom it's best for* (pp. 215–223). San Francisco: Jossey–Bass.

Dundas, E. (1992). Sandplay therapy. *Association for Play Therapy Newsletter, 11*(3), 1–3.

Evans, C., & Street, E. (1995). Possible differences in family patterns in anorexia nervosa and bulimia nervosa. *Journal of Family Therapy, 17,* 115–131.

Goss, S., & Campbell, M. A. (2004). The value of sandplay as a therapeutic tool for school guidance counsellors. *Australian Journal of Guidance & Counseling, 14*(2), 211–220.

Grubbs, G. A. (1994). An abused child's use of sandplay in the healing process. *Clinical Social Work Journal, 22*(2), 193–209.

Homeyer, L. E., & Sweeney, D. S. (1998). *Sandtray: A practical manual.* Canyon Lake, TX: Lindan Press.

Hunter, L. B. (1998). *Images of resiliency: Troubled children create healing stories in the language of sandplay.* Palm Beach, FL: Behavioral Communications Institute.

Johnston, A. (1996). *Eating in the light of the moon: How women can transform their relationships with food through myths, metaphors, and storytelling.* Carlsbad, CA: Gurze Books.

Kalff, D. M. (2003). *Sandplay: A pychotherapeutic approach to the psyche.* Cloverdale, CA: Temenos Press.

Kestly, T. (2001). Group sandplay in elementary schools. In A. A. Drewes, L. J. Carey, & C. E. Schafer (Eds.), *School–based play therapy* (pp. 329–349). New York: John Wiley & Sons.

Koplow, B. (1993). Mustn't bite the hand that feeds: The boy who refused to eat. *Journal of Child Psychotherapy, 19*(2), 23–36.

Levine, M., & Smolak, L. (2006). *The prevention of eating problems and eating disorders: Theory, research and practice.* Mahwah: NJ: Lawrence Erlbaum Associates.

Lowenfield, M. (1935/1967). *Play in childhood.* New York: Wiley.

Maine, M., & Kelly, J. (2005). *The body myth: Adult women and the pressure to be perfect.* Hoboken, NJ: John Wiley & Sons, Inc.

Miller, C., & Boe, J. (1990). Tears into diamonds: Transformation of child psychic trauma through sandplay and storytelling. *Arts in Psychotherapy, 17*(3), 247–257.

Minuchin, S., Rosman, B. L., & Baker, L. (1978). *Psychosomatic families: Anorexia*

Nervosa in context. Cambridge, MA: Harvard University Press.

Ogden, J. (2003). *The psychology of eating: From healthy to disordered behavior.* Malden, MA: Blackwell Publishing.

Pearlman, L. A., & Saakvitne, K. W. (1995). *Trauma and the therapist.* New York: Norton.

Pole, R., Waller, D., Stewart, S., & Parkin–Feigenbaum, L. (1988). Parental caring versus overprotection in bulimia. *International Journal of Eating Disorders, 7,* 601–606.

Strober, M. & Humphrey, L.L. (1987). Familial contributions to the etiology and course of anorexia nervosa and bulimia. *Journal of Consulting and Clinical Psychology, 55,* 654–659.

Tennessen, J., & Strand, D. (1998). A comparative analysis of directed sandplay and therapy and principles of Ericksonian psychology. *The Arts in Psychotherapy, 25*(2), 109–114.

Wells, H. G. (1911/1975). *Floor games.* New York: Arno Press.

White, J. (1992). Women and eating disorders: II. Developmental, familial, and biological risk factors. *Health Care for Women International, 13,* 363–373.

Wu, P. (2003). Sandplay therapy. *Nevada Association for Play Therapy Newsletter, 2*(3), 3.

Zerbe, K. (1993). *The body betrayed: Women, eating disorders, and treatment.* Washington, DC: American Psychiatric Press, Inc.

Biographies

Charles Edwin Myers, M.A., LPC, LMHC, NCC, NCSC, RPT–S is a Licensed Professional Counselor in the State of Texas, a Licensed Mental Health Counselor and Certified School Counselor in the State of Florida, a National Certified Counselor and National Certified School Counselor, and a Registered Play Therapist–Supervisor. Mr. Myers is currently a doctoral student at the University of North Texas specializing in play therapy and works for the Center for Play Therapy as Coordinator for Training and Development. Charles has presented at the local and state levels on play and filial therapy, sandtray therapy, and elementary counseling. In addition, Charles has served as a school counselor in rural and inner city schools using play and sandtray therapy, as well as providing play and filial therapy in a homeless shelter in Tampa and crisis counseling in the hurricane shelters in Dallas. Charles has also served in leadership roles for a number of state and local level professional organizations and is currently on the Ethics and Practice Committee of the Association for Play Therapy.

Kathryn Noel Klinger is currently a master's level student at the University of North Texas specializing in play and filial therapy. Ms. Klinger is interested in and well–versed in the literature pertaining to eating disorders. Kathryn currently uses play therapy in working with children with interpersonal trauma under supervision at the University of North Texas counseling clinics. Kathryn plans to utilize play and sandtray therapy in working with individuals with eating disorders as well as individuals who have experienced trauma. Kathryn is currently a member of the Texas Counseling Association.

Chapter 7

HEALING HUNGER THROUGH PLAY: AN OVERVIEW OF PLAY THERAPY TECHNIQUES FOR COUNSELING CHILDREN WITH EATING DISORDERS

BRIAN L. BETHEL

Nowhere could I have a greater sense of tragedy than when I consider the complexity of eating disorders. Within the past few decades, research has attempted to examine the diagnosis and treatment of this unique population. However, little research exists regarding the treatment of males with eating disorders (Anderson, 1999) Similarly, only a limited amount of research has documented the use of creative therapies when counseling individuals with eating disorders (Dokter, 1994). This chapter will attempt to provide an overview of the current literature in the treatment of eating disorders. Additionally, a case illustration will be offered to assist clinicians in implementing play therapy techniques in the course of treating individuals with eating disorders.

Although cases of eating disorders have been documented for hundreds of years, it has only been with in the last twenty years that a great deal of research has alerted mental health professionals to the severity and dangers involved in treating the unique population of individuals with eating disorders (Reijonen et al., 2003). Each year, millions of individuals confront the complex disease of eating disorders. Estimates suggest the prevalence of Anorexia Nervosa is between 0.5 to 2 percent of the general population (Roth & Fonagy, 1996).

There are numerous obstacles in both diagnosing and treating individuals with eating disorders. Levitt and Sansone (2003) reported that there is no greater challenge in community mental health than the treatment of individuals with eating disorders. Although the eating–disordered population presents significant challenges, clinicians must explore available treatment options as the prevalence of eating disorders has increased over the last several years (Roth & Fonagy, 1996). As recently as 2003, literature suggested that professionals in the community mental health setting are challenged with increasing numbers of persons needing treatment for eating disorders (Levitt & Sansone, 2003).

This increase of identified persons with eating disorders has precipitated saturation in the literature regarding the topic of eating disorders (Crosscope–Happel et al., 2000). Tragically, only a fraction of the published literature has examined the diagnosis and treatment of males with Anorexia Nervosa. Zebre (1993) reported that the male population has been understudied in the area of eating disorders. Likewise, Keel, Fulkerson, and Leon (1997) found that as recently as 1997, no studies of eating disorders of early adolescent males were found in a review of the literature. Only in recent years have efforts been made to examine this unique population of males with eating disorders (Crosscope–Happel et al., 2000; Keel et al., 1998; Levitt & Sansone, 2003).

Despite the deficiencies in the literature, it is estimated that Anorexia Nervosa impacts over one million males annually (Crosscope–Happel et al., 2000). Similarly, Walcott, Pratt, and Patel (2003) reported that males comprise ten to fifteen percent of the eating disorder population. However, studies have also cited the belief that exact estimates of eating disorders among males may be difficult to determine and are likely higher than what current research estimates (American Psychiatric Association, 2000).

Additional obstacles to for the identification of males with eating disorders include the societal stigma commonly associated with eating disorders as this can often encourage males to go to great lengths to keep their eating disorders secret. Consequently, making the diagnosis difficult (Patel et al., 2003). Additionally, Crosscope–Happel and colleagues (2000) reported that mental health clinicians and medical professionals often misdiagnosis males with eating disorders due to the common misconception that these disorders are exclusively present in females. Braun (1997) also reported that males with anorexia often exhibit symptoms consistent with other mental and emotional disorders including obsessive–compulsive disorders, dependent and passive aggressive personality disorders as well as avoidant features.

Levitt and Sansone (2003) found additional complications of diagnosing an individual's underlying eating disorder as persons often present with multiple mental health diagnosis. Reijonen and colleagues (2003) supported this hypothesis as they identified co–morbid disorders as a significant risk factor for adolescent males developing an eating disorder. Therefore, the diagnosis of an eating disorder can be a complex task for clinicians.

Regardless of the controversy surrounding estimates of males with eating disorders, the diagnostic criterion is synonymous for both sexes. According to the *Diagnostic and Statistical Manual of Mental Disorders* (APA, 2000) the diagnostic criteria includes an individual's refusal to maintain a normal body weight as defined by less than 85 percent of what would be expected for the person's height. Additionally, the individual has an extreme fear of weight gain. Specific to females with Anorexia is the condition of amenorrhea or the absence of at least three consecutive expected menstrual cycles.

Seligman (1998) listed two types of Anorexia Nervosa. The most common type of the disorder is the restrictive type that involves individuals severely limiting their food intake. The second classification includes an individual's pattern of binge eating and/or purging behavior. Common examples include: self–induced vomiting and the use of laxatives or diuretics.

Crosscope–Happel et al. (2000) alerted mental health clinicians to several differences between females and males with anorexia. Specifically, unlike females with anorexia, males with the disorder have a history of being over-weight prior to the development of the disease. In addition, sexual orienta-tion and sex role identification issues are typically more apparent for males with anorexia. Walcott and colleagues (2003) suggested that homosexual males are also at an increased risk to developing an eating disorder. In con-trast to the effect of a female's menstrual cycle, men with anorexia experi-ence a decrease in testosterone levels as the result of starvation (Cross-cope–Happell et al., 2000).

Like the diagnosis of Anorexia, the treatment for this eating disorder can prove to be particularly challenging. Levitt and Sansone (2003) reported that individuals with eating disorders often need intense and extensive treatment. Similarly, due to the potential medical complications of anorexia, research has encouraged clinicians to work collaboratively with medical professionasl so that the physical effects of the disease can be monitored appropriately (APA, 2000; Seligman, 1998). Furthermore, Levitt and Sansone (2003) also encouraged a multi–dimensional perspective in outpatient treatment for indi-viduals with anorexia. Crosscope–Happell and colleagues (2000) encouraged the use of a multidisciplinary approach when working with males who are suspected to have anorexia. This philosophy includes an emphasis on med-ical interventions, education, weight restoration, as well as psychotherapy. Despite these guidelines, the American Psychiatric Association (2000) indi-cated that no specific form of counseling is more effective than any other in treating anorexia.

However, several sources have supported the implementation of behav-ioral counseling as an effective intervention for treating individuals with anorexia. Thompson and Rudolph (2000) cited the use of positive reinforce-ment and punishment as specific techniques for counseling persons with anorexia. Additionally, Seligman (1998) reported behavioral therapy as the core of treatment for eating disorders. Techniques including behavioral contracting, promoting self–awareness, reinforcement, and relaxation techniques for anxiety reduction have been found to be beneficial. Moreover, cognitive techniques of positive self–talk and psycho–education have provided positive outcomes in the treatment of individuals with anorexia.

More recent literature has supported other counseling theories for the treatment of eating disorders. O'Halloran (1999) examined the use of a solution–focused brief therapy family based approach when counseling individuals with anorexia. Specifically, family members can prove to be essential in providing resources with the ongoing support for individuals with eating disorders. Levitt and Sansone (2003) also supported family therapy as an effective tool for counseling individuals with anorexia and have cited that families are routinely integrated into partial hospitalization programs that treat individuals with eating disorders.

Although research appears to support a number of counseling approaches in serving persons with eating disorders, a limited amount of literature has addressed the use of creative therapies in treating this population. Levitt and Sansone (2003) recommended that counseling approaches be implemented on an individual basis and used to meet an individual's unique needs in therapy. Due to the complexity of eating disorders and the individual variables involved, creative therapies should be examined as an additional tool for strengthening treatment regiments for persons who confronts eating disorders. This chapter will specifically explore the application of play therapy in the treatment of Anorexia Nervosa.

Rationale for Play Therapy

Unlike traditional therapeutic models, play therapy does not require children to cognitively re–visit past traumatic events. Therefore, clinicians can use play therapy as an avenue for children to regain a sense of mastery and control over their environment without necessarily reliving the trauma that they have experienced (Hall, 1997). The following case illustration provides examples of how play therapy techniques can be implemented in the successful treatment of individuals with eating disorders.

Play therapy offers a unique approach for working with children and adolescents by offering individuals a non–threatening environment in which children can work to regain some sense of stability. With the specialization of play therapists and play therapy techniques, these theories have been popularly implemented over the last fifty years (Kauson et al., 1997). Similarly, Landreth, Homeyer, Glover, and Sweeney (1996) concluded that play therapy is an effective tool for counseling children with a variety of issues. Gil (1994) also stated that most child therapists agree that play therapy is the most effective medium for treating children.

While there are varying theories of play therapy, this chapter will focus on three specific types of play therapy including child–centered play therapy or non–directive, directive play therapy, and filial play therapy. Landreth (1991) defined play therapy as "the dynamic interpersonal relationship between a child and a therapist trained in play therapy procedures who provides select-ed play materials and facilitates the development of a safe relationship for the child to fully express self through the child's natural medium, play" (p. 14).

The history of play therapy dates back to as early as 1920 (Gil, 1991). However, Virginia Axline is perhaps the most commonly recognized for the application of child centered therapy techniques via play in her work with children (Axline, 1947). Child–centered therapy or nondirective therapy grew out of the work of Carl Rogers. This model emphasized the philoso-phies of unconditional positive regard and being present with the child as foundations of this theory (Rogers, 1980).

Landreth expanded on Axline's work and identified the term child–cen-tered play therapy using these same standards. Similar to the work of Rogers, child–centered play therapy focuses on the relationship between the clinician and the child (Landreth, 1991). Thus, clinicians should be cautioned that establishing rapport with individuals is essential for utilizing play therapy.

Conversely, directive play therapy techniques are typically best imple-mented to address specific therapeutic goals. Literature has suggested the implementation of directive play therapy techniques to assist children with a variety of issues. Specifically, Gil (1991) reported techniques of story telling, puppet play, and certain board games as directive therapies for children who are survivors of sexual abuse. Namka (1995) also discussed cognitive restruc-turing and directive techniques to assist individuals in actively disputing irra-tional beliefs. Kauson and colleagues (1997) cited a number of directive play therapy techniques in *The Playing Cure*.

Filial play therapy is an additional intervention when working with chil-dren and families. Guerney (1964) first developed filial play therapy as a means of involving parents in the treatment of children with emotional and behavioral difficulties. Yet, this practice has been applied in treating a vari-ety of issues. Gil (1991) cited filial play therapy as a successful intervention for parents of sexuality abused children. Costas and Landreth (1999) also noted the importance of filial play therapy as it allows children to gain parental support via play. The following case illustration will provide exam-ples of how each of these theories of play therapy that have been imple-mented in the treatment of a young male with Anorexia Nervosa.

Case Illustration

Erik was twelve years old when he was first brought to the attention of mental health professionals. I first heard Erik's story when I received a telephone call from a local children's psychiatric hospital. Hospital officials reported that Erik was admitted to their facility after significant weight loss and he was consequently diagnosed with Anorexia Nervosa. Social workers from the hospital were attempting to secure outpatient counseling services for Erik upon his discharge from the hospital.

A few days later, I was again reviewing Erik's discharge summary while making my way to the lobby to meet Erik and his mother. Despite being armed with this clinical information, nothing could have prepared me for this upcoming meeting. At twelve years of age, one would have expected Erik to be a strong active teenager. Yet, his fragile frail body seemed to tell an entirely different story. After introducing myself, I could not help but to notice that his light gray t–shirt did little to conceal his rib cage underneath his shirt. As we began to make our way to my office, I began to question if this teenager would have the strength to make the short commute back down the hallway.

Although the first session focused on obtaining a psychosocial history, important clinical information was revealed. First, Erik's mother provided a detailed account of a horrific childhood for her son which included being sexually victimized, allegedly perpetrated by his father. Erik remained relatively quiet simply responding with short answers and keeping his eyes lowered. This seemed to substantiate his mother's theory of her son's low self–esteem. I met with Erik privately at which time he endorsed suicidal ideation in the past and acknowledged self–induced vomiting during the course of the last twelve months. Even though Erik participated in the session and provided honest responses, it was obvious that he was somewhat resistant to outpatient counseling services.

It was Erik's initial resistance that prompted me to explore the use of play therapy in the course of his treatment. Rapport is a key element in most counseling situations. However, the literature clearly has defined the importance of establishing a solid rapport with individuals being treated for eating disorders. Seligman (1998) noted a strong therapist–client rapport as integral in the treatment of those with eating disorders and reported that a great deal of support and approval need to be present in the therapeutic relationship. For these reasons, I determined the use of child–centered play therapy techniques would be appropriate for the initial phase of Erik's treatment.

Upon his arrival for the second session, Erik again presented with some initial resistance. However, Erik began to explore the various items in my office and started to ask questions regarding the sandtray that is standard in my office. When I described to Erik what other children have chosen to do with the sandtray, he immediately asked if he could complete a sandtray. I simply responded by stating that he could choose to do any task or activity he wanted during the session.

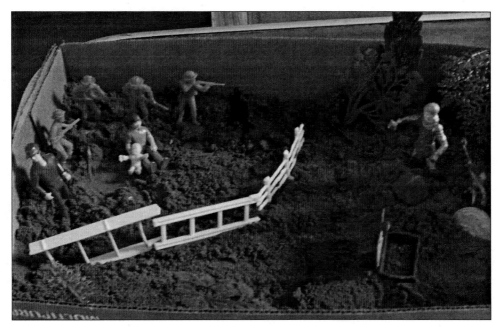

Figure 1. Erik's Sandtray

Sandtrays have been widely used in counseling with children. Numerous studies have supported the use of client–centered sandtrays with traumatized children and reported positive outcomes (Grubbs, 1994). This also proved to be the case for Erik. The only directive provided to Erik was to use the toy miniatures provided to create his world in the sand. I simply reflected Erik's activity through verbal statements. Once completed, Erik voluntarily offered an explanation of his world in the sand. The picture below shows Erik's portrayal of his world.

Themes in Erik's sandtray appeared consistent with unique aspects of male anorexic behavior. First, Erik reported the use of army men placed around him as the war of feelings he had experienced while in the hospital. Research has reported that males with eating disorders often have an inability to control their emotions (Crosscope–Happell, Hutchins, Getz, & Hayes, 2000). Second, Erik stated that the knights shown in the sandtray were "strong people" who could protect themselves. Due to the knights being placed far away from Erik this seemed to support Erik's belief of being vulnerable and having a less than masculine image. Last, issues of gender identity confusion were also evident in Erik's sand tray. Anderson (1999) discussed identity confusion as a common theme for males with anorexia. Erik informed me that the baby placed near him in the sandtray was his child and appeared to be nurturing the child. Likewise, Erik chose a strong masculine figure also placed in close proximity to the baby and identified this figure as "the baby's father."

The completion of Erik's sandtray provided important clinical themes to address in future sessions. Most importantly, however, was the process that allowed Erik to complete this task. As the clinician, I simply reflected Erik's activity with statements of acceptance and understanding and identified key emotions that Erik was demonstrating via the miniatures in the sand. I think this was essential in strengthening rapport with Erik. This process allowed Erik the freedom act out his hurtful emotions using play in a non–threatening, non–judgmental environment.

For the next four sessions Erik completed additional sandtrays with each one being a little different. The final sandtray involved Erik conquering the soldiers around him and talking with the knights on the opposite side of the sandtray. I found this particular sand tray to signify clinical importance in that Erik had portrayed a sense of control and mastery. Likewise, Erik and I had developed a good rapport and I think through the child–centered play therapy technique, an environment of trust and support was established. Therefore, I began to prepare for more directive techniques to implement in the next session.

There are common themes that have been documented for males with eating disorders. Specifically, males with eating disorders most often will present with low self–esteem and engage in all or nothing thinking. Like females, males with eating disorders will present with issues of body dissatisfaction and have a poor body image (Crosscope–Happell et al., 2000). These key themes along with the information obtain through Erik's sandtrays provided a clinical framework in determining specific directive play therapy techniques.

Crisci, Lay, and Lowenstein (1998) identified several directive play therapy techniques for counseling sexually traumatized children in *Paper Dolls and Paper Airplanes*. This publication proved to be a valuable resource in addressing Erik's feelings of vulnerability, low self–esteem, and poor body image. This clinician adapted various techniques from this publication to address Erik's clinical needs.

It was during the fifth session that I introduced *The Feeling Good Every Day Game*, a technique that was adapted from the *Paper Dolls and Paper Airplanes* (Crisci, Lay, & Lowenstein, 1998). Erik was provided a blank calendar with specific directives given for each day. For example, Erik was asked to fill–in one day with things that he liked about himself, and another day with three things that he could do to make himself feel better when he was feeling sad. Throughout the next month, this technique generated a great deal of discussion involving Erik's irrational thoughts and served to promote a more pos-

itive self–image. This technique parallels some cognitive–behavioral ap–
proaches by utilizing play to promote discussion and identify irrational belief
systems.

I had suspected that Erik's sexual abuse history had contributed to his low
self–esteem and poor body image. Therefore, I adapted the paper dolls tech–
nique from *Paper Dolls and Paper Airplanes* (Crisci, Lay, & Lowenstein, 1998).
Erik was asked to identify specific hurts that he had experienced and label
them on the body outline. I strongly encouraged Erik to not only focus on
physical pains but also the challenging and difficult emotions that he had
experienced. Erik was then asked to place band aids over the various hurts
and identify things that would help to cope with each specific hurt. This tech–
nique aided in discussions which served to normalize Erik's feelings. Addi–
tionally, this enabled Erik to begin to generate some of his own solutions and
thereby promoted Erik's gaining mastery over his environment. Erik's paper
doll is identified in the picture below.

Other directive play therapy techniques included assisting Erik with iden–
tifying supportive resources in his life. Erik identified his mother as the pri–
mary support person in his life. This is not uncommon for males with eating
disorders. Crosscope–Happell and colleagues (2000) reported that males with
eating disorders commonly tend to have close relationships with their moth–

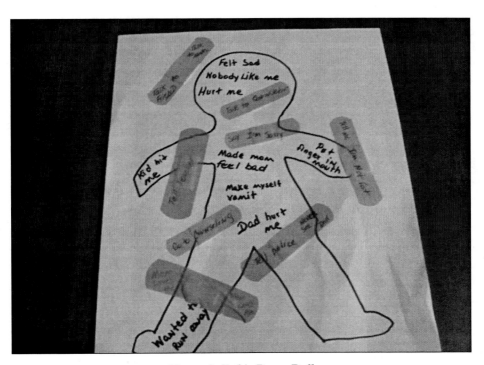

Figure 2. Erik's Paper Doll

ers. It was Erik's strong relationship with his mother that greatly influenced the decision to incorporate her into Erik's treatment.

I began to include Erik's mother in sessions after approximately ten sessions. I had provided Erik's mother with clear instructions regarding her role for the session. I simply asked that Erik's mother do nothing but observe the interactions between Erik and myself. Erik again decided to complete his sand tray with his mother present. Once more, I remained completely child–centered and simply reflected Erik's activities and emotions. I made particular efforts to validate Erik's feelings as exhibited in his play.

At the conclusion of the session, I met with Erik's mother individually and discussed the process. I then instructed Erik's mother to observe his play at home. After two sessions with Erik's mother observing, I then instructed her to begin to identify Erik's emotions in his play at home. I cautioned Erik's mother that she must remain non–judgmental and simply reflect his feelings and activities. Although Erik had a close relationship with his mother prior to treatment, it was noted that at times this relationship was inappropriate. Erik would always defer to his mother to solve problems and Erik's mother herself reported she often would attempt to solve Erik's dilemmas without validating his emotional experiences. I think this proved to be valuable in strengthening the child–parent bond.

Eliana Gil (1994) developed specific play techniques for use in family therapy and outlined these techniques in *Play in Family Therapy.* I included one such technique in my work with Erik and his mother. It was near termination of Erik's treatment that I suggested Erik and his mother choose puppets from a collection that I frequently use in my office. As Gil (1994) suggested, I then asked both Erik and his mother to make–up a story using the puppets. The story had to contain a beginning, middle, and an end. After providing the pair several minutes to prepare their story, I then asked them to act out the story using the puppets.

Ironically, the portrayal provided by Erik and his mother provided a good illustration of Erik's progression in therapy. Unlike the miniatures Erik used in his first sandtray, Erik chose a lion puppet which typically symbolizes strength. However, in the story, Erik reported that the lion had been injured by an alligator which he had also chosen for his second puppet.

Erik's mother used a princess and reported that the princess cried when the lion was hurt by the alligator. However, Erik's mother continued by reporting that the injured lion and the princess went to see a wise wizard which she chose for her second puppet. Erik continued by telling the story that the wizard helped the lion by teaching him how he can care for himself and teaching the princess what she could do to help the lion. Erik and his mother stated that the lion and the princess after learning valuable skills lived happily ever after.

This puppet story provided information to support the fact that Erik had progressed in therapy. Issues of body safety and vulnerability were easily resolved within the context of the story. The puppet story served as an excellent analogue for on–going safety planning and termination in therapy. This also served as an avenue for Erik to communicate his specific needs for safety to his mother.

The above identified play therapy techniques are only a few examples of how play therapy can be used effectively in the treatment of individuals with eating disorders. Through the twelve months of Erik's therapy, these techniques provided a non–threatening approach to therapy and assisted in the discovery of important clinical information. It should be noted that these play therapy techniques were used in conjunction with additional services. Specifically, I maintained on–going contact with Erik's primary care physician, nutritionalist, and psychiatrist. Collaboration with all treatment providers is vitally important.

In summary, counseling children can be extremely challenging. As Gil (1991) stated the work with children can be both very rewarding and yet challenging. Therefore, clinicians should be strongly advised to establish appropriate boundaries and utilize appropriate self–care practices. This is especially noteworthy in treating individuals with eating disorders.

The treatment of individuals with eating disorders is a complex and often challenging task. It is important that clinicians explore all available options when counseling this challenging population. Play therapy provides one theory for the treatment of children with eating disorders. However, play therapy offers a variety of techniques to assist clinicians with individuals diagnosed with eating disorders. Limitations in the literature as previously discussed seem to support additional research for the diagnosis and treatment of persons with eating disorders. Yet, as clinicians who are dedicated to serving children, we all have a responsibility to heal the hunger within.

References

American Psychiatric Association. (2000). *Diagnostic and statistical manual of mental disorders.* Washington, DC: Author.

Anderson, A. E. (1999). Eating disorders in gay males. *Psychiatric Annals, 29,* 206–212.

Axline, V. (1947). *Play therapy: The inner dynamics of childhood.* Cambridge, MA: Houghton Mifflin Company.

Braun, D. (1997). What objective criterion for diagnosing anorexia nervosa is absent in males? *Medscape Mental Health, 2*(4). Retrieved June 15, 2006 from the World Wide Web: http://www.medscape.com/medscape/question/1997/apr/q190.htm.

Costas, M. & Landreth, G. (1999). Filial Therapy with nonoffending parents of ahildren who have been sexually abused. *International Journal of Play Therapy, 8*(1),

44–66.

Crisci, G., Lay, M., & Lowenstein, L. (1998). *Paper dolls and paper airplanes therapeutic exercises for sexually traumatized children.* Indianapolis, IN: Kidsright Publishing.

Crosscope–Happell, C., Hutchins, D. E., Getz, H. G., & Hayes, G. L. (2000). Male Anorexia Nervosa: A New Focus. *Journal of Mental Health Counseling, 22,* 365–370.

Dokter, D.(1994). *Art therapies and clients with eating disorders.* UK: Jessica Kingsley Publishers.

Gil, E. (1994). *Play in family therapy.* New York: Guilford Press.

Gil, E. (1991). *The healing power of play.* New York: Guilford Press.

Grubbs, G. A. (1994). An abused child's use of sandplay in the healing process. *Clinical Social Work Journal, 22,* 193–209.

Guerney, B. G. (1964) Filial therapy: Description and rationale. *Journal of Counseling Psychology, 28*(4), 303–310.

Hall, P. E. (1997). Play therapy with sexually abused children. In H. D. Kauson, D. Cangelosi & C. E. Schaefer (1997). *The playing cure.* Northvale, NJ: Jason Aronson, Inc.

Kauson, H. G., Cangelosi, D., & Schaefer, C. E. (1997). *The playing cure.* Northvale, NJ: Jason Aronson, Inc.

Keel, P., Fulkerson, J. & Leon, G. (1997). Disordered eating precursors in pre– and early adolescent girls and boys. *Journal of Youth and Adolescence, 26*(2), 203–215.

Keel, P., Klump, K., Leon, G., & Fulkerson, J. (1998). Disordered eating in adolescent males from a school–based sample. *International Journal of Eating Disorders, 23,* 125–132.

Landreth, G. L. (1991). *Play therapy: The art of the relationship.* Muncy, IN: Accelerated Development, Inc.

Landreth, G. L., Homeyer, L. E., Glover, G., & Sweeney, D. S. (1996). *Play therapy interventions with children's problems.* Northvale, NJ: Jason Aronson, Inc.

Levitt, J. L., & Sansone, R. A. (2003). The treatment of eating disordered clients in a community–based partial hospitalization program. *Journal of Mental Health Counseling, 25,* 140–151.

Namka, L. (1995). Shame busting: Incorporating group social skills training, shame release and play therapy with a child who was sexually abused. *International Journal of Play Therapy, 4,* 81–98.

O'Halloran, M. S. (1999). Family involvement in the treatment of Anorexia Nervosa: A solution–focused approach. *The Family Journal: Counseling and Therapy for Couples and Families, 7,* 389–398.

Patel, D. R., Greydanus, D. E., Pratt, H. D., & Phillips, E. L. (2003). Eating disorders in adolescent athletes. *Journal of Adolescent Research, 18,* 244–260.

Rogers, C. L. (1980). *On becoming a person.* Boston: Houghton Mifflin.

Roth, A., & Fonagy, P. (1996). *What works for whom?* New York: Guilford Press.

Reijonen, J. H., Pratt, H. D., Patel, D. R., & Greydanus, D. E. (2003). Eating disorders in the adolescent population: An overview. *Journal of Adolescent Research, 18,* 209–222.

Seligman, L. (1998). *Selecting effective treatments: A comprehensive guide to treating mental disorders.* San Francisco, CA: Jossey–Bass, Inc.

Thompson, C. L., & Rudolph, L. B. (2000). *Counseling children* (5th Ed.). Belmont,

CA: Brooks/Cole.

Walcott, D. D., Pratt, H. D., & Patel, D. R. (2003). Adolescents and eating disorders: Gender, racial, ethnic, sociocultural, and socioeconomic issues. *Journal of Adolescent Research, 18,* 223–243.

Zerbe, K. J. (1993). *The body betrayed: A deeper understanding of women, eating disorders, and treatment.* Carlsbad, CA: American Psychiatric Press.

Biography

Brian L. Bethel is the Director of Outpatient Services for Scioto Paint Valley Mental Health Center in Chillicothe, Ohio. As a Professional Clinical Counselor (PCC) and a Licensed Chemical Dependency Counselor (LCDC), Mr. Bethel specializes in providing clinical services to children, adolescents, and families. Mr. Bethel earned Master's degrees in clinical counseling and rehabilitation counseling from Ohio University. In addition to providing mental health services Mr. Bethel serves as an independent trainer and consultant for a variety of human services organizations.

Chapter 8

DISCOVERY AND RECOVERY THROUGH MUSIC: AN OVERVIEW OF MUSIC THERAPY WITH ADULTS IN EATING DISORDER TREATMENT

ANNIE HEIDERSCHEIT

Historically and similarly popular belief continues to hold that eating disorders are a "teenage girl's disease." Despite the fact that the average age of onset of an eating disorder is 15 years of age (Rome et al., 2003), recent research indicates a higher prevalence of anorexia nervosa and bulimia nervosa among adult samples compared to previous years (Hoek & van Hoeken, 2003; Streigel–Moore, Franko & Ach, 2006). Researchers estimate that in the United States as many as 10 million females and 1 million males are diagnosed with either anorexia or bulimia nervosa (Crowther et al. 1992; Fairburn et al., 1993; Gordon, 1990; Hoek et al., 1995; Shisslak et al., 1995).

Treating adults with eating disorders introduces clinical issues and challenges that may and often are not present in treating adolescents. Adults diagnosed with an eating disorder (ED) can present a longer history with the ED, various mental health diagnoses, medical complications due to engaging in symptom use and malnutrition, financial struggles, employment related issues, and marital tensions. Additionally, the adult patient may also have caregiver responsibilities and entering treatment leaves them to find others to manage these duties. In cases where the adult patient has engaged in previous treatment episodes, re–entering treatment may feel like a failure or they may feel little hope in the treatment process.

This multitude of factors adds to the complexity and the necessity of treatment the whole person and not the disorder. Implementing treatment modalities that provide opportunities for a new perspective and a safe, non–threatening method of addressing the myriad of treatment related issues is imperative to the success of treatment for the adult patient. Music therapy is a creative modality that allows the patient to engage at their current level, and as they progress in treatment, deepen their engagement in the therapeutic process. The clinical illustrations in this chapter will further help demonstrate how the adult patient engages in the music therapy session and how this translates into the overall treatment process.

Psychiatric Comorbidities

There are many issues and challenges that are unique to treating adults with eating disorders. Clinical and epidemiological data support the strong comorbidity between eating disorders and various other mental health diagnoses (Braun, Sunday, & Halmi, 1994). Research suggests that well over half of the women diagnosed with anorexia nervosa report the presence of an anxiety disorder, most commonly generalized anxiety disorder, obsessive compulsive disorder, and social phobia (Bulik, 2002, Bulik, Sullivan, Fear, & Joyce, 1997; Kaye et al., 2004). Clinical studies also suggest a high prevalence of anxiety disorders in women with bulimia nervosa (Brewerton et al., 1995; Bushnell et al., 1994).

Research suggests a wide range of estimates (20%–98%) for the percentage of women that espouse depressive disorders (Braun, Sunday, & Halmi, 1994; Bulik, 2002). Additionally, rates of substance abuse are significantly higher in clinical and community samples of individuals with eating disorders (Holderness, Brooks–Gunn, & Warren, 1994; Wilson, 2002). Additionally, the research exploring the comorbid relationship between eating disorders and personality disorders shows higher rates of obsessive–compulsive personality disorders, borderline personality disorder (Dennis & Sasone, 1991), dependent personality disorder (Ames–Frankel et al., 1991), and impulsive and narcissistic personality traits in individuals with eating disorders (Lilenfeld et al., 2000).

Another prevalent diagnosis with adults in eating disorder treatment is post–traumatic stress disorder (PTSD). Individuals that have been the victim of sexual abuse or another form of trauma may meet the diagnostic criteria of PTSD (Brooke, 2007). Research suggests a range in the prevalence of specifically sexual abuse with individual with eating disorders, ranging from 10–55 percent (Ackard et al., 2001; Fallon & Wonderlich, 1997; Thompson & Wonderlich, 2004). Whether the abuse occurred during childhood or was a recent event, whether it was a single assault or years of abuse, the issues still become areas to address in the course of treatment and therapy.

The diagnoses addressed in the previous sections are not the only psychiatric diagnoses evident in individuals with eating disorders, they simply have a higher prevalence rate in this clinical population. Individuals with eating disorders may also present with a variety of diagnoses include various bipolar disorder, social anxiety disorder, somatization disorder, and body dys-morphic disorder. (For more details and diagnostic criteria on the various mental health diagnoses, please refer to the *DSM–IV–TR*, APA, 2000.)

Medical Complications

In addition to the many psychiatric comorbities, another complicating fac-tor is the myriad of medical complications that can arise in conjunction with, and as a result of, the eating disorder. Decreased oral intake and purging behaviors can lead to renal and electrolyte abnormalities which can progress to cardiovascular abnormalities. Gastrointestinal (GI) complications can occur in any and every portion of the GI tract, ranging from mild esophagi-tis to esophageal rupture (Pomeroy & Mitchell, 2002). Endocrine abnormal-ities also occur as a result of the eating disorder, resulting in high cortisol (stress hormone) levels to abnormal thyroid functioning. Metabolic abnor-malities can also arise. Loss or decrease of bone density (osteopenia) is com-mon with an eating disorder (Pomeroy, 2004).

Additional medical complications include pregnancy and reproductive function. Clinical data suggest that eating disorders are a cause of infertility (Pomeroy, 2004). When an individual is pregnant, this can be a challenging period of time. Research suggests higher rates of miscarriage, obstetric com-plications and postpartum depression (Pomeroy & Mitchell, 2002). Struggles with body image may be exacerbated due to the weight gain during preg-nancy. This in turn can prompt symptom use (restricting, over exercising or purging) to cope with these stressors, thus interfering with the fetal weight gain and the risk of low birth weight (Pomeroy & Mitchell, 2002).

The neurological system is also affected by the eating disorder. Individuals with anorexia suffer both structural and functional complications. Imaging studies have documented the loss of gray and white matter and a "pseu-do–atrophy" in the brain (Addolorate et al., 1998, 2001). These structural abnormalities manifest in the way of impaired cognitive functioning (Pomeroy, 2004).

The hematological and immune systems are also impacted by eating dis-orders, resulting in depressed cell mediated immune response and an increased risk for bacterial infections (Pomeroy, 2004). Dermatological abnormalities including hair loss, hypercarotenemia (orange discoloration of the skin), brittle nails, and dry skin frequently occur in individuals with eat-ing disorders. Lastly, dental complications can arise as a result of the eating disorder, erosion of the surface of teeth and loss of dental enamel occurs as a result of self–induced vomiting (Pomeroy & Mitchell, 1997).

The medical complications of the eating disorder reviewed in the previous section are not by any means a comprehensive review. It touches on each of the systems of the body and gives the reader only a glimpse of the impact the eating disorder has on the body. Please refer to a medical or eating disorder sourcebook to obtain a complete comprehensive overview of the medical complications associated with eating disorders. It is important to note that the serious medical complications associated with eating disorders can be fatal. Anorexia nervosa carries a high mortality rate, ranging from 6–20 percent of patients succumbing to the disorder, whether due to starvation or suicide (Crisp et al., 1992; Mitchell, Pomeroy & Adson, 1997).

Adults in Eating Disorder Treatment

Adults that enter treatment for their eating disorder may have recently developed their eating disorder or it may be a reoccurrence or a continuation of their eating disorder. For those in which it is a reoccurrence or a continuation, there may be a long and extensive eating disorder and treatment history. This can also mean the eating disorder is well established in the life of the individual (Vitousek, 2002). This extended eating disorder history can translate into multiple treatment attempts at various levels of care (inpatient, partial hospitalization, intensive outpatient, outpatient, or residential) as well as the eating disorder as a habitual part of life. The thought of changing behavior patterns and letting go of the eating disorder can be overwhelming. Additionally, returning to treatment can leave an individual feeling hopeless, as if they have failed in the recovery process again.

Since the age range of an adult is broad (18 and up), this can include a young adult just emerging into adulthood, exploring or entering a vocation, or beginning college, to an adult that is well established, highly educated, and a successful professional. Despite their vocation or location in the working world, entering treatment disrupts and interrupts life, whether interfering with college studies or employment. This in turn can create financial strains due to taking a medical leave/leave of absence from work, or needing to drop out of college, or suspend studies.

Another unique aspect for adults entering and engaging in treatment is that they are often engaged in multiple relationships in their life: i.e. spouse, children, parents, siblings, colleagues, coworkers and friends. These many relationships bring added dimensions and issues into the therapeutic process including marital difficulties (divorce, or separation), behavior problems (a child acting out or with special needs), sibling or parent conflict. Additionally, these relationships can bring added responsibilities, such as caring for children, spouse, or parents. Entering treatment means finding other ways and allowing other people to take over these responsibilities for a period of time.

It is evident that when an adult enters into eating disorder treatment, there are many complicating and confounding factors that come into the process. This requires clinicians to espouse a holistic approach, treating the whole person and all of the issue that present with the individual as they enter the treatment process. Effectively addressing these complex issues requires a multifaceted approach in a treatment program.

Psychotherapeutic Approaches

A wide variety of therapeutic interventions are employed to address the symptoms of the eating disorder and treatment for the individual. Despite the various methods employed, only a few of these psychotherapeutic approaches have been consistently and extensively studied. These approaches will be outlined to further demonstrate how music therapy incorporates principles from these various methods.

Cognitive behavioral therapy (CBT) is most widely utilized in eating disorder treatment (Devlin, Jahraus & Dobrow, 2005). CBT targets two broad areas of the eating disorder symptoms: cognitive and attitudinal disturbances (over emphasis on body image, distortion, weight and shape, or low self esteem), and behavioral aspects of eating and weight regulation (purging, restricting food intake). Further, CBT works to challenge the rigid rules about eating and weight that patients with eating disorders impose on themselves. This in turn develops healthier behaviors and cognitions (Pike, Devlin & Loeb, 2004)

Psychoeducation is often a component of CBT. Psychoeducation is based on the assumption that an individual is less likely to engage in self–defeating behaviors if they are aware of the factors that perpetuate the eating disorder (Garner, Vitousek & Pike, 1997). An important and basic tenet of psychoeducation is that the responsibility for change rests with the individual. The aim is to increase motivation and decrease defensiveness in the recovery process. In the process of treatment, psychoeducation may appear in the form of nutritional management, stress management, and socio–cultural factors related to eating disorder (Fairburn, 2005).

Interpersonal psychotherapy (IPT) is a short–term therapeutic approach in which the focus is addressing the interpersonal difficulties and conflicts that arise and can hinder recovery (Fairburn, 1997). The premise is that these conflicts within relationships are a strong contributing factor to the onset and continuation of a myriad of issues including depression, eating disorder symptoms, substance use, and marital discord (Weissman & Markowitz, 1994). Therefore, addressing these issues assists the individual caught in these self–perpetuating patterns to identify and deal with the problems that contribute to the eating disorder.

Within the last few years, Dialectical Behavior Therapy (DBT) has been explored and researched within the treatment and recovery process for individuals with eating disorders. DBT functions under the premise that the individual (due to past invalidation) does not possess the coping skills necessary to deal with and manage the sudden and intense emotions that arise in response to everyday and challenging issues (Linehan, 1993). DBT works to decrease responses that interfere with therapy, decrease behaviors that interfere with quality of life, develop distress tolerance, and enhancing respect for self, develop emotion regulation, develop coping skills that improve interpersonal relationships and functioning (Wisniewski & Kelly, 2003).

The approaches outlined above are the traditional therapies implemented in eating disorder treatment. There is a growing trend to provide multidisciplinary care and incorporate a variety of therapies to fully address the needs of the wide variety of patients that enter eating disorder treatment. Experiential therapies, including music therapy, are part of this trend. Frisch, Franko and Herzog (2006) found that of the 19 residential programs surveyed, all offered arts based therapies at least once a week and 26 percent offered an art–based therapy once a day. The programs surveyed reported they offered these types of therapies to facilitate self–discovery, self–exploration, and self–expression, allow patients to face and challenge issues related to body image, self–esteem, depression and isolation.

In exploring the traditional psychotherapies and the reasons why treatment programs are incorporating arts–based therapies into treatment process, it is clear to see there is a commonality in the issues addressed in all the approaches, despite the fact the medium in which they are addressed differs. The use of creative means provides a different perspective than the traditional verbal approach of the psychotherapeutic modalities.

The next section will further explore and explain how music therapy relates to the various psychotherapeutic approaches. The illustrations and case example will assist in clarifying how music therapy is being implemented to meet the needs of the individual or group in the treatment process.

Music Therapy

Music is a universal experience in which individuals from all backgrounds and cultures create, experience, perform, and engage in the art form. Everyone has experiences with music and has developed their own specific music preferences (Davis & Gfeller, 1999). Music therapy is the prescriptive use of music to address the needs of an individual or group (Heiderscheit, 2006). In the music therapy process, music is the applied medium which facilitates the achievement of the therapeutic goals.

A music therapist utilizes music in a therapeutic manner to address physical, emotional, cognitive, and social needs. Music therapy sessions are designed to address the following needs (AMTA, 2006; Heiderscheit, 2006): improve and facilitate communication, manage stress and anxiety, facilitate expression of feelings, explore and resolve emotional issues, improve self–esteem, develop new insights, develop self–acceptance and self–concept, and discover and develop new ways of coping.

Music therapy techniques vary greatly among clinical settings and with clinical populations. Music can be meaningful in a variety of ways to a variety of individuals because it is a flexible art form (Thaut & Gfeller, 1999). Music therapists implement support–oriented interventions that require active engagement in the here and now, insight and process–oriented sessions that facilitate problem solving, self–awareness and emotional expression, or catalytic experiences that uncover and resolve subconscious conflicts (Houghton et al., 2005).

Rationale for Music Therapy

Due to the fact that a myriad of complications and comorbities can accompany an individual diagnosed with an eating disorder, the treatment process must be able to address the wide array of needs this can present. The complexities of each individual and their clinical presentation support and require utilizing a modality that is equally complex and yet easily approachable. This ultimately requires matching the client to the appropriate therapy medium and intervention. The flexibility of music as a therapeutic agent allows the therapist to individualize the process and also meet a wide variety of needs simultaneously.

Music offers a unique means of expression at a time when feelings and emotions may be fragmented, elusive, and inaccessible to language. Parente (1989) suggests that music therapy improvisation allows the client to explore and express emotions in a non–verbal manner and that this act of musical expression serves as a bridge between the conscious mind and the expression of those feelings. Nolan (1989) also states that "improvisation is useful in facilitating psychotherapy because it stimulates the awareness and expression of emotions and ideas on an immediate level" (p. 167).

Sloboda (1993) writes of her work with an adult male diagnosed with bulimia and anorexia. She reports that the eating disorder functioned as a "visible symptom of painful feelings and also served as a defense against experiencing them" (p. 105). The process of individual music therapy details how music facilitated the expression of these emotions, thus bringing them to a conscious awareness. Hilliard (2001) describes his use of cognitive–behavioral music therapy in the treatment of women with eating disorders. He outlines how music therapy interventions help to manage stress, decrease anxiety at meal times, manage physical discomfort and address therapeutic issues such as self–esteem, empowerment, and issues surrounding body image.

Although the literature on the application of music therapy in the treatment of clients with eating disorders is sparse, the references and literature are still noteworthy. The illustrations outlined in the previous paragraphs support the clinical implementation of music therapy with eating disorder clients. The case examples that follow will further demonstrate how music therapy is an integral component of the recovery process and how music uniquely meets the vast and complex needs of the individuals in treatment.

Clinical Illustrations

The names of the individuals utilized in the case illustrations have been changed to protect their identity. Additionally, specific identifying details have been altered or deleted to further protect their identity. The details of the therapeutic process have not been altered to illustrate the role of music therapy in the overall treatment process.

The Case of Joanie and Song communication

Joanie is a 31–year–old woman with a successful career in marketing, diagnosed with anorexia nervosa. She holds a master's degree in business and was working for a prominent marketing firm at the time of admission. Her eating disorder began around age 15 and was persistent. She had experienced multiple hospitalizations on the inpatient eating disorder unit and the partial hospitalization program. This particular admission was prompted by the fact that Joanie was terminated from her position. She had been leaving her work for hours at a time to work out at the fitness center. Her workout time per day would range between 4–6 hours. She held memberships at three local fitness centers and she would rotate her workouts to avoid generating suspicion by the fitness center staff.

Joanie was devastated by the loss of her dream job. The stress that resulted from the job loss exacerbated the symptoms of her eating disorder. She then increased her amount of exercise and severely restricted her food intake. Joanie entered treatment medically compromised and emotionally closed off. She was isolated and quiet in group therapy sessions. Then one day in a music therapy session, each member of the group was asked to find a song that described what life was like with an eating disorder. Joanie discovered a song that identified with her experiences.

When each member of the group had completed their selection, one by one the group listened to each song. Joanie selected a song by Tracy Chapman entitled "Remember the Tin Man" from her 1995 album entitled, "New Beginning" (the lyrics that follow are only a portion of the song).

There are locks on the doors
And chains stretched across all the entries to the inside
There's a gate and a fence

And bars to protect from only God knows what lurks outside
Who stole your heart left you with a space
That no one and nothing can fill
Who stole your heart who took it away
Knowing that without it you can't live
Who took away the part so essential to the whole
Left you a hollow body
Skin and bone
What robber what thief who stole your heart and the key

Who stole your heart
Did you know but forget the method and moment in time
Was it a trickster using mirrors and sleight of hand
A strong elixir or a potion that you drank
Who hurt your heart

If you tear down the walls
Throw your armor away remove all the roadblocks barricades
If you can forget there are bandits and dragons to slay
And don't forget that you defend an empty space
And remember the tin man
Found he had what he thought he lacked
Remember the tin man
Go find your heart and take it back

The song is written in a minor key, which give it an austere and eerie sound. The vocalist is accompanied solely by an acoustic guitar, with a repetitive chord progression. This simplistic accompaniment gives the song an intimate and personal feeling. The chorus repeats again and again . . . "who stole your heart," questioning over and over; relentlessly asking the listener for an answer to this question.

When the group had listened to the song in its entirety, Joanie was asked by the music therapist why she had selected this song. She shared that she felt the eating disorder had robbed her, taking away her heart (the essence of who she is) her self-worth, her life's ambitions and desires, and pushed her loved ones away. She felt the eating disorder deceived her, lied to her, tricked her, leaving her to feel like she was victimized by an intruder. The end of the song left her with a sense of hope that maybe if she explored deep within herself she would find remnants of who she was, as well as begin to discover who she is, and reclaim those aspects of her life.

This song gave a voice to the complex feelings Joanie felt in being ravaged by her eating disorder. The song was able to express her experiences and her feelings of powerlessness. In her process of acknowledging her powerlessness, she discovered hope. The hope that the eating disorder did not take the essence of who she is, the hope that if she began to look inside herself she would rediscover who she is and reclaim her life. She approached the remainder of her treatment with renewed energy. Also, she successfully completed her stay on the inpatient unit and was discharged to outpatient services. She has been able to maintain her success on an outpatient level and return to her career.

The Case of Sara and Song Analysis

Sara was a 45–year–old woman diagnosed with anorexia nervosa, who was attending the partial hospitalization program (PHP). She entered the PHP following a six–week stay on the inpatient eating disorder (ED) unit. She reported a long eating disorder history, with the onset of her disorder in her late teens. Despite her long ED history, this was her first treatment episode. Sara was married and was a stay at home mom. She and her husband had three children, ages 17, 19 and 23. She was soon to be a grandmother and very excited about that new venture. Her treatment episode was prompted by the fact that she was feeling overwhelmed by the changes in her life (children growing up and depression worsening). This seemed to increase her symptom use which included restricting her food intake and over exercising. She also noted that when her symptoms were exacerbated, she tended to isolate herself from her friends and loved ones.

While in the PHP, Sara attended music therapy sessions with the other members of the group. The group she was a part of consisted of women ranging from ages 29 to 57. During this particular session, the music therapist utilized a song analysis intervention. This entails the therapist bringing a song into the session that she feels has therapeutic value for the group and the group process. The song that was introduced to the group was "Little Butterfly" by Esther Alvarado, Ginger Baker and Jana Stanfield, from Jana Stanfield's 1999 album entitled "Little Butterfly." The song is performed by a solo voice, accompanied on acoustic guitar. Again this instrumentation gives the song a close, intimate feeling, accenting the personal nature of the struggle. Below are excerpts from the song:

> *I have lived all alone in a world without light*
> *I have lived in a cell without bars, without sight*
> *While longing for meadows, and fields full of flowers*
> *Pain and confusion have filled lonely hours*

I wanted to fly, to soar over green fields
But the hard shell around me would not crack, would not yield
I felt bound to the earth, wrapped in ribbons of steel
It hurt when I hoped, it hurt when I'd feel
Yet even as I yearned so much for release
Something inside spoke softly of peace
A whisper was there each time that I cried

Saying, "Don't give up child, keep hope alive"
Hope seemed a thing as distant and far as the most distant galaxy the most distant star
I did not believe I would ever be free of the heavy cocoon that was covering me
Then slowly, so slowly, came a glimmer of light
It scared me at first, this first bit of sight
There were others around me
Why had they come
Why had they entered my dark, lonely home
And then, one by one, they reached out a hand
And lifted the ribbons of steel strand by strand
When their hands touched the ribbons, the steel fell away
And I began to feel different in this lightness of day
They smiled and rejoiced, and I heard a song
One that had played in my heart all along

These are the words the song sings to me
This is what it says:
I can feel a change is coming, I can feel it in my skin
I can feel myself outgrowing this life I've been living in
And I'm afraid, afraid of change
Butterfly, please tell me again, I'm gonna be alright
And I know, I know, I'm going to be all right
And I know, I know I will take flight

After the group listened to the song in its entirety, the music therapist asked the group to share any thoughts they had about the song. Several individuals in the group highlighted various lyrics that resonated with them. The song had a more profound impact on Sara. Also, she shared that the whole song seemed to encapsulate her life with the eating disorder. She shared line by line the lyrics of the song that spoke to her experiences. She acknowledged, "I have been living in a cell, it was a self-imposed cell, there were no bars, I just allowed my eating disorder to keep me there. It has been so lonely, I have shut everyone out for all these years and as much as I wanted to escape I was totally terrified of what that meant. But now that I am in treatment and I have disclosed to my friends and family that I have an eating disorder, they are all reaching out and caring for me. And I can feel that things are different for me, it is scary and I feel uncertain, but I don't want to go back into that prison. I have to keep telling myself I am going to be alright."

This song generated an "ah-hah" moment for Sara. It shed light on her experience with the eating disorder in a way she had never examined. She realized she had been living a life she did not want to live, but she was terrified of the uncertainty of what life without the eating disorder would be. Sara was so moved by this song, she asked the music therapist for the details on where she could purchase this recording and by the following session she had obtained her own copy. She also reported she was sharing this song with her family and friends to help them understand what her life has been like, living all these years with the secret of her eating disorder.

Case Illustration of Group Songwriting

The process of writing a song can feel like an overwhelming task for an individual. However when incorporated into the therapeutic process under the guidance of a music therapist, the experience can be empowering. The following is a song that was written by a group of individuals attending the PHP. The group consisted of young women ranging in age from 18–23. The group had requested writing their own composition to the melody of a song by the Dixie Chicks called "Goodbye Earl." They wanted to entitle their song "Goodbye ED" (to represent the eating disorder). During the session the music therapist sang the original song, "Goodbye Earl" for the group, so they could gather of sense of how the song tells a story. The song is about two friends, one of whom is in an abusive marriage. The two friends devise a plan to resolve this abusive relationship. This song had prompted the group to discuss the similarities between an abusive relationship and life with an eating disorder.

Since the group had already determined the theme of the song, it was now time to discuss how the story should unfold. Through the course of the group discussion, it was determined that the song should start from the point at which the eating disorder began, evolved and progressed. What follows is the song that was written by this group within a one–hour therapy session.

I ate ice cream bars and doughnuts too all through my carefree days
Until all the other girls where skipping lunch and then I changed my ways.
If the scale and the weight didn't suit my taste I went back to bed.
And when all the other girls were getting boyfriends I hooked up with ED.
Well it wasn't two weeks until ED started saying, "You gotta lose more weight".
So put the Oreos and cheesecake down or you'll never get a date.
I started getting crabby and irritable, I couldn't concentrate.
I got skinnier and skinnier and ED kept saying, "You gotta lose more weight."
CHORUS
I started losing my hair and people got scared,
But I didn't give a damn.
My friends held my hand and we worked out a plan,

And it didn't take long to decide
That ED had to die.
Na, Na...
Goodbye ED
Na, Na...
That mac–n–cheese tastes alright to me, ED.
You wanna put up a fight?
I'll take another bite.,
I went to the clinic for my regular check up the doctor said I had to stay.
They talked with my parents and then they locked ED and I away.
I was mad that I had to gain weight 'cause my BMI was low.
They started feeding me fats and all kinds of snacks and I could not say no.
Well as time went on my support stood by and helped me stand up to ED.
My clothes started fitting and now I find that ED's not always in my head.
Well the meals went by and spring turned to summer and summer faded into fall.
And it turns out ED was a cruel disorder that nobody missed at all.

CHORUS
So I held my head high and reclaimed my life,
And ED doesn't win the fight.
I eat three meals a day and snacks are okay,
And I don't lose any sleep at night.
'Cause ED had to die.
Na, Na...
Goodbye ED
Na, Na...
We need a break.
ED's such a big fake.
We'll pack a lunch and stuff ED in the trunk.
Na, Na...

The therapeutic process of songwriting is not about producing an end result (a song). It is a process in which a group describes and shares their experiences. As they talk about the feelings related to these experiences the song becomes the vehicle for carrying this information. This song describes various aspects of the eating disorder, the desire to be thin, the medical complications associated with the disorder, and the psychological issues (body image struggles, mood disturbances, and resistance to treatment). Finally, the song focuses on the process of reclaiming life and how life can and does begin to be different as recovery from the eating disorder is envisioned and achieved.

When the group completed their song they were very excited to share it with staff, family, and friends. Within moments of completion, staff had gathered to hear the song and the group sang their words proudly. They sang with a new confidence having completed a task they never considered doing before treatment. If writing a song was an insurmountable task they could achieve, what more lay ahead that they could overcome? This sense of empowerment is a valuable by product of the songwriting process and a vital force in the process of treatment and recovery.

Case Illustration of Improvisation and Meeting Your Needs

The use of active drumming and improvisation is a way to actively engage a group in the here and now. In the improvisational music experience, the music therapist brings a variety of drums (djembes, tubanos, frame drums, bongos, and congos) and a wide variety of rhythm instruments (egg shakers, rainstick, cabasa, maracas, finger cymbals, guiro, claves, frog rasp, shekere, and triangle). Consideration must be given to the group and their process. The therapist must be mindful of the level of medical stability of each individual in the group. If an individual is severely medically compromised, the level of activity in an improvisation experience may require expending too much energy. Care must be given in determining the physical readiness of a group to engage in improvisation, this is of primary consideration for patients on an inpatient unit. Individuals in a residential care setting are required to have achieved medical stability.

This group of women were in a residential eating disorder program and ranged in age from 21 to 35. Of the eight participants, only one had previously engaged in a music improvisation or drumming experience prior to this session. For those individuals that struggle with perfectionism, engaging in something new can feel overwhelming and stir up a feeling of fear of failure.

This session began with the therapist asking the group to develop a list describing what they need to succeed in their recovery. The list the group developed included the following: peace, comfort, love, hope, calmness, self–acceptance, and patience. The therapist then asked the group how to musically create the needs included on the list. The group then talked about the need to hear a consistent rhythm, harmony rather than dissonance, rhythms that complemented one another and felt cohesive, soft to moderate dynamics, and consistency within the dynamic levels.

Each member of the group was then asked to select an instrument they would like to play. They were instructed to begin playing as they felt ready and what they chose to play should fit within the framework outlined by the group. As the group began to play, they listened to each other, at times matching rhythms and other times struggling to play cohesively. The dynamic level remained consistently muted to create the feelings they had listed. As the improvisation progressed the group began to listen to each other more intently finding where each fit and what felt comfortable. Each kept playing until the group hit a "groove," or a moment when all the rhythms seemed to come together and ease into one another. At this moment, you could see the group collectively relax into the experience. The group maintained this for several minutes, playing and engaging with one another in the moment and in the music, creating what they all needed.

The music therapist signaled the end of the improvisation. When everyone had set down their instrument, she asked the group, "How did that feel?" "Did you create what you needed?" The group identified feeling calm and more relaxed then they did at the start of the session. They recognized how in listening to one another they created wonderful rhythms and felt listened to and cared for by each other. They recognized how they worked beyond the fear of failure, took the risk and tried something new. The group was struck by a comment by one of the women. In the process of talking about the improvisational experience, she remarked, "While we were playing together and creating music, my eating disorder was not present. How great it feels to have time away from it."

The process of actively making music pushed them to take a risk, confront the fear of failure and help them to see within the moment that they could meet their own needs. The ultimate benefit was that by placing their full presence in the here and now, they were able to step away from the eating disorder. They could capture a glimpse of life free of the eating disorder. And for a moment in time, experience that life without the eating disorder.

Conclusion

The universality of music lends itself to the therapeutic process in that it can meet each person wherever they are on their journey of recovery. The complexities within music speak to the subconscious, connecting to our emotions and providing the outlet for those feelings that have been unresolved. The process of music therapy can empower the individual to discover the answers within rather than grasp for answers outside themselves. Music and music therapy can help them recognize what they have not been able to see or hear in any other way before. This process of discovery that takes place within the therapeutic application of music can hold the keys the individual needs to unlock the door to their own recovery.

Appendix–Terms

Bongo–Bongo drums or bongos are a percussion instrument made up of two small drums attached to each other. Bongo drums produce high–pitched sounds, and should be held between the knees. They are traditionally played by striking the drumheads with the fingers, although some contemporary classical compositions require sticks or brushes.

Cabasa–The Cabasa, is a percussion instrument that is constructed with loops of steel ball chain wrapped around a wide cylinder. The cylinder is fixed to a long, narrow wooden or plastic handle.

Claves–Claves is a percussion instrument consisting of a pair of short (about 20–30 cm), thick dowels. Normally they are made of wood but nowadays they are also made of fiberglass or plastics due to the longer durability of these materials. When struck, they produce a bright clicking noise.

Conga–The conga is a tall, narrow, single–headed drum that is meant to be played with bare hands. Although ultimately derived from African drums made from hollowed logs, the Cuban conga is staved, like a barrel. These drums were probably made from salvaged barrels originally.

Djembe–A djembe (pronounced *JEM-bay*) is a skin covered hand drum shaped like a large goblet and is meant to be played with bare hands. It is a hollow drum and is open at the bottom.

Egg shaker–Small egg-shaped shakers that fit easily into any size hand. They are typically made of plastic in a variety of bright colors. They can make a multitude of sounds, depending on how hard they're shaken, how much hand is holding them, and how fast they're going.

Finger cymbal–Finger cymbals are tiny cymbals. Each cymbal has an elastic band to attach it to a finger. A set of finger cymbals consists of four cymbals, two for each hand.

Frame drum–A frame drum has a drumhead diameter greater than its depth. It can be played with bare hands or a soft mallet.

Frog rasp–The frog rasp is a wooden percussion instrument that looks like a frog with ridges on its back. Scrape, rasp, or croaking–type sounds are produced when the wooden stick is scraped across the ridges.

Guiro–The güiro is a percussion instrument consisting of an open–ended, hollow gourd with parallel notches cut in one side. It is played by rubbing a wooden stick along the notches to produce a ratchet–like sound.

Maraca–Maracas are simple percussion instruments usually played in pairs, consisting of a dried calabash or gourd shell, or coconut shell filled with seeds or dried beans. They may also be made of leather, wood, or plastic. Often one maraca is pitched high and the other low.

Rainstick–A rainstick is a long, hollow tube which is filled with small baubles such as beads or beans and has small pins arranged helically on its inside surface. When the stick is upended, the beads fall to the other end of the tube, making a sound reminiscent of a rainstorm as they bounce off the pins. The rainstick is generally used to create atmospheric sound effects or as a percussion instrument.

Shekere–The shekere is a percussion instrument consisting of a dried gourd with beads woven into a net covering the gourd. The shape of the gourd determines the sound of the instrument. To play, it is shaken and/or hit against the hands.

Tubano–A tubano is a tall, narrow drum with a cutout at the bottom of the drum which allows the player to project at full volume from a sitting position.

References

Ackard, D. M., Neumark–Sztainer, D., Hannan, P. J., French, S., & Story, M. (2001). Binge and purge behavior among adolescents: Associations with sexual and physical abuse in a nationally representative sample: The Commonwealth Fund survey. *Child Abuse and Neglect, 6,* 771–785.

Addolorate, G., Taronto, C., Capristo, E., & Babarrini, G. (1998). A case marked cerebellar atrophy in a woman with anorexia nervosa and a review of the literature. *International Journal of Eating Disorders, 24,* 443–447.

American Music Therapy Association. (2006). *2005 Music Therapy Sourcebook.* Washington, D.C.: American Music Therapy Association.

American Psychiatric Association. (2000). *Diagnostic and statistical manual of mental disorders* (4th ed.). Text Revision (*DSM–IV–TR*). Washington, D.C., American Psychiatric Association.

Ames–Frankel, J., Devlin, M. J., Walsh, B. T., Strasser, T. J., Sadik, C., Oldham, J. M., & Roose, S. P. (1992). Personality disorder diagnoses in patients with bulimia nervosa: Clinical correlates and changes in treatment. *Journal of Clinical Psychiatry, 53,* 90–96.

Braun, D. L., Sunday, S. R., & Halmi, K. A. (1994). Psychiatric comorbidity in patients with eating disorders. *Psychological medicine, 24,* 859–867.

Brewerton, T., Lydiard, R. Herzog, D., Brotman, A., O'Neil, P., Ballenger, J. (1995). Comorbidity of Axis I psychiatric disorders in bulimia nervosa. *Journal of Clinical Psychiatry, 56,* 77–80.

Brooke, S. L. (2007). *The use of the creative therapies with sexual abuse survivors.* Springfield, IL: Charles C Thomas, Publisher, Ltd.

Bulik, C. (2002). Anxiety, depression, and eating disorders. In C. G. Fairburn & K. D. Brownell (Eds.), *Eating disorders and obesity: A comprehensive handbook* (pp. 193–198). New York: Guilford.

Bulik, C., Sullivan, P., Fear, J., & Joyce, P. (1997). Eating disorders and antecedent anxiety disorders: A controlled study. *Acta Psychiatrica Scandinavica, 96,* 101–107.

Bushell, J. A., Wells, E., McKenzie, J. M., Hornblow, A. R., Oakley–Browne, M.A., & Joyce, P. R. (1994). Bulimia comorbidity in the general population and in the clinic. *Psychological Medicine, 24,* 605–611.

Chapman, T. (1994). Remember the Tin man. On *New Beginnings:* (CD). New York: Elektra Entertainment.

Crisp, A. H., Callender, J. S., Halek, C., & Hsu L. K. G. (1992). Long–term mortality in anorexia nervosa. *British Journal of Psychiatry, 161,* 104–107.

Crowther, J., Crawford, P., & Shepherd, K. (1992). The Stability of the Eating

Disorder Inventory. *International Journal of Eating Disorders, 12*(1), 97–101.

Davis, B., & Gfeller, K. (1999). Clinical practice in music therapy. In W. Davis, M. Thaut & K. Gfeller (Eds.), *An introduction to music therapy: Theory and practice* (pp. 3–15). Boston: McGraw–Hill.

Dennis, A. B., & Sasone, R. A. (1991). The clinical stages of treatment for eating disorder patients with borderline personality disorders. In C. L. Johnson (Ed.), *Psychodynamic treatment of anorexia nervosa and bulimia nervosa* (pp. 126–164). New York: Guilford Press.

Devlin, M., Jahraus, J., & Dobrow, I. (2005). Eating disorders. In J. L. Levenson (Ed.), *Textbook of psychosomatic medicine* (pp. 311–334). Arlington, VA: American Psychiatric Publishing.

Fairburn, C. (2005). Evidence–based treatment of anorexia nervosa. *International Journal of Eating Disorders, 37*, S26–S30.

Fairburn, C. (1997). Interpersonal psychotherapy for Bulimia Nervosa. In D. Garner & P. Garfinkel (Eds.), *Handbook of treatment for eating disorders* (2nd ed.), (pp. 278–294). New York: Guilford Press.

Fairburn, C., Welch, S., & Phillipa, J. (1992). The classification of recurrent overeating: The "binge eating disorder proposal." *International Journal of Eating Disorders, 13*(2), 155–159.

Fallon, P., & Wonderlich, S. (1997). Sexual abuse and other forms of trauma. In D. Garner & P. Garfinkel (Eds.), *Handbook of treatment for eating disorders* (2nd ed.), (pp. 394–414). New York: Guilford Press.

Frisch, M., Frank, D., & Herzog, D. (2006). Arts–based therapists in the treatment of eating disorders. *Eating Disorders, 14*, 131–342.

Garner, D., Vitousek, K., & Pike, K. (1997). Cognitive behavioral therapy for anorexia nervosa. In D. Garner & P. Garfinkel (Eds.), *Handbook of treatment for eating disorders* (pp. 94–144). New York: Guilford Press.

Gordon, R. (1990). *Anorexia and bulimia: Anatomy of a social epidemic.* Cambridge, MA: Basil Blackwell.

Heiderscheit, A. (2006) in production. *Music Therapy*, cited February 13, 2007 in http://www.takingcharge.csh.umn.edu

Hilliard, R. (2001). Cognitive–behavioral music therapy and eating disorders. *Music Therapy Perspectives, 2*, 109–113.

Hoek, H., Bartelds, A., Bosveld, J., van der Graaf, Y., Limpens, V., Maiwald, M., & Spaaij, C. (1995). Impact of urbanization on detection rates of eating disorders. *The American Journal of Psychiatry, 152*(9), 1272–1278.

Hoek, H. & van Hoeken, D. (2003). Review of the prevalence and incidence of eating disorders. *International Journal of Eating Disorders, 34*, 283–396.

Holderness, C. C., Brooks–Gunn, J., & Warren, M. P. (1994). Comorbidity of eating disorders and substance abuse: Review of literature. *International Journal of Eating Disorders, 16*, 1–34.

Houghton, B., Scovel, M., Smeltekop, R., Thaut, M., Unkefer, R., & Wilson, B. (2005). Taxonomy of clinical music therapy programs and techniques. In R. Unkefer & M. Thaut (Eds.), *Music therapy in the treatment of adults with mental disorders: Theoretical bases and clinical interventions* (pp. 181–206). Gilsum, NH: Barcelona Publishers.

Kaye, W., Bulik, C., Thornton, L., Barbarich, N., & Masters, K. (2004). Comorbidity of anxiety disorders with anorexia and bulimia nervosa. *American Journal of Psychiatry, 161*(12), 2215–2221.

Lilenfeld, L. R., Stein, D., Devlin, B., Bulik, C., Strober, M., Plotnicov, K., Pollice, C., Rao, R., Merikangas, K. R., Nagy, L., & Kaye, W. H. (2000). Personality traits among currently eating disordered, recovered, and never–ill first degree female relatives of bulimic and control women. *Psychological Medicine, 30*, 1399–1410.

Linehan, M. M. (1993b). *Skills training manual for the treatment of borderline personality disorder.* New York: Guilford Press.

Mitchell, J., Pomeroy, C., & Adson, D. (1997). Managing medical complications. In D. Garner & P. Garfinkel (Eds.), *Handbook of treatment for eating disorders* (2nd Ed.), (pp. 383–393). New York: Guilford Press.

Nolan, P. (1989). Music therapy improvisation techniques with bulimic patients. In L. M. Hornyak & E. K. Baker (Eds.), *Experiential therapies for eating disorders* (pp. 167–187). New York: Guilford Press.

Parente, A. B. (1989). Music as a therapeutic tool in treating anorexia nervosa. In L. M. Hornyak & E. K. Bake (Eds.), *Experiential therapies for eating disorders* (pp. 305–328). New York: Guilford Press.

Pike, K., Devlin, M., & Loeb, K. (2004). Cognitive behavioral therapy in the treatment of anorexia nervosa, bulimia nervosa and binge eating disorder. In K. Thompson (Ed.), *Handbook of eating disorders and obesity* (pp. 130–162). New York: Guilford Press.

Pomeroy, C. (2004). Assessment of medical status and physical factors. In K. Thompson (Ed.) *Handbook of eating disorders and obesity* (pp. 81–111). New York: Guilford Press.

Pomeroy, C., & Mitchell, J. (2002). Medical complications of anorexia nervosa and bulimia nervosa. In C. Fairburn & K. Brownell (Eds.), *Eating disorders and obesity: A comprehensive handbook* (2nd ed.), (pp. 278–329) New York: Guilford Press.

Rome, E., Ammerman, S., Rosen, D., et al. Children and adolescents with eating disorders: The state of the art. *Pediatrics, 111*, 98–108.

Shisslak, C., Crago, M., & Estes, L. (1995). The spectrum of eating disturbances. *International Journal of Eating Disorders, 18*(3), 209–219.

Sloboda, A. (1993). Individual therapy with a man who has an eating disorder. In M. Heal & T. Wigram (Eds). *Music therapy in health and education* (pp. 103–111). London: Jessica Kingsley Publishers.

Stanfield, J., Alvarado, E., & Baker, G. (1999). Little Butterfly. (Recorded by Jana Stanfield.) *On Little Butterfly* (CD).

Streiger–Moore, R., Franko, D., & Ach, E. (2006). Epidemiology of eating disorders: An update. In S. Wonderlich, J. Mitchell, M. de Zwaan, & Steiger (Eds.), *Annual review of eating disorders, part 2* (pp. 65–80). United Kingdom: Radcliffe Publishing, Inc.

Thaut, M., & Gfeller, K. (1999). Music therapy in the treatment of mental disorders. In W. Davis, M. Thaut & K. Gfeller (Eds.), *An introduction to music therapy: Theory and practice* (pp. 93–132). Boston, MA: McGraw-Hill.

Thompson, K., & Wonderlich, S. (2004). Child sexual abuse and eating disorders. In K. Thompson (Ed.), *Handbook of eating disorders and obesity* (pp. 679–694). New

York: Guilford Press.

Vitousek, K. (2002). Cognitive–behavioral therapy for anorexia nervosa. In C. Fairburn & K. Brownell (Eds.), *Eating disorders and obesity* (2nd Ed.), (pp. 308–313). New York: Guilford Press.

Weissman, M. M., & Markowitz, J. C. (1994). Interpersonal psychotherapy: Current status. *Archives of General Psychiatry, 51*, 599–606.

Wilson, G. (2002). Eating disorders and addictive disorders. In C. Fairburn & K. Brownell (Eds.), *Eating disorders and obesity: A comprehensive handbook* (2nd ed.), (pp. 199–203). New York: Guilford Press.

Wisniewski, L., & Kelly, K. (2003). The application of dialectical behavior therapy to the treatment of eating disorders. *Cognitive and Behavioral Practice, 10*, 131–138.

Biography

Annie Heiderscheit, Ph.D., MT–BC, FAMI, NMT is a board–certified music therapist with 16 years of clinical experience. Dr. Heiderscheit is an adjunct faculty member in music therapy at the University of Minnesota and is a lecturer in the Center for Spirituality and Healing. She maintains a private practice in music therapy, specializing in the use of music therapy in medicine and music psychotherapy. She also continues her clinical practice at Methodist Hospital in the Eating Disorder Institute, providing music therapy services in the inpatient, partial hospitalization, and residential programs. She also serves as an internship supervisor for the internship program at Park Nicollet Health Services. Dr. Heiderscheit also provides clinical music therapy services at the University of Minnesota Children's Hospital on the Pediatric Bone Marrow Transplant Unit and Pediatric Intensive Care Units.

Chapter 9

MUSIC THERAPY IN THE TREATMENT OF EATING DISORDERS

Marah Bobilin, MA, MT–BC

The National Eating Disorders Association (NEDA) reports that an estimated 5–10 million people have eating disorders in the United States alone. Due to the unprecedented growth of eating disorders in the past twenty years, there is also an increased likelihood of creative arts therapists providing services to patients with eating disorders in a variety of settings including private practice, mental health facilities, hospitals, and specialized inpatient facilities. However, the eating–disordered population is also considered one of the most difficult populations to treat due to high treatment resistance and the complex, often paradoxical, nature of the pathology. Therefore, it is imperative that creative arts therapists understand the complexity of the disorder and the dynamics of therapy in order to provide the best treatment for the patient and to evaluate the efficacy of our interventions.

Currently, most of the literature on music therapy with eating disorders is comprised of individual work written from a psychoanalytic perspective in which the primary intervention is musical improvisation (Frederiksen, 1999; Robarts, 1995; Robarts, 2000; Robarts & Sloboda, 1994; Smejsters, 1996; Smejsters & van den Hurk, 1993). Less has been written about group music therapy work and/or the use of alternative music therapy interventions with clients with eating disorders with the exception of Justice (1994), Loth (2002), and Nolan (1989). As of yet, only case studies and anecdotal writings have been published. No comprehensive evaluation of music therapy treatment with clients with eating disorders has been conducted. Much more information is needed regarding the therapy implementation, demographic parameters of the field and client population, and therapeutic dynamics.

In order to examine the current practice of music therapy with clients with eating disorders, a national survey of music therapists listed in the national registry as working with the mental health and eating disorder patient populations was conducted (Spring, 2006). The survey sought to establish the demographic parameters of the patient population served by music therapists and also to investigate various aspects of the music therapy process including the use of clinical improvisation and the interpersonal and musical dynamics.

The results of the survey revealed that although music therapists found the use of clinical improvisation to be the most effective therapeutic intervention to use with clients with eating disorders, they experienced difficulty in implementing this intervention, and used it less often than others including song writing and lyric analysis. Several areas of interest also emerged from the results including: the resistance of the patient population to active music making, manifestations of the eating disorder in the music, and the implications of the therapeutic dynamics, and are discussed in the sections to follow.

The purpose of this chapter is two–fold: (1) to describe the complex nature of the pathology of eating disorders and treatment goals, and (2) to present a discussion of the outcomes from a recent survey of music therapists working with the client population. It is hoped that the results of the study may assist other creative arts therapists in establishing treatment protocol, increasing treatment efficacy and evaluation, and to stimulate new areas of research and treatment for the client population.

Etiology and Symptoms of the Pathology

Much of the music therapy literature has conceptualized the etiology from the disorder from the psychoanalytic framework. The etiology of the disorder will be described briefly from the psychodynamic and cognitive theoretical paradigms in order to better understand the origins of the core issues and the nature of the patient's resistance to treatment.

Psychoanalytic Model

Psychoanalytic theorists believe trace the roots of the disorder to a dysfunction during the early childhood developmental stages of symbiosis and separation–individuation, wherein the individual fails to develop the ability to self–soothe and achieve object constancy. This dysfunction is thought to occur because the child internalizes the caregiver's anxieties, rather than feelings of security and safety (Loth, 1988). Therefore, in order to attain a sense of well–being, the child strives to meet the needs of the caregiver and to express herself in ways that will elicit approval from the caregiver. As a result of this enmeshment, the child may experience difficulty in successfully individuating from the caregiver and achieving autonomy.

Further, the cycle of "perfectionism" becomes established as this behavior often yields considerable praise from parents and teachers, and then becomes perpetuated until adolescence when symptoms of the disorder usually manifest. However, at this time, the individual is confronted with changing social roles and expectations for which she is ill–prepared to cope.

Goodsitt (1997) writes that the eating–disordered individual "negates her selfhood. Instead, she directs her attention to pleasing, accommodating, and being sensitive to others. The guiding rule is to serve others by meeting their needs. She strives to become a self–object (i.e., a function for others) and not a self" (p. 212). He mentions the "self–guilt" that individuals with eating disorders experience for having feelings and needs that are different from that of the caregivers, or wanting to have a separate identity. He writes, "An act of occupying psychological space is experienced as an immoral, hostile, and destructive act that deprives others of their psychological space" (p. 213). The concept of self–guilt also helps to explain the self–starvation or the bingeing experience, in which the individual with an eating disorder reverses her obligation to care for others and is intensely devoted to her self–experience (Goodsitt, 1997).

Cognitive–Behavioral Model

The cognitive–behavioral theory states that the individual develops an eating disorder because of her perceived overall ineffectiveness in other areas of functioning and turns to the eating disorder as the only successful experience (Fairburn, Shafran, & Cooper, 1998). The individual with anorexia has a need for control and views the eating disorder as the aspect in life that can be controlled. The eating disorder thus becomes very important to the individual, as one client with anorexia exclaimed, "If I let go of my eating disorder, what will I have left?" (Sloboda, 1993, p. 105). An example of distorted thinking resulting from low self–esteem includes the following, "I was not giving anything to the world, so I did not have the right to eat" (Bruch, 1988, p. 175).

Patient Resistance

Consequently, many patients who enter treatment for an eating disorder may display a high level of resistance to therapy because the eating disorder represented their coping mechanism, means of self–esteem, and essentially, their identity (Fairburn et al., 1999; Goodsitt, 1997; Zerbe, 1998). This resistance to treatment is illustrated by anorexics' acute denial of their illness (Bruch, 1988; Zerbe, 1998). Bruch (1988) warns that many therapists consider the clients to be deceitful or dishonest because they do not consider themselves suffering from an illness nor profess to view themselves as emaciated. Such suspicions are indeed likely to be detrimental to the client's treatment as it may reinforce a vicious cycle Bruch defines as 'systematic training in dishonesty.' She explains that many therapists fail to acknowledge that these patients entire existence has been founded on false experiences wherein others acknowledge only "good" behavior and other feelings including misery and depression are ignored.

Goodsitt (1997) writes that resistance may be better understood if the therapist understands the role of the eating disorder in the client's life and that the eating disorder protects the client from not feeling difficult or unpleasant emotions and therefore represents security and identity. Because emotions are communicated and understood as bodily impulses, the individual with an eating disorder attempts to control difficult emotions by controlling physical impulses and bodily needs via maladaptive eating behaviors. In this manner, the individual becomes disengaged from their emotional state and sense of self (Dokter, 1995).

Rationale for Music Therapy

Goodsitt (1997) writes that clients with eating disorders are driven to constant activity in order to avoid difficult emotions. While verbal therapies use language and thinking in anticipation of action and provide an *indirect* intervention, music therapy is active and process oriented by nature (Bruscia, 1998). In addition, the use of music as emotional communication may be a viable use in treatment for individuals with eating disorders who customarily use the body as a symbol of emotional distress and/or have the tendency to intellectualize emotions.

Because music making is a physical manifestation of one's emotions and thoughts as they flow through time, music therapy improvisation offers a unique opportunity for clients with eating disorder to gain insight into their emotional state and sense of self. Stephens (1983) writes "In the act of playing, we release physical energy. We may express a specific emotion or emotions at any moment in our playing; our playing reflects who we are, how we organize ourselves, and how we feel as we move through time. . . . In improvising with others we are also dealing in a fundamental way with our relatedness to other people" (p. 30).

Loth (2000) describes the use of musical improvisation in a group of patients with eating disorders, in which the members were instructed to "play what they came in with." Loth remarked that it was common for patients to move around between various instruments "restlessly," with "little interaction between group members," with the music fading out prior to the end;

however, in this instance, the group "fell into a slow beat that was shared by all" (p. 98). In this manner, patients were not only able to obtain relief through the playing, but to move towards group cohesion by finding a new way to relate and interact with each other through the music.

Nolan (1989) describes how musical improvisation can function as a transitional object to disrupt the binge–purge cycle. When patients began to experience overwhelming affect during the group improvisation, he encouraged them to stay "with the beat," and found that many patients reported feeling "safety" instead of "a loss of control" (p. 111). Nolan (1984) also describes how the use of a tape recording during the verbal processing following an improvisation can be used to facilitate new self–awareness and insight into the cognitive distortions. For example, prior to listening to the playback, clients' statements often reflected expressions of low self–esteem and negative connotations regarding their individual sound in the group. One client said, "It sounded fine until I started playing the tambourine too loud" (p. 180). Following the objective feedback of the tape, many patients expressed great surprise over the difference between their perception of their function in the group and their actual effect.

Sloboda (1995) describes how the technique of thematic improvisation can be used to enable clients to make connections between aspects of their playing and their emotions, as well as the function of the eating disorder. Her work also includes the use of musical role play, an improvisational technique in which patients are asked to play the music of specific character or persons in their life. She describes how a discussion of the "character's" music may enable the client to develop insights regarding the roles of these individuals and emotional content of these relationships. She writes, "the immediacy of the experience of free improvisation helped them become more conscious of their emotional state" (p. 252).

Frederiksen's (1999) work focuses on the use of clinical improvisation to facilitate emotional expression and the development of autonomy in a client with anorexia. She uses a variety of rhythmic "grounding" techniques to provide an environment for the client to explore and separate musically (p. 222).

Task of Therapy

The complex task of therapy involves guiding the client in her search for identity through the discovery of natural impulses and repressed emotions (Bruch, 1988). Goodsitt (1997) writes that the therapeutic task is to find a way to engage the client's individuality, encouraging them to "Let go and take a chance on life. . . . Therapy is an endeavor that gives the patient an opportunity to occupy more psychological space" (p. 208). The concept of musical space has particular significance when viewed in this manner. Loth (2002) writes that, "It is the task of music therapist help the client through their defenses in order to find the creative possibilities of the music and the group" (p. 103).

The following section will describe the nature of the patient's resistance in music therapy improvisation and the dynamics of implementing clinical improvisation with the patient population. Areas of specific focus in the survey concern manifestations of pathology in the music, group interaction, and client/therapist transferences. These sections will be followed by a brief discussion of these results and future implications for therapists.

Survey Results: Music Therapists Working in Eating Disorder Rehabilitation Participants

Although 36 music therapists participated in the survey, only four, or 8 percent, stated that they worked primarily with patients with eating disorders. Since the researcher used a sample of convenience derived from the national listing, it is possible that music therapists who are not registered members of the national registry are working with clients with eating disorder and were excluded from the sampling frame. Due to this factor, the results of this survey may not be representative of the practice of music therapists that do specialize in eating disorder rehabilitation. In addition, out of the 36 music therapists participating in the survey, only 18 stated that they were currently working with patients with eating disorders while 18 based their answers on work done in the past. In addition, the section on clinical improvisation were answered by only a third of respondents.

According to the results of the survey, the majority of clinicians treated patients with eating disorders in the inpatient treatment facility wherein music therapy was provided as part of the milieu therapy program. Frequency statistics revealed that the majority of music therapists used a psychodynamic framework, followed by the eclectic, humanistic, and cognitive theoretical paradigms. Clinicians stated that their goals for clients were to gain more awareness of the eating disorder, to identify cognitive distortions underlying the disorder, and to provide an outlet for emotional expression. To accomplish this, clinicians used a variety of interventions listed by order of frequency: lyric analysic, songwriting, improvisation, music and imagery, and group singing. Clinicians were also asked to share which interventions were the most successful in meeting their treatment goals.

Although clinical improvisation was considered the most effective therapeutic intervention to use with clients with eating disorders, it was not the most frequently utilized intervention according to clinicians taking part in the survey, and followed the use of both lyric analysis and songwriting. The discrepancy between the less frequent use of clinical improvisation compared to its perceived effectiveness also stands in contrast with the majority of music therapy literature that has describes the successful use of clinical improvisation with this patient population.

Some of factors that may have contributed to this outcome include the client's characteristic resistance to treatment and the clinicians' treatment of clients with more advanced disease, as well as the number of clinicians participating that did not specialize in treating the disorder. One clinician succinctly describes an example of client resistance to active music making, "These critical clients seemed to have spread the word of their discontent with the group and resistance was high. The interventions that required effort on their part were discontinued and music listening became the group's focus. As a result, I did not feel that music was the medium of best expression for these clients."

Clinical Improvisation

Participants were then asked to describe various aspects of clinical improvisation, including the musical behavior of clients, their role as facilitator, and the dynamics of the group improvisation. While several clinicians used group drumming and structured rhythmic improvisations, the majority of clinicians responded that they provided the least amount of structure needed in order to facilitate the improvisation. While clients were encouraged to assume as much responsibility for the music as possible, their narratives revealed that those clients that were more advanced into the disorder exhibited more signs of resistance and therefore needed more musical structure for successful participation.

One clinician specified that a higher level of structure was used for patients that were "new to the group" to create a "safe environment" for participation, while another described most of the improvisations as "very structured, but not so that the clients become defensive because the task is too childish." Clinicians used more or less structure depending on the clients' level of functioning, as one participant mentioned that the structure of the improvisation was kept pretty loose. Other clinicians remarked that the level of structure depended on the group's needs and stating that, "If there is an inherent leader in the group, I minimize my role in the improvisation," and another participant wrote that her accompaniment would, "Depend on what the group needs . . . sometimes its good to be a strong musical presence, other times it is more beneficial for clients to be the prevalent musical presence."

Participants were asked to describe the client's response to being asked to musically improvise. One participant wrote, "Some were open and excited, while others appeared fearful and reluctant. Many times, their reaction was dependent on their openness to receive treatment." While some clinicians reported that they did not observe any signs of resistance to musical improvisation, other clinicians mentioned ways that patients would "minimize" the activity, either by "rolling their eyes," or making fun of the group behind her back. One participant noted, "Clients with bulimorexia were more resistant to anything but supportive level of therapy. The more advanced the disease, the more pronounced the resistance to the musical participation."

Musical Manifestations of Pathology

Music therapists reported that the balance or expressive breath of the musical expression with regard to tempo, dynamics, phrasing, and rhythmic organization, could be used to indicate the client's degree of pathology or well–being. According to clinicians, signs of pathology were indicated by music that was expressively "polarized," for example, either very loud or very soft, or "lacking in control" versus "very restricted." The majority of participants (67%) described manifestations of pathology in terms of music that was very restrictive in its expression. For example, music that was "restrictive" lacked variation, sounded "repetitious," and exhibited little contrast when asked to play music of different emotions. The limited range of expressivity was also exhibited by the use of simple and unchanging rhythms, and playing at either a very soft or very loud volume.

Other clinicians (30%) described signs of pathology in terms of "dissociative" characteristics in the music, evidenced by the patient's difficulty maintaining a stable pulse, and difficulty connecting rhythmically to other group members. One participant indicated that dissociation was also illustrated by the client's inability to make connections between their playing and their emotions, and another clinician recalls a client that reported that she felt she were "somewhere else" during the verbal processing. Four participants, or 45 percent, defined musical manifestations of pathology as resistance to the activity or nonparticipation. Other examples of musical manifestations of pathology became evident during the group interaction and will be discussed in the following section.

Interactional Styles

Participants were also asked to describe the musical interaction of clients with various eating disorders in a group, and to report any differences in the musical behavior between patients with different diagnoses. While a little over half, or 54 percent, of participants acknowledged differences in musical behavior between patients with different diagnoses, when asked to specify these differences, their responses suggested that these differences could best be interpreted as reflecting a range of musical behaviors that indicated the patient's level of psychopathology and willingness to receive treatment, more so than due to characteristic differences based on diagnosis. In fact, the majority of participants described more similar manifestations of pathology among the two groups than between them. For example, participants mentioned that individuals with both diagnoses tended to isolate from each other, i.e. not join each others rhythms and that their musical patterns were often compulsive and repeating. The majority of clinicians stated that the major difference between the musical behavior of anorexic and bulimics was that individuals with anorexia were more "restrictive" and rigid towards change in their playing, while those with bulimia presented as more "outgoing," "challenging," and "gregarious."

However, despite the consistency of the more "outgoing" bulimic tendencies to the more "restrictive" playing of the anorexic, both subtypes did exhibit signs of rhythmic instability and isolated from others musically. One participant wrote:

> *Those with bulimia sometimes were not aware of the effect of their playing upon the music of the group; all clients seemed generally concerned about mistakes and therefore the group improvisations would focus on simple and rhythmic groupings as phrases. Limited dynamics, unless insights emerged, then sudden dynamic changes of rageful proportions. Most often these were ultimately a breakthrough from the person. Dissociative qualities emerged as sounding "out of touch," the musical ideas didn't fit in well with the group.*

Another participant described a similar dynamic: "Those with bulimia tend to be more easily motivated towards full expression, but vacillate in their emotive and rhythmic playing." One participant described that differences in the musical behavior were "Hard to say based on diagnosis . . . as with any mixed diagnosis group, there is the same jealously of the BN pts of the AN patients (I want to be that skinny), and the AN patient's fear of the BN patients (I never want to be that out of control) some of these issues come up musically."

Therapist/Client Dynamics

Music therapists participating in the survey also reported that patients with eating disorders tended to respond to them in a polarized manner and formed "very positive or very negative" transferences towards them. One clinician described the reactions of patients to her as either "love or hate," and their projection onto her as that of a "good mother or a withholding mother." Two participants noted that the reactions of patients were "very positive overall; rapport is built easily with these patients" and "usually comfortable, trusting." Another participant described that the reaction of patients towards her was polarized in terms of attachment strategies, stating that clients had "very intense or very aloof" ways of relating towards her.

One participant describes a scenario in which several patients appeared to be "kind/amiable–then I hear them making fun of the music group with peers on the unit." This example may illustrate the complexity of providing therapy to patients with eating disorders as well as the difficulty in assessing patients based on overt musical participation. In addition to primary or explicit resistance to the activity, patients may covertly "resist" the activity, while appearing outwardly compliant to treatment.

Countertransference

Clinicians were asked to share their reactions towards the client population and their answers revealed a similar dialectic in terms of both the intensity of the reaction and polarized positive/negative valence of the response, with clinicians experiencing feelings of "frustration," "defensiveness," "anger," and "rejection," as well as feelings of "responsibility/caregiving." One participant's response indicates the intensity of her countertransference in the following statement, "my reaction usually requires more self–exploration than the ones I notice with other populations."

These reactions can also be understood as reactions engendered from the client or "projective identifications," that can also serve to enable clinicians to better understand the emotional content of the patient's issues. A clinician describes this process: "I try to use my emotions in my work with clients–I understand that quite often my response is typical of what the patients elicit from people . . . so I try to use that in the musical process. Its [sic] often a balance between control, letting go, listening, initiating change, encouragement, expression. . . . Many layers are happening musically. I may not have the answers for them, but I can offer my experience and understanding as a tool for them–modeling healthy anger, modeling healthy confrontation, etc."

Many clinicians reported experiencing feelings of "caregiving/responsibility" exhibited by the following excerpts, "I had a feeling of responsibility to ease their pain and contain their feelings . . . and wanted to help them and let them know that they could live without the eating disorder." Another participant shared that "I found myself wishing to help foster a warm, family–like group environment via the opening musical experiences." Another clinician remarked that how she "didn't have time to get bogged down with her own stuff with the client, I work hard to keep it separate so that I can be there for them," while another felt, "helpless at not being able to extend treatment time."

Several clinicians remarked that the nurturing response triggered their need to create expressive music for the group. One participant stated that she made, "use of various timbres (not just piano, but recorder, xylophone, cello, violin,; use of tempo and dynamics contrasts (high energy, slow easy energy, etc.); long improvised melodic lines usually in major modes with many modulations." Another remarked that, "I use the drum circles and improvisations to release my frustrations, anger, and sense of being stuck. I have an excuse to be a bit more wild . . . to free up the clients."

Discussion

Patient Defenses

When asked to describe manifestations of pathology, the participants described ways that patients restricted their musical output in order to defend against experiencing emotions, and even instances when patients were so threatened that they exhibited dissociative behaviors in the group. Another example of patient defenses were exhibited by the fixed, yet polarized styles of interaction. According to the participants, clients with eating disorders tended to employ two particular styles of interaction, the first of which is characterized by "moving away" behaviors: emotional withdrawal and musical isolation by patients with eating disorders towards others. The second interpersonal style is characterized by "moving towards": caretaking/supportive behaviors and approval–eliciting behaviors.

Isolation

Both participants and the review of the literature indicate that clients with eating disorders are often "isolated" from musical contact with others. Several clinicians remarked that it was difficult for members to connect to each other's musical rhythms, and also that sometimes the musical expression would function as a wall of noise to keep others out. The musical isolation from others and the lack of emotional expression may indicate the client's need to control or avoid difficult emotions that may aroused from contact with others. If the client avoids contact with others, she may avoid experiencing uncomfortable reactions from others, including rejection. Patients with eating disorders may also feel threatened to let others in to share their experience because they feel they will lose some of their "specialness." Perhaps this is because isolative behaviors, including the solitary act of dieting and restriction, have provided the source of self–esteem for these patients and therefore represents their superiority to others. However, because this inflexible interpersonal style is based on being "special," it prevents the client from understanding and integrating other emotional states.

Caretaking

Interestingly, when participants were asked to describe the musical interaction of patients with eating disorders in the group, the common response by participants was that clients had a hard time musically connecting to others. However, when participants were asked to describe the group dynamic, the most common response was that clients with eating disorders sought to care for and support the music of others in the group. However, the music therapists participating in this study interpreted this "caregiving" as the cohort effect; as one participant describes the patients, "helped each other stay sick."

One participant describes how this dynamic was characteristic of patients with eating disorders because they tended to be "very agreeable to the suggestions of other, and do not assert themselves." Another participant discusses that, "Usually there is one or two 'leaders' in the group who set the pace for the others . . . the other group members may support this and join in or may resist and attempt not to conform. There is almost always a lack of attempt to encourage those more bashful, quiet group members to become more expressive."

These polarized interpersonal styles may indicate the nature of the client's conflict. Both the literature review and the results of the study suggest that the client's tendency to care for the needs of others indicates a maladaptive coping strategy in which her self–esteem is based on her ability to be sensitive to the needs of others. For the client with an eating disorder, being supportive and taking care of others enables her to feel virtuous, and therefore provides the client with a false sense of self–esteem and identity.

However, these inflexible interpersonal styles are maladaptive because they prevent the client from integrating and experiencing various levels of emotional experience. The task remains for the music therapist to gently challenge these rigid rules of interaction in order to help the client to discover ways of relating to others that are not based on avoiding contact with others or eliciting approval.

Therapeutic Dynamics

Zerbe (1998) writes that when working with eating disordered patients "having strong feelings is the rule rather than the exception" and that many clinicians often experience "self–vilifying internal criticism and personal vulnerability" (p. 32). As the therapist helps the patient to uncover repressed emotions, he/she may also begin to experience a number of physical and emotional reactions garnered by the therapeutic process. In addition, because the client's transferences towards the therapist may reflect early developmental issues, a variety of raw emotions may emerge during the therapeutic process. In tandem with other patient behaviors, patient transferences were often polarized into extremely positive or extremely negative reactions. Therefore, it is extremely important to consider the implications of the therapist/client dynamics.

Patients with eating disorders may form intensely negative transferences towards the therapist, reactions that could reveal their fear of being controlled or dominated by the primary caretaker. Zerbe (1998) writes that one severely ill anorexic shouted to her from the bedside, "I don't want you taking over my body!" (p. 36). Loth (2002) writes, "I often feel I am being experienced as the mother, who is trying to feed them the music that they are rejecting, the one that 'makes' them play" (p. 103). Because the goal of treatment is to help the client to express and tolerate difficult emotions as well as to develop autonomy, allowing and tolerating this negative transference builds the therapeutic relationship and can be helpful for the client who has been previously unable to express these difficult emotions within her family of origin and/or other relationships. While these countertransferential reactions may provide the therapist with insight into how the client is feeling, they may be difficult to musically "contain" as well as emotionally endure, and may seem almost impossible as when the patient refuses to participate in the group.

Conversely, patients may also experience the therapist as the "good mother," and attempt to elicit approval and compassion. Evidence of this dynamic was revealed in the therapist's musical countertransference or desire to imbue the music with expressive qualities, or to facilitate a "warm" family–like group experience. A common reaction for the therapists was to "nourish" the group sound with expressive musical qualities. These instances reveal the very real difficulty of maintaining a balance between meeting the client's need for structure, expression, and reflection, while still allowing the client to maintain responsibility for the emotional content of the music. The therapist, through maintaining this balance in the improvisation, can best assist the patient in developing an awareness of her own impulses and emotions. Frederiksen (1999) suggests that the therapist meet the client's expression "cautiously and with respect, but also challenging them a little" (Loth, 2002, p. 102). Because patients with eating disorder may become easily overwhelmed, it is important that the therapists not "force–feed" emotional content into the musical expression but, instead, remain open to detecting any subtle change in the music in order to facilitate this expression. Although the music may be emotionally restrictive, the therapist should strive to respect this resistance while remaining attuned and responsive to these subtle changes in expression.

Closing Remarks

Music therapy represents a viable form of treatment that can contribute to a greater understanding of the patient and his or her abilities: including their degree of insight and cognition regarding the disorder as well as their emotional experience. This information can be brought to the treatment team and help provide a fuller portrait of the client. The survey results also reveal the very real difficulty of using clinical improvisation with the client population, and represents an area that warrants more exploration.

Because it is so multifaceted, music therapy may be used on all levels in the treatment of clients with eating disorders. However, depending on the severity of the disorder, clients may be extremely resistant to participating in active musical experiences in which these painful experiences can be evoked. Loth (2002) describes the importance of preparing individual members prior to the group by explaining the purpose of music therapy, exploring the patient's relationship to music, and also invited the patient to explore the musical vocabulary of the instruments. This preparation may facilitate the development of a therapeutic alliance and "lessen the potency of her fear in the group" (p. 97).

In addition, it may be helpful to begin with structured musical activities in which the client can participate with a great deal of success. Further, successful participation in these musical experiences may help to reduce the resistance and empower the client to explore the deeper issues. While lyric analysis may be used to help patients develop an awareness of the disorder, more active musical experiences such as improvisation may be a good means to engage the client's individuality and to help patients to integrate deeper levels of emotional experience. Finally, several of the music therapists who participated in the survey described how easily rapport was built with clients. As human beings, we all enjoy being admired and adored, and it may be tempting to believe this veneration. However, this dynamic may also reflect the characteristic preoccupation that individuals with eating disorders have with pleasing others. Therefore, a possible pitfall may be to interpret a client's pleasing, attentive behavior or openness to participation levels as healthy, "good," or adaptive, and resistance or lack of participation as "bad", or maladaptive. This tendency may reinforce a destructive cycle of thinking and reinforce what Hilde Bruch (1988) has referred to as "systematic training in dishonesty."

As arts therapists we provide an environment via an artistic medium wherein patients can "take a chance" and experiment with different ways of being and expressing different emotions. In order to achieve this, we must stay vigilant to meeting our own needs for approval, lest we merely recreate old scenarios with the client population and limit their development. We must also be creative in order to adapt our artistic medium in ways that can be utilized most effectively by the patients.

Finally, patients with eating disorders may present as extremely compliant and pleasant, and it may be difficult to provide the gentle confrontation they may need in order to explore their own issues. The nature of the work require intense self–awareness so that we can best understanding the client's dynamics, and an openness to explore often painful and raw emotions with the client. Due to these intense transferential dynamics, music therapists working with clients with eating disorders may find it helpful to process these reactions in supervision. A peer supervision group with other clinicians or music therapist who work with eating disorders may provide and invaluable means of support for the clinician and provide a forum where the therapist can explore and process these issues.

References

Bruch, H. (1988). *Conversations with anorexics.* New York: Basic Books.

Bruscia, K. E. (1987). *Improvisational models of music therapy.* Springfield, IL: Charles C Thomas, Publisher, Ltd.

Dokter, D. (1995). Fragile board: Arts therapies and clients with eating disorders. In D. Dokter (Ed.), *Arts therapies and clients with eating disorders* (pp. 3–22). London: Jessica Kingsley Publishers.

Fairburn, C. G., Shafran, R., & Cooper, Z. (1999). A cognitive–behavioural theory of Anorexia nervosa. *Behavior Research and Therapy, 37,* 1–13.

Frederiksen, B. V. (1999). Analysis of musical improvisations to understand and work with elements of resistance in a client with anorexia nervosa. In T. Wigram & J. De-Backer (Eds.), *Clinical application of music therapy in psychiatry* (pp. 211–231).

Goodsitt, A. (1997). Eating disorders: A self–psychological perspective. In D. M. Garner, & P. E. Garfinkel (Eds.), *Handbook of treatment for eating disorders* (pp. 205–229). New York: Guilford Press.

Justice, R. W. (1994). Music therapy interventions for people with eating disorders in an inpatient setting. *Music Therapy Perspectives, 12,* 104–110.

Loth, H. (1988). There's no getting away from anything in here: A music therapy group within an inpatient program for adults with eating disorders. In A. Davies & E. Richards (Eds.), *Music therapy and group work: Sound company* (pp. 90–104). NY: Hogarth Press.

Loth, H. (2002). There's no getting away from anything in here: A music therapy group within an inpatient program for adults with eating disorders. In A. Davies & E. Richards (Eds.), *Music therapy and group work: Sound company* (pp. 90–104).

National Eating Disorder Association's (NEDA) Facts for activists. Retrieved September 1, 2006, from http://www.nationaleatingdisorders.org/p.asp?WebPage_ID=286& Profile_ID=95634.

National Association for Music Therapy. (1980). *A career in music therapy*, brochure. Washington, DC: National Association for Music Therapy.

Nolan, P. (1989). Music therapy improvisation techniques with bulimic patients. In L. M. Hornyak & E. K. Baker (Eds.), *Experiential therapies for eating disorders* (pp. 167–186). New York: Guilford Press.

Nolan, P. (1989). Music as a transitional object in the treatment of bulimia. *Music Therapy Perspectives, 6*, pp. 49–51.

Robarts, J. Z. (1995). Towards autonomy and a sense of self: Music therapy and the individuation process in relation to children and adolescents with early onset anorexia nervosa. In D. Dokter (Ed.), *Arts therapies and clients with eating disorders* (pp. 229–244). London: Jessica Kingsley Publishers.

Robarts, J. Z. (2000). Music therapy and adolescents with anorexia. nervosa. *Nordic Journal of Music Therapy, 9*(1), 3–12.

Robarts, J., & Sloboda, A. (1994). Perspectives on music therapy with people suffering from anorexia nervosa. *Journal of British Music Therapy, 8*, 1.

Sloboda, A. (1993). Individual therapy with a man who has an eating disorder. In M. Heal & T. Wigram (Eds.), *Music therapy in health and education* (pp. 103). London: Jessica Kingsley Publishers.

Sloboda, A. (1995). Individual music therapy with anorexic and bulimic patients. In D. Dokter (Ed.), *Arts therapies and clients with eating disorders* (pp. 247–261). London: Jessica Kingsley.

Smejsters, H. (1996). Music therapy with anorexia nervosa : An integrative theoretical and methodological perspective. *British Journal of Music Therapy, 10*(2), 3–13.

Smeijsters, H. & Hurk, J. van den. (1993). Research in practice in the music therapeutic treatment of a client with symptoms of anorexia nervosa. In M. Heal & T. Wigram (Eds.), *Music therapy in health and education.* London: Jessica Kingsley Publishers.

Stephens, G. (1983). The use of improvisation for developing relatedness in the adult client. *Music Therapy, 3*, pp. 29–42.

Zerbe, K. J. (1998). Knowable secrets: Transference and countertransference manifestations in eating–disordered patients. In W. Vandereycken & P. Beumont (Eds.), *Treating eating disorders: Ethical, legal, and personal issues* (pp. 30–55). New York: New York Universities Press.

Biography

Ms. Marah Bobilin is currently working at the Institute for Music and Neurologic function at Beth Abraham Health Services in Bronx, New York under the auspices of Dr. Concetta Tomaino. She recently completed her thesis on the use of music therapy in the treatment of eating disorders and is currently specializing in neurologic rehabilitation and the dementia program and treatment.

Chapter 10

CULTURALLY COMPETENT GROUP THERAPY WITH LATINA ADOLESCENTS AND YOUNG ADULTS WITH EATING DISTURBANCE: THE USE OF POETRY AND MUSIC

GENEVA REYNAGA–ABIKO

Introduction

Latinos are the largest ethnic minority group in the U.S., currently comprising 12.5 percent of the population. They are the fastest–growing group in the U.S. and are often poor, with 22 percent living at poverty levels (compared to 7.7% of European Americans). There exists tremendous heterogeneity among Latinos along racial and ethnic lines, meaning that they may be of any "race," or skin color. Most Latinos possess some degree of fluency in Spanish, although there are many different dialects spoken in the U.S. Several different subgroups are included among those commonly labeled "Latino," including Mexican Americans (58.5%), Puerto Ricans (9.6%), Cubans (3.5%), Central Americans (4.8%) and South Americans (3.8%) (U.S. Census Bureau, 2001). Although there are several different terms used for this group, "Latino" (male) and "Latina" (female) are used throughout this chapter.

Eating disturbance (ED), including but not limited to diagnosable eating disorders, is increasingly common in the U.S. The age of onset is usually during adolescence (Mussell, Binford, & Fulkerson, 2000). It is estimated that 1–3 percent of adolescent and young adult females, and 1–5 percent of college–aged females, binge and/or purge. Self–starvation is present in 0.5–1.0 percent of adolescent females and compulsive eating affects nearly 20 percent of the population, including males and females (Harris & Kuba, 1997). A range of ED exists in "normal" women as well, including dieting in rough-

159

ly 90 percent of U.S. females, binge eating at least once a month in 20 percent of women, and vomiting or laxative abuse in 10 percent of women (Dolan, 1994). Some estimate that subclinical forms of eating disorders are two to five times more common than diagnosable conditions, affecting 4–16 percent of the general population (Mussell et al., 2000.). There are a variety of factors leading to ED, including sociocultural, psychological, and political pressure (Gold, 2000).

Eating disturbance is a serious and growing concern within the Latino community, although the stereotype that ED affects only European American females continues to exist in the mental health community (Root, 1990). This can lead to mis- or under–diagnosis in ethnic minority clients (Thompson, 1996). It has been surmised that people of Color do not seek treatment at the same rates as European Americans but a recent study found no differences in treatment seeking among women of Color and European Americans who were struggling with ED (Cachelin et al., 2000). Given the fact that most experts on ED are European American (Root, 1990), and women of Color often do not receive appropriate treatment referrals when struggling with ED (Cachelin et al., 2000), it seems that many clinicians remain at a loss with how to deal with this potentially life–threatening continuum of disorders with Latinas and other women of Color.

This chapter focuses on the use of poetry and music in group therapy with Latina adolescents and young adults with ED. Most symptoms of ED begin in adolescence (Mussell et al., 2000), and it seems appropriate to provide treatment as early as possible in order to prevent symptoms worsening with age. The approaches recommended herein may be used independently or in combination with verbal psychotherapies (Leijssen, 2006). The use of poetry and music in therapy with Latinas represents culturally sensitive practice because it builds on cultural phenomena that already exist in Latino culture. For example, there is a history in Latino culture of using poetry and song lyrics to educate people on social issues (McDonald, Antunez, & Gottemoeller, 2003). Further, poetry and music are activities that many adolescents and young adults already use to communicate their feelings and experiences, which allow a seamless transition into their use as therapeutic tools.

This chapter will begin with a review of the available literature to provide the reader with information on how symptoms and causes of ED differ among Latinas compared to other groups. This is followed by recommendations to use when forming therapy groups with Latinas and exercises to use in poetry and music therapy with this group. Very little has been written on using art therapy with Latinas, and nothing has been published on poetry or music therapy with Latina clients suffering from eating disturbance. It is the author's hope that this chapter will broaden the scope of culturally sensitive clinical techniques with members of the largest and fastest–growing ethnic group in the U.S.

Review of Available Literature

It is important to understand culturally specific aspects of ED among Latinas, as it is unethical to consider European Americans as the standard against which all other groups are compared (Smolak & Striegel–Moore, 2001). Few theories of ED include Latinos, or any people of Color (Harris & Kuba, 1997), and the stereotype that ED affects only European American, middle class females remains a common belief among many clinicians (Root, 1990). The studies on ED among Latinas that exist have been published primarily in the last two decades. Most focus on the question of whether there are differences in eating pathology among Latinas when compared to other ethnic groups in the U.S. Some studies show no differences among Latinas and other groups, including European Americans, with regard to symptoms of ED (Hiebert et al., 1988; Shaw, Ramirez, Trost, Randall, & Stice, 2004; Snow & Harris, 1989). Others provide evidence that Latinas have greater levels of problematic eating behaviors compared to African Americans (Grabe & Hyde, 2006; Vander Wal & Thomas, 2004), African Americans and European Americans (Miller et al., 2000), Asian Americans and European Americans (Robinson et al., 1996), European Americans (Pidcock et al,, 2000), and all groups combined (Story et al., 1995). One study had mixed results, showing that Latinos binge and purge less than European Americans and Native Americans, but are more terrified of gaining weight than European Americans (Smith & Krejci, 1991).

Other studies attempt to explain what contributes to ED among Latinas. Root (1990) argues that racism and oppression are key factors, with which Thompson (1996) agrees. Root conducted detailed life history interviews and found that symptoms of ED were associated with trauma, racism, poverty, acculturation, and abuse. Pumariega (1986) found that lower levels of acculturation were related to less distorted attitudes about eating in a non–clinical Latino population, although a later study showed that acculturation was not associated with ED (Granillo, Jones–Rodriguez, & Carvajal, 2005). Pidcock and colleagues (2000) showed that high levels of family dysfunction ultimately put Latinas at increased risk for developing Bulimia Nervosa, which was supported by Kuba and Harris (2001), who found that inflexible interactions among family members and poor socialization were the most significant predictors of bulimic symptoms and over concern with weight control among Mexican Americans.

These studies demonstrate the complex nature of ED with all clients, with additional layers added for Latinas, given their sociocultural status as an ethnic minority in the U.S. The role of racism, oppression, poverty, trauma, and acculturation, among others, remain largely misunderstood and under–studied in the formation and maintenance of ED among Latinas. While causal factors remain unclear, it is likely that "the relationship between ethnocultural identity, eating practices, and cultural convergence is a complex one that crosses boundaries of nationality, ethnicity, culture, and immigration status" (Harris & Kuba, 1997, p. 341). In other words, ED can affect anyone, and there is no clear way to prevent it.

Culturally Competent Therapy with Latinas with Disturbed Eating: The Use of Poetry and Music

There are many therapeutic skills that transcend the sociocultural background of the client, but working with Latinas requires serious consideration of several sociocultural factors that are not always included in the psychotherapeutic enterprise. While a fuller discussion is beyond the scope of this chapter, when working with Latina adolescents and young adults, it is helpful to remember that, in addition to the expected pressure to be thin that bombards all females, they must also manage a host of other potential stressors that are not relevant for European Americans (Smolak & Striegel–Moore, 2001). This includes the experience of racism, the stress of acculturation, and becoming bicultural (Root, 1990), bilingualism, increased incidence of poverty (U.S. Census Bureau, 2001), and traditional family values that are often not supported in a dominant culture that supports rugged individualism (see Santiago–Rivera, Arredondo, & Gallardo–Cooper, 2002 for more information on working with Latinos).

When treating ED, the goal is to help the client "understand why the symptoms, food, eating and body image are a preferable means of communication to language and feeling, helping them to find both the individual and cultural explanations" (Gold, 2000, p. 136). Group therapy often helps clients feel less pressured or vulnerable, as there are several members and alliances among them slowly develop over time. There exist many approaches to treatment for clients with ED, including medical interventions, pharmacological treatment, and talk therapies (Dokter, 1995). This chapter adds to the variety of treatment options by discussing art therapy with clients with ED, specifically poetry and music therapy.

Art therapy may be defined as the use of art during psychotherapy "as an alternate path for exploration and communication" (Leijssen, 2006, p. 137). While there exist distinct fields of art therapy and formally trained art therapists, psychotherapists who traditionally employ verbal therapy modalities may use a variety of art techniques as a supplement (Leijssen). This helps access material that the client may not otherwise share because it is too painful or difficult to verbalize (Levens, 1994), it lies outside of conscious awareness (Leijssen), or the client is otherwise unwilling to participate in talk therapy (Jones, 2005). Clients with ED often approach the process of creating and/or using art materials in the same way they approach food. For example, those with restrictive tendencies may approach materials with an inflexible style, whereas those with binge disorders may become easily overwhelmed (Dokter, 1995). However, if the client is sincerely unable to participate for any reason, it is important to respect her decision and find another therapeutic style that will be more effective.

Poetry therapy and music therapy are the two types of art therapy that will be the focus of this chapter. For example, poetry therapy includes the use of metaphor, storytelling, and other types of writing (Mazza, 2003). It stimulates honesty and self–disclosure (Stepakoff, 1997), as the client is able to communicate her voice in the poem. Music therapy is the planned use of music to promote healing and personal growth (Jones, 2005). It is not necessary to possess formal training in music (Sloboda, 1995), as the process and personal meaning of the music to the client are what hold therapeutic value.

In order to provide poetry and music therapy to Latinas with ED in the most culturally sensitive manner possible, we will discuss the unique issues to consider when forming the therapy group. Practical exercises to use in these groups will then be provided. These recommendations work equally well with groups that are solely comprised of Latinas, or groups with members from a variety of ethnic backgrounds. The exercises may be used within the context of verbal psychotherapy as an adjunct, or in groups devoted exclusively to art therapy.

Forming the Group

The first step when forming a therapy group with Latinas is recruiting group members. This will differ based on the clinical setting, but may include networking with leaders in the local Latino community, including clergy, directors of community centers, or school counselors; receiving referrals from other providers, including nutritionists, medical doctors, and other mental health professionals; or posting flyers around a college campus or treatment center. Once potential group members have been identified, it may be helpful to conduct screenings to establish which individuals meet pre–selected criteria. This may include identification as a Latina, proficiency with written and/or oral communication styles, willingness to participate in treatment for ED, or other factors deemed to be important by the group leader. If possible, ensure that a range of ED symptoms are present among group members, including at least one individual who has successfully managed her symptoms (Dokter, 1995).

Once members have been screened, form a therapy group with a minimum of two and a maximum of 8–10 members at a setting and time that is convenient for the group. Keep in mind that Latinas may have other responsibilities, such as family concerns, a job, or strict rules about how late they can be out after school. It may be helpful to conduct the group in a place that is familiar to its members, such as a school, church, or community center. Decide beforehand if the group will continue accepting new members and if it will be open or time–limited in nature.

Rules, or group norms, should be discussed as soon and as often as necessary. This may include issues of confidentiality, with an agreement to not discuss what occurs in group with any family or friends. Dual relationships should also be discussed, given the potential for outside contact that is common among ethnic minority groups, especially if their numbers are relatively small within the larger community. For example, will contact be allowed outside of the group? How should the therapist or other group members act if they see each other in public? Another issue worthy of discussion is what language to speak in the group. Groups may be conducted in English, Spanish, or Spanglish (a combination of English and Spanish; Altarriba & Santiago–Rivera, 1994), which allows members to share information in the language that is most relevant to them. It also prevents denial of mental health services based on inability to speak English.

Racism is inevitable in any group interaction, given that "people come with all sorts of attitudes absorbed from the racist culture around them" (Weston, 1999, p. 182). Among Latinos, racist themes that may emerge may be related to differences in ethnic background (i.e., Mexican American, Puerto Rican, etc.), language fluency (in either English or Spanish), skin tone, class, acculturation level, or other sociocultural factors. When these issues surface, they must be confronted directly (Weston) so that the group will not become fragmented. It is also helpful for the group members to witness a productive method of dealing with racism, given the impact racism and discrimination may have on their ED symptoms (Root, 1990; Thompson, 1996).

Music and Poetry Exercises

When choosing poems to include in treatment, the therapist may consult anthologies of poetry and creative writing (see Appendix A) and should have a variety of work, modeling an appreciation of diversity. Music that is popular among adolescents and young adults should be used to maximize participation, and it is most helpful to receive recommendations from the members themselves. Include material that focuses on topics relevant to the Latino community, which may not be well represented in "mainstream" work (Stepakoff, 1997). Relevant topics with this group are the variety of pressures facing adolescents and young adults, including that of family, friends, Latino culture, and dominant U.S. culture; competing images of attractive women in Latino and U.S. cultures (e.g., a curvaceous figure vs. ultra–thin representations); the influence of poverty on how food is approached (Thompson, 1996); and how to establish a healthy sense of self while managing these stressors.

The following exercises have been adapted to fit clients with ED as well as clients from a Latino background. They can be changed as necessary, but it may be helpful to consult with an expert in Latino culture before doing so (see Appendix B) to prevent unintentional cultural insensitivity. Most exercises may be used with poems, song lyrics, or short stories.

1. Read a poem and hand out a copy of the poem for visual reference. Explore the reactions each member has to the poem and what it meant to her. Invite the client(s) to change the ending of the poem, or rewrite it so that it makes more sense to her (Mazza, 2003).

2. Read a poem. After reading it, ask the client(s) to write down her experiences in a stream of consciousness style. Construct a poem with the material and discuss what thoughts or memories the process brought up (Stepakoff, 1997).

3. Provide words or phrases and ask the clients to write down whatever comes to mind (Mazza, 2003). Then ask the clients to construct a poem based on what they wrote. Relevant words may include: food, fat/skinny, culture, racism, peer pressure, obligation/duty, family, etc.

4. Ask the client to write an autobiographical poem (Mazza, 2003) or story. The following questions should be addressed: Is it possible to identify as a Latina while maintaining a healthy body image? Can you be successful in the dominant culture while having a curvaceous figure? Does your family get offended if you do not eat a certain amount of food? How do popular images of Latinas influence your ideal body image?

5. Play a song. The song may be in English or Spanish and from any genre. Ask the group members to describe the relationship between their mood and the song (Mazza, 2003). Why was this song chosen? What is the artist trying to say? How does this song make you feel?

6. Break the group into smaller parts and have them write a piece of music. It may be song lyrics, drum beats, or anything else of their choosing, though it is important to illustrate how they feel about themselves. When this is complete (and it may take a couple of sessions),

each subgroup performs for the rest of the group. Process what the experience was like for both artist and audience and what messages were conveyed through the song.

While the exercises presented above are not an exhaustive list, they provide a list of possible exercises that are relevant tools for use in therapy with Latinas suffering with ED. There are no specific rules for what the outcome of each exercise should be, as it is most important that the client access their personal experience in the process. An example of some poetry are as follows.[1]

In Magazines (I Found Specimens of the Beautiful)
Once
I looked for myself
between the covers of
Seventeen
Vogue
Cosmopolitan
among blue eyes, blonde hair, white skin, thin bodies,
this is beauty.
I hated this shroud of
Blackness
that makes me invisible
a negative print
some other one's
nightmare.[2]

I Give You Back
I release you, my beautiful and terrible
fear. I release you. You were my beloved
and hated twin, but now, I don't know you
as myself. I release you with all the
pain I would know at the death of
my daughters.

...

I take myself back, fear.
You are not my shadow any longer.
I won't hold you in my hands.
You can't live in my eyes, my ears, my voice
my belly, or in my heart my heart
my heart   my heart

---

1. Due to the confidential nature of poems created in the course of individual and/or psychotherapy, the author has chosen to use published work relevant to themes commonly seen in work with ED clients.
2. Excerpt from Omosupe, E. (1990).

But come here, fear
I am alive and you are so afraid
of dying.[3]

The Three Tongues

Tied to the backs
of some women are
bloody sorrows,
leech–like troubles
that make them weak.

In every strong woman
there are three tongues
all in contradiction,
silenced during the day
by a heavier hand.

At night minutes before bed
the strong woman
must unbraid
the three tongues
and let them speak.
Only then can she sleep.[4]

Conclusion

This chapter discusses the use of creative therapy modalities, specifically poetry and music, as a means to transcend cultural barriers and provide effective treatment to the largest ethnic minority group in the U.S. It is clear that Latinas suffer from ED, often at levels greater than other ethnic groups. However, we still do not know what contributes to this trend and there may be distinct pathways to ED with this group, pointing to a need for further consideration (Smolak & Striegel–Moore, 2001). It is also important to study prevention and treatment efforts, as it is erroneous to assume that the methods that work with European Americans will be similarly effective with Latinos (Grabe & Hyde, 2006). The use of poetry and music in therapy with Latinas represents one form of culturally sensitive practice not only because of the focus on themes relevant to the community, but also because it builds on the open communication style flowing through traditional Latino culture. The fact that the group is comprised of all Latinas allows them to share information that they may not be comfortable sharing in front of elders, males, or

3. Excerpt from Harjo, J. (1990).
4. Rios, C. (1990).

family members. Group therapy is also more economically feasible than individual therapy, and may take place in a variety of settings, thereby diminishing the stigma associated with mental health settings. If the mental health profession hopes to effectively address the needs of Latinas with eating concerns, clinicians must adopt a culturally sensitive style.

Appendix A–Poetry and Creative Writing Sources

African American Anthologies

Angelou, M. (1986). *Poems.* New York: Bantam Books.
Angelou, M. (1993). *Wouldn't take nothing for my journey now.* New York: Bantam Books.
Bell–Scott, P. ((1994). *Life notes: Personal writings by contemporary Black women.* New York: W. W. Norton & Company.
Bell–Scott, P. (1998). *Flat–footed truths: Telling Black women's lives.* New York: Henry Holt and Company.
Jordan, J. (1997). *Kissing God goodbye: Poems 1991–1997.* New York: Anchor Books.
Lorde, A. (1984). *Sister outsider.* Freedom, CA: The Crossing Press.

Asian American Anthologies

Asian Women United of California. (1989). *Making waves: An anthology of writings by and about Asian American women.* Boston: Beacon Press.
The Women of South Asian Descent Collective. (1993). *Our feet walk the sky: Women of the South Asian diaspora.* San Francisco: Aunt Lute Books.

Latina/o Anthologies

Anzaldua, G. (1990). *Making face, making soul/Haciendo caras: Creative and critical perspectives by feminists of Color.* San Francisco: Aunt Lute Books.
Anzaldua, G. (1999). *Borderlands/La Frontera: The new Mestiza* (2nd ed.). San Francisco: Aunt Lute Books.
Anzaldua, G. E., & Keating, A. (2002). *This bridge we call home: Radical visions for transformation.* New York: Routledge.
Augenbraum, H., & Stavans, I. (1993). *Growing up Latino, memoirs and stories: Reflections on life in the United States.* Boston: Houghton Mifflin Company.
Castillo–Speed, L. (1995). *Latina women's voices from the borderlands.* New York: Simon and Schuster.

Heide, R. (2002). *Under the fifth sun: Latino literature from California*. Berkeley, CA: Heyday Books.

Moraga, C. (1993). *The last generation: Prose and poetry*. Boston: South End Press.

Moraga, C. L., & Anzaldua, G. E. (2002). *This bridge called my back: Writings by radical women of color* (3rd ed.). Berkeley, CA: Third Woman Press.

Multicultural Anthologies

Hernandez, D., & Rehman, B. (2002). *Colonize this! Young women of color on today's feminism*. New York: Seal Press.

Linthwaite, I. (1990). *Ain't I a woman! A book of women's poetry from around the world*. New York: Peter Bedrick Books.

O'Hearn, C. C. (1998). *Half and half: Writers on growing up biracial and bicultural*. New York: Pantheon Books.

Native American Anthologies

Harjo, J., & Bird, G. (1997). *Reinventing the enemy's language: Contemporary Native women's writings of North America*. New York: W. W. Norton & Company.

Sanchez, C. L. (1997). *From spirit to matter: New and selected poems 1969–1996*. San Francisco: Taurean Horn Press.

Appendix B–How to Seek Consultation from a Cultural Expert

It is ideal to seek consultation from local professionals, as they will likely possess information about the specific Latino subgroups in the area. In order to find a consultant, contact professional organizations and ask for names of experts in Latino psychology. These include:

1. Local and/or state psychological association(s)
2. The National Latina/o Psychological Association (NLPA) (http://www.nlpa.ws)
3. California Latino/a Psychological Association (CLPA) (http://www.latinopsych.org)
4. New Jersey Latina/o Psychological Association (NJLPA) (http://www.lpanj.org)

5. Society for the Psychological Study of Ethnic Minority Issues (Division 45 of the American Psychological Association) (http://www.apa.org/divisions/div45/homepage.html)

If local experts are not available, there are many resources available online. These include:

1. Latino Behavioral Health Institute (http://www.lbhi.org)
2. Latino Mental Health (http://www.latinomentalhealth.net)
3. National Latino Behavioral Health Association (NLBHA) (http://nlbha.org)
4. EthnicCounselors.com, a web–based referral network whose purpose is to help people find culturally, religious, and linguistically appropriate counseling resources (http://ethniccounselors.com)

References

Altarriba, J., & Santiago–Rivera, A. L. (1994). Current perspectives on using linguistic and cultural factors in counseling the Hispanic client. *Professional Psychology: Research and Practice, 25*(4), 388–397.

Cachelin, F. M., Veisel, C., Barzegarnazari, E., & Striegel–Moore, R. H. (2000). Disordered eating, acculturation, and treatment–seeking in a community sample of Hispanic, Asian, Black, and White women. *Psychology of Women Quarterly, 24*, 244–253.

Dokter, D. (1995). Fragile board – Arts therapies and clients with eating disorders. In D. Dokter (Ed.), *Arts therapies and clients with eating disorders: Fragile board* (pp. 7–22). London: Jessica Kingsley Publishers.

Dolan, B. (1994). Why women? Gender issues and eating disorders: Introduction. In B. Dolan & I. Gitzinger (Eds.), *Why women? Gender issues and eating disorders* (pp. 1 – 11). London: The Athlone Press.

Gold, B. (2000). Group–analytic psychotherapy in the treatment of eating disorders. In T. Hindmarch (Ed.), *Eating disorders: A multiprofessional approach* (pp. 135–156). London: Whurr Publishers.

Grabe, S., & Hyde, J. S. (2006). Ethnicity and body dissatisfaction among women in the United States: A meta–analysis. *Psychological Bulletin, 132*(4), 622–640.

Granillo, T., Jones–Rodriguez, G., & Carvajal, S. C. (2005). Prevalence of eating disorders in Latina adolescents: Associations with substance use and other correlates. *Journal of Adolescent Health, 36*, 214–220.

Harris, D. J., & Kuba, S. A. (1997). Ethnocultural identity and eating disorders in women of Color. *Professional Psychology: Research and Practice, 28*(4) 341–347.

Hiebert, K. A., Felice, M. E., Wingard, D. L., Munoz, R., & Ferguson, J. M. (1988). Comparison of outcome in Hispanic and Caucasian patients with Anorexia Nervosa. *International Journal of Eating Disorders, 7*(5), 693–696.

Jones, P. (2005). *The arts therapies: A revolution in healthcare.* New York: Brunner–Routledge.

Kuba, S. A., & Harris, D. J. (2001). Eating disturbances in women of color: An exploratory study of contextual factors in the development of disordered eating in Mexican American women. *Health Care for Women International, 22,* 281–298.

Leijssen, M. (2006). Validation of the body in psychotherapy. *Journal of Humanistic Psychology, 46*(2), 126–146.

Levens, M. (1994). Psycho–social factors in eating disorders explored through psychodrama and art therapy. In B. Dolan & I. Gitzinger (Eds.), *Why women? Gender issues and eating disorders* (pp. 79–90). London: The Athlone Press.

Mazza, N. (2003). *Poetry therapy: Theory and practice.* New York: Brunner–Routledge.

McDonald, M., Antunez, G., & Gottemoeller, M. (2003). Using the arts and literature in health education. In M. I. Torres, & G. P. Cernada (Eds.), *Sexual and reproductive healthy promotion in Latino populations: Parteras, promotoras, y poetas, Case studies across the Americas* (pp. 161–174). New York: Baywood Publishing Co., Inc.

Miller, K. J., Gleaves, D. H., Hirsch, T. G., Green, B. A., Snow, A. C., & Corbett, C. C. (2000). Comparisons of body image dimensions by race/ethnicity and gender in a university population. *International Journal of Eating Disorders, 27*(3), 310–316.

Mussell, M. P., Binford, R. B., & Fulkerson, J. A. (2000). Eating disorders: Summary of risk factors, prevention programming, and prevention research. *The Counseling Psychologist, 28*(6), 764–796.

Pidcock, B. W., Fischer, J. L., Forthun, L. F., & West, S. L. (2000). Hispanic and Anglo college women's risk factors for substance use and eating disorders. *Addictive Behaviors, 25*(5), 705–723.

Root, M. P. P. (1990). Disordered eating in women of Color. *Sex Roles, 22*(7/8), 525–536.

Santiago–Rivera, A. L., Arredondo, P., & Gallardo–Cooper, M. (2002). *Counseling Latinos and la familia: A practical guide.* Thousand Oaks, CA: Sage.

Shaw, H., Ramirez, L., Trost, A., Randall, P., & Stice, E. (2004). Body image and eating disturbances across ethnic groups: More similarities than differences. *Psychology of Addictive Behaviors, 18*(1), 12–18.

Sloboda, A. (1995). Individual music therapy with anorexic and bulimic patients. In D. Dokter (Ed.), *Art therapies and clients with eating disorders: Fragile board* (pp. 247–261). London: Jessica Kingsley Publishers.

Smith, J. E., & Krejci, J. (1991). Minorities join the majority: Eating disturbances among Hispanic and Native American youth. *International Journal of Eating Disorders, 10*(2), 179–186.

Smolak, L., & Striegel–Moore, R. H. (2001). Challenging the myth of the golden girl: Ethnicity and eating disorders. In R. H. Striegel–Moore & L. Smolak (Eds.), *Eating disorders: Innovative directions in research and practice* (pp. 111–128). Washington, DC: American Psychological Association.

Snow, J. T., & Harris, M. B. (1989). Disordered eating in South–western Pueblo Indians and Hispanics. *Journal of Adolescence, 12,* 329–336.

Stepakoff, S. (1997). Poetry therapy principles and practices for raising awareness of racism. *The Arts in Psychotherapy, 24*(3), 261–274.

Story, M., French, S. A., Resnick, M. D., & Blum, R. W. (1995). Ethnic/racial and socioeconomic differences in dieting behaviors and body image perceptions in adolescents. *International Journal of Eating Disorders, 18*(2), 173–179.

Thompson, B. W. (1996). "A way outa no way": Eating problems among African American, Latina, and White women. In E. N–L. Chow, D. Y. Wilkinson, & M. B. Zinn (Eds.), *Race, class, and gender: Common bonds, difference voices* (pp. 52–69). Thousand Oaks, CA: Sage Publications, Inc.

U. S. Census Bureau. (2001). *The Hispanic population: Census 2000 brief.* Washington, DC: U.S. Government Printing Office.

Vander Wal, J. S., & Thomas, N. (2004). Predictors of body image dissatisfaction and disturbed eating attitudes and behaviors in African American and Hispanic girls. *Eating Behaviors, 5*, 291–301.

Weston, S. (1999). Issues of empowerment in a multi–cultural art therapy group. In J. Campbell, M. Liebmann, F. Brooks, J. Jones, & C. Ward (Eds.), *Art therapy, race and culture* (pp. 177–191). London: Jessica Kingsley Publishers.

Biography

Geneva Reynaga–Abiko is a clinical psychologist who earned a Doctorate of Psychology (Psy.D.) degree from Pepperdine University in West Los Angeles, CA. She specializes in working with Latina/o clients and enjoys clinical work, teaching, research, and supervision. She is the Chair of Latina/o Student Outreach as well as the Primary Instructor for the paraprofessional program at the University of Illinois, Urbana–Champaign Counseling Center. Her interest in difficulties related to eating began during her undergraduate education. She currently co–leads an eating disturbance group and maintains an active caseload of clients from diverse backgrounds. Dr. Reynaga–Abiko enjoys volunteering her time to further the field of multicultural psychology, which includes a position on the editorial board of PsycCRITIQUES: APA Review of Books as well as the Diversity Issues Section Editor for the Depth Psychotherapy Network (http://www.depth–psychotherapy–network.com/). She has authored several articles on working with Latinas/os that are currently in press and is working on a book about culturally relevant assessment with Mexican Americans.

Chapter 11

WOMEN, FOOD AND FEELINGS: DRAMA THERAPY WITH WOMEN WHO HAVE EATING DISORDERS

SHEILA RUBIN

Introduction

The treatment of eating disorders can be highly complex and needs to be addressed on multiple treatment levels. Many women with an eating disorder have emotional dysregulation as well, and are trying to use food and other compulsions to try to regulate their emotional system or cope with their world. Because it is active and experiential, clinical use of drama therapy can support embodied learning of important self–regulatory skills, increase mindfulness, self–awareness, and appropriate self expression that can help clients learn to identify and express feelings in an appropriate setting, rather than deny or suppress emotions with food. Drama therapy can be an effective modality to use with this population if done with structure and great care in tandem with other parts of treatment.

When I tell fellow clinicians that I use drama therapy with patients with eating disorders, many are incredulous. They assure me that patients with an eating disorder won't get out of their chairs and won't do role–plays. In fact, drama therapy is not only possible, it can be very effective with this population. In this chapter and supplement, I will describe a series of steps that can lead safely into the drama therapy process. I will show how to invite clients with an eating disorder to participate; and I will show how powerful these techniques can be with this population.

My work is gentle and supportive, providing a psycho–educational frame around each exercise, and progressing in a series of small steps that lead gradually to an appropriate drama therapy exercise. Since most clients with eating disorders may be anxious and easily frightened, it is clinically appropriate to provide predictability, structure, support, and explanations about each exercise. I am respectful and let patients know that participating at their own comfort level in the group is the first step toward developing their internal sense of what is safe and what is not. I use humor, playfulness, and my skills as a drama therapist to use exercises that include support, a series of successes, and build with logical progression.

I have developed these drama therapy techniques and interventions over ten years of working with patients who have eating disorders. They include ways of teaching many skills including the psychosocial skill sets presented in Dialectical Behavioral Therapy (DBT; Linehan, 1993). These skill sets provide structure for the development of the self. Skills taught include core mindfulness, interpersonal effectiveness, distress tolerance, emotional regulation, "wise mind" and increased sense of self. I also draw on Fairburn (1995) for the psycho–education about eating disorders, the food log, awareness of hunger/fullness, and the connection between bingeing and feelings. The tools offer understanding, coping skills, and choices to clients coping with compulsive eating, disordered thinking, unhealthy behaviors, and offer alternative healthier choices. This is a hopeful and positive approach that builds skills for the patient's journey with her eating disorder.

Drama Therapy

Drama therapy is the intentional and systematic use of drama and theater processes to achieve psychological growth and change (Emunah, 1994, p. 3).The power of this healing modality is that the exercises are active and experiential. They can be adjusted and finely tuned to fit each individual and group. The drama therapist directs with great sensitivity, artfulness, and clinical awareness. Dramatic enactment can create a bridge between human limitations and human aspirations, between who we are and who we want to become (Emunah, 1994, p. 27). Addtionally, drama therapy exercises by their nature frequently evoke positive feelings and positive qualities in the participant including: spontaneity, playfulness, expressiveness, resourcefulness, imagination, humor, and empathy (p. 28). These are often the very qualities that are frozen in the individual with an eating disorder. Other therapeutic benefits of drama therapy can include expression and containment of emotion, increased in role repertoire, development of an observing ego, an increased sense of self, and increased interpersonal skills gained through structured exercises.

Some drama therapy exercises use the externalization process to help the client to separate themselves from the problem so they can stand back and look at it and see the problem, as a separate entity and not as a part of themselves (Emunah, 2000, p. 114). Some externalizing drama therapy exercises used with this population include the patient writing letters to her eating disorder, making collages, choosing symbolic objects to represent the eating disorder or different internalized voices. These activities allow participants to feel separate from their eating disorder – sometimes for the first time in their lives. Many have commented, "I thought I was my eating disorder, now I realize I have an eating disorder." (Please note: A partial list of drama therapy exercises is in the appendix that supplements this chapter.)

DBT – Dialectical Behavioral Therapy

Marcia Linehan's groundbreaking work of DBT (Dialectical Behavioral Therapy) is an integration of eastern psychological and spiritual practices (Zen practices) and western approaches to therapy (Linehan, 1993, p. 5). Dialectical Behavioral Therapy offers Cognitive Behavioral Therapy (CBT) treatment developed specifically for patients with borderline personality disorder. The work provides for multiple levels of learning, beyond the cognitive for people who suffer from trauma and states of emotional dysregulation. I chose this model because it speaks of skill deficits that can be taught through skills modules. Many of the skills that are needed to treat borderline personality disorder are the same skills needed for working with women with eating disorders. Linehan states that the core disorder in borderline personality disorder (BPD) is emotional dysregulation. Most women with eating disorders also have emotional dysregulation as well, and are trying to do use food and other compulsions to try to regulate their emotional system or cope with their world.

Linehan (1993) writes about the "the invalidating environment" being the crucial developmental circumstance in the creation of the disorder. Either parents or caregivers responded erratically or inappropriately to patient's feelings, thoughts, and sensations, or simply ignored the child's communications. A person in this environment, especially someone who is highly sensitive to begin with learns to invalidate her own experience and learns to scan the environment to figure out how to respond (p. 3).

She goes on to say that "the inability to regulate emotional arousal also interferes with the development and maintenance of a sense of self" (Linehan, 1993, p. 4). The holding back of the individual's responses, as with women with eating disorders, may contribute to an absence of a sense of identity. Since relationships depend on a stable sense of self and spontaneous emotional expression, these individuals develop chaotic relationships. Skills in distress tolerance and interpersonal effectiveness offer the training to these skill deficits in the clients.

Linehan "reframes" her client's suicidal and dysfunctional behaviors as part of a problem–solving repertoire (Linehan, 1993, p. 5). In my work with clients with an eating disorder, I reframe the eating disorder behaviors as part of client's problem–solving repertoire. As patients begin to see that binging, purging, restricting, and food rituals are attempts to self–sooth or cope with overwhelming feelings, the group offers new, healthier choices.

Drama Therapy and Adult Survivors of Eating Disorders

The program that I created was initially for the eating disorder portion of the Partial Hospitalization Program for Adults and the PHP for Adolescents at Mills Peninsula Hospital in Burlingame, CA when I was the eating disorder specialist from 1998–2003. My groups were a mixture of women who had a diagnosis of bulimia, binge eating disorder, and anorexia. Co–morbid conditions included body dysmorphic disorder, depression, anxiety, OCD, diabetes, and other health issues related to their eating disorder. Some had sub–clinical symptoms. It also included a 12–week outpatient group for women with eating disorders at that hospital. I have since adapted this work and continue to offer weekly "Woman, Food, and Feelings Groups" in my private practice in San Francisco and Berkeley, CA and through a local Women's Resource Center.

In addition to this group, patients in the partial hospitalization program also attended in addition to this group, a full program of psychotherapy and other groups, as well as having a case manager and psychiatrist. Patients in the 12–week outpatient group did not necessarily have a psychiatrist and did not attend other groups. The outpatient group met 2 hours a week for 12 weeks with the option of taking the group a second time and third time. The partial hospitalization eating disorder group met twice a week for an hour. Clients taking the "Woman Food, and Feelings" groups in my private practice sometimes have a treatment team and sometimes do not. The work is adjusted to fit each particular configuration of psychological needs of the members of each group.

How the Groups Worked

Groups had a predictable weekly structure that clients could count on. We would begin with a body scan, followed by a check in, followed by presentation and discussion of the topic, followed by a creative process, and ending with another check in and goal setting for the week and closure. Before the initial check in, patients were led through a brief meditation to achieve a state of mindfulness which included a body scan to help them notice body sensations, emotions, and thoughts. To check in, patients reported first on what they noticed when scanning their bodies, then on their homework. The middle part of the group focused on a particular topic or skill from DBT, Fairburn, or the author's themes to discuss and explore. Exercises were constructed to allow each person to participate at her own level of comfort and safety. The exercises led gradually from discussion to writing to drawing to choosing roles to enacting. Although the themes were set, each group was entirely different due to the individual nature of each participant's relationship to her eating disorder, her level of relative ego strength, the length of time the group had been meeting, new members just joining the group, etc. Issues and successes from clients' homework discussions could be further explored through poetry, drawing, or active techniques. Over time there was a playfulness developed in the group from simple drama therapy exercises like category ball and partner exercises (see supplement).

Creative Approach

Developing Core Mindfulness and an Internal "Wise Mind"

In order to teach self–awareness and core mindfulness, in addition to using meditation and somatic body sensing exercises, I also adapted Marcia Linehan's model of Reasonable Mind, Emotional Mind, and Wise Mind (Linehan, 1993). In DBT, a person is in the state of Reasonable Mind when she is approaching knowledge intellectually and is cool in her approach to problems. A person is in her Emotional Mind, when cognitions are hot, facts are amplified, or distorted. Wise Mind is the integration between Emotional Mind and Reasonable Mind, adding intuitive knowing to emotional experiencing and logical analysis (Linehan, 1993). I used a series of drama therapy exercises to teach this experientially (see supplement). Using large brightly colored drama therapy scarves, I led clients through guided visualizations and role plays to identify and be able to talk to their Emotional Mind (that may want to buy cookies for a binge) and their Reasonable Mind (that demands they stay on a strict diet), and their Wise Mind (that can hold both the desire for cookies and the need for structure/control with compassion and lead the person to make a healthy choice). My gentle and supportive guidance led clients to gradually move from discussion and visualization to actually role–playing one or all of the roles.

The series of exercises about the three minds also allowed them to get in touch with the inner boondoggle and begin to see how much of their energy was involved in the struggle, and hear the arguments that they've heard in their head over and over, now externalized in the room where it can be seen, heard, talked to, and reduced. Hidden shame would be diffused as group members realized that their peers also had similar absurd conversations in their minds about food and body image. These exercises also allowed each member to hear, sense, interact with, and eventually embody her Wise Mind. It also led to increased connection to Wise Mind and encouraged women to begin to seek out a state of mindfulness more and more of the time in her life (see supplement).

Interpersonal Effectiveness Skills

A woman with an eating disorder needs to learn to be in relationship with others in a way that nourishes rather than drains her, a woman must be able to listen to others without loosing her own voice (Linehan, 1993). She needs "balance between the need to be in relationship with others and the need to remain true to herself, remain aware of her inner thoughts and feelings even when interacting with others" (Johnson, 1996, p. 63). She needs to begin to change the inner dialogue and the questions she asks herself. Instead of asking, "What will he think if I do this?" One can ask, "How do I feel about what he said? What is my reaction?" A woman learns to be able to say "No", or "That may be OK with you, but it's not OK with me" (Linehan, 1993, p. 63). The clients can practice this through drama therapy exercises in group.

When women disconnected from themselves, they cling desperately to their relationships with others hoping to get the attention, love, and support they are not able to give themselves" (Johnson, 1996, p. 63). Further, "By failing to respect and respond to their own needs they become depleted rather than nourished in their relationships. They have become so adept at listening to the needs, wishes, and values of others, they have forgotten their own" (Johnson, 1996, p. 62). Drama therapy exercises and mindfulness help women to realize this and to install an inner coach or wise internal mother. They can develop a strong, mature inner mother to provide them with nourishment and guidance, not only to survive, but also to grow and flourish (Johnson, 1996, p. 81).

Interpersonal effectiveness has to do with obtaining the change one wants, maintaining the relationship, and maintaining self–respect. Problems that clients have with distress tolerance make it difficult to tolerate fears, anxieties, or frustrations that are typical in situations with conflicts that arise in relationships (Linehan, 1993). Interpersonal effectiveness skills taught include awareness of the need to identify and track personal needs and to also attend to relationships and keep both in balance. The ability to balance priorities, balancing wants and shoulds and building mastery and self–respect are other areas.

Body Image

Body image issues were addressed through discussion about societal pressures for women to be thin and perfect. This was followed by art work making a collage about what society thinks women should look like and making another collage about what were the true strengths and beauty inside. Women who have an eating disorder often have the associated body dysmorphic disorder, a severe distortion of what their body looks like. During eating disorder assessments I conducted, over 99 percent of women who had eating disorder symptoms reported "hating" or "strongly disliking" their bellies, and thought they were "too fat." Others dislike their whole body and had a distorted view of their size. Many reported they began restricting or binging and purging in high school or college because they feared becoming overweight. Drama therapy exercises that are helpful here are the drawing of mirrors: the distorted mirror and the "reality check mirror." This parallels the images on this book's cover. Another exercise involves the therapist or one of the patients standing behind a mirror frame and taking the role of the positive voice or wise mind of her fellow patient (see supplement for exercise).

Food Logs

Food logs are introduced in the second or third session. They are from Fairburn's book *Treating binge eating* (Fairburn, 1995). They serve as a tool to help clients begin to observe their eating patterns and the connection between food and feelings. It is important to remind clients to be in a state of mindfulness or be a neutral observer when observing and writing down what they ate. If they are in a place of self judgment, the information will be used to beat themselves up instead of for information for deeper healing. Food logs can initially be a practice in mindfulness and self–acceptance, simply observing. Later skills can be taught to distinguish between physical hunger and emotional hunger and to identify coping skills.

Family, Food, and Body Image

Family and food relationships are a very important part of the work. Often it is an internalized voice of a parent or teasing friend that the client experiences as judging and demanding perfection which can lead to disordered eating. Family dynamics can be explored first through discussion, then drawing a genogram, and finally through role–play. The genogram is drawing of the family. The client is asked to write a line or phrase for each family member about what she learned about food or weight from that person. If the person wants to work further, I might set up chairs in the room to represent her family members. She can choose an object or a peer from the group to take on the role of each family member and place them in the chairs. I then led the person slowly from one chair to another and ask her to give a line to each family member to say to her about food or weight from her genogram. Then we go through one by one and she listens to what each one tells her. She reclaims herself by telling them that what they believe is not true for her body and her food choices. Group members may say things like, "I know you were always working on diets to stay thin, Mom, but I don't want to have to be on a diet in order to like myself." "It's not ok with me that you make fun of my body when I go to family picnics by saying, 'Are you really going to eat that!'" This can be further explored through psychodrama and then integrated through drawing or journaling new insights from the work.

Family dynamics need to be discussed because the eating disorder is often an unconscious way for a person to separate from her family or refuse to separate from her family. Family dynamics can be addressed under interpersonal effectiveness and also under emotional regulation topics. Lists can be made, letters written that are not to be sent to help clients identify feelings, and role–plays can be enacted using interpersonal effectiveness skills. Drama therapy can offer opportunity for group members to try on new roles that they can use in their families.

Emotional Regulation

Clients discuss the importance of feelings and the fallacy that some feelings are good and some are not allowed. Discussion provides psycho–education about anger and other misunderstood feelings. Clients learn that an emotion is a communication that something is not right. Through story and metaphor women can discover their anger, then through drama therapy women can express and explore their anger, moving beyond the victim role. DBT skill sets offers modules that teach each of the emotions that lend themselves to storytelling and role play.

Feelings are like fluid waves of energy. They have a natural cyclical rhythm like the ebb and flow of the tides, the waning and waxing of the moon. Women with eating disorders build dams to stop the natural flow using compulsive behavior with food to distract themselves from their feelings. Feelings are not the cause of the eating disorder, but rather the attempt to control the feelings (Johnson, 1996). As the women become adept at riding out their feelings instead of blocking them, an inner relationship can be established in which the feelings become allies and guides in one's life journey. "Acceptance of all feelings without judgment requires an acknowledgment of the idea that feelings don't have to make sense or be liked, but simply have to be accepted" (Johnson, 1996, p. 59) and expressed.

Self-Expression

Self-expression is vital to help a woman step beyond her eating disorder by helping her find a glimpse of herself. Most women with an eating disorder often do not have a sense of self, are "other focused," preferring to get their sense of safety and well being from grades, positive comments from men, or looking for the expression on another person's face. They may only know when they have done enough by the praise or lack of praise from a relative, boyfriend, or person in authority. Self-expression may begin simply with uttering one word in the group. This word is often the word, "No." When, "no" is spoken, I respect this absolutely. This is the client setting a boundary, and in order to set a boundary, this "no" is a creative act. It is an act of self-definition. This "no" may be representative of the role that the eating disorder plays in the person's life. This is usually saying no to process or group exercise that I suggest. I tell them all through the group that each person is able to choose when to participate and when to observe. They are also able to track their sense of relative safety by using mindfulness to scan their body and thoughts and feelings after saying "no" and having the therapist accept and respond to their setting a boundary. They are invited to observe other group members trying the exercise and they may later say "yes" and participate in the exercise or later in the group or in the next group, with my guidance to observe how it feels inside to participate.

Other means of self-expression are the collages we do, writing poems, and participating in a small or large way in the drama therapy exercises, at their own pace. Most women and teen girls with an eating disorder have a hard time speaking their thoughts and feelings. Often this is because they are not aware of what their thoughts or feeling are. Discussion can focus on reasons for not speaking up for oneself: not wanting to offend someone, not knowing oneself, not knowing the right words, being afraid, and it is ineffable. To move beyond this stuck place, it is helpful to be able to create a story about someone who was able to talk for herself or remember a friend who was good at that. Eventually we move into role-plays about this. The self expression exercises gradually helped women move from deep shame and self loathing to realize that "every woman is gorgeous."

Embodiment

Women in these groups usually hated their bodies and not only didn't want to get out of their chairs, they really didn't want to feel their bodies at all. I created a number of exercises to assist with this. I would play music, ask each woman to choose one of the large colorful scarves and then to move the scarves to the music. While moving the scarves, some would discover the rhythm of the music and begin to move off the chair as well. Once one woman started moving slightly to the music others might join in. It was much easier to move when their focus was on moving the scarf, not their body. Some beautiful group dances resulted from slowly guiding one direction and then another, "notice how your scarf flows forward and back, long pause, see if you want to expand that, long pause, see if you want to move in other directions, long pause, how slowly can your scarf move, long pause, how fast can it move? Can your scarf dance with the scarf of the woman next to you?" The exercise would end with mindfulness, tuning into what they felt inside and noticing if this was different than what they felt at the beginning of the group. After the exercise we would discuss what they noticed, using mindfulness, about their scarf, the music, the movement, and what sensations they might have noticed in their bodies.

Using mindfulness and body mind exercises, I would offer short guided visualizations to help each woman begin to feel sensations inside her body. We might begin with feeling the breath, the heart, the pulse, and lead into observing sensations of emptiness and fullness so that each woman could have access to more mindfulness about when she feels hungry and when she feels full.

Binge Buster

When a client feels they are going to binge she can do the Binge Buster as homework. This is a one–page list of brief questions designed to help her evoke a state of mindfulness and explore her inner experience. The first direction asks her to sit quietly and tune inside herself, using breathing or mindfulness exercises from the group, and then ask the following questions.

1. Am I hungry?
2. What am I feeling?
3. What am I thinking?
4. What do I really want?
5. What coping skills can I do now instead of binge?
6. Choose a coping skill that you will use after the exercise.
7. Is there something else that I need to address later, a larger issue?

If she still feels hungry, she can eat two bites and then sit and sense if her body wants more. They are learning to listen to what their body wants. The

Binge Buster is adapted from Tannis Hugill's Binge Buster from Belmont Hills Hospital.

Anita Johnson writes that once a woman recognizes that her urge to eat when she's not physically hungry is a signal of a different hunger she needs to address, she can begin to discover ways of feeding herself the nourishment she really desires (Johnson, 1996, p. 54).

Fear of Change

The eating disorder is often an unconscious way for a woman to keep her life, growth, and development on hold. As she begins to find her self, the self that has been hidden beneath the symptoms and obsessions of the eating disorder, something in her may begin to unfreeze. There will be changes, small changes at first and then larger ones. She may choose to make healthy changes such as making new food choices, making healthy thought choices, even new patterns and new routines, talking differently to parents or to her spouse, meeting new people, and even eventually coping with life transitions i.e. going off to college, making a decision to interview for a new job, etc. Drama therapy processes can support the client's changes through enactments and role plays that acknowledge the client's fear of change, remind her of her many strengths, new coping skills, and can even help role play the potentially scary situations, and role play rehearsals and positive outcomes (see supplement).

Humor and play are vital elements in the psyche of a healthy person. Drama therapy can invite humor and play into therapy in subtle and more profound ways. When laughter is heard for the first time in these groups, it is a balm for the soul. Having the ability to laugh, just a little, at one's behavior or one's need for perfection creates a little space for self acceptance and eventually perhaps even for change. Clients are learning to be able to check in with each of the three minds to help access feelings and make decisions and they are learning to reduce perfectionism and increase flexible thinking.

Conclusion

Because treatment of eating disorders needs to address many clinical issues on a variety of levels at the same time, drama therapy can be a very effective modality. It allows for embodied learning of DBT skill sets, and other theoretical teachings and expressive activities. Benefits of drama therapy offers experiential learning of core mindfulness, emotional regulation, and interpersonal effectiveness as well as easier bonding between group members, expanded role repertoire, increased comfort with play, access to intuition and creativity, and increased flexibility of thinking. As participants practice accessing their "wise minds," and expressive activities they can experience embodied access to emotions and sensations and even more of a sense of "self." Role play about mindfulness practices and life changes is an important way to begin to transfer what is learned in the group into their life in the world.

One of the benefits of drama therapy is the increase in the client's role repertoire. By practicing being able to play the role of another group member's Wise Mind or positive voice in the mirror (or annoying boss or parent), each person in the group tries on new roles. Rigidity about how they hold themselves and express themselves is being opened to new embodied experience. They can also practice new communication skills to develop interpersonal effectiveness and cope with fear of change, challenging automatic thoughts and rigid patterns.

Another benefit of drama therapy is that of engagement in the activity and sometimes even a sense of pleasure and play. Groups can address issues of body image through levels of exercises. Drama therapy also offers a large number of exercises with many steps so that clients can slowly move into the drama therapy activities because it is often a long journey from the frozen, terrified place a client comes in with to the place of participating in a role–play in an engaged way and laughing with peers about what used to be their deepest fears.

Appendix

Category Ball

Category ball is a phase–one drama therapy exercise. I use a small hand–size rubber koosh ball that can be easily tossed and caught. I ask a question and the ball is tossed from one group member to another in no particular order, as the group sits around the table. The person catching the ball says the first thing that comes to mind that answers the question. The subject being discussed can be broken down into themes to explore and the category ball was a great way to break up structure, get "the energy moving" in the group, and include everyone in discussion and even bring a bit of humor into what might be a very heavy discussion. For instance, when discussing what a binge is, I might say, "When you catch the ball, say the first thing that you think of when you hear the word food." Responses may range from, "scared, comfort, control, too much, need, friend, to not allowed." The next question might be, "What is the first thing you think of when you hear the word, "self–sooth." Responses may range from, "None, comfort, caring, for others, to need." Then I might say, "What is the first thing that comes into your mind when I say the word binge?" Responses might be, "reward, earned, respite, time out, secret, alone, private, uncontrollable, and temper tantrum." I might write these responses on the board or continue the discussion about any of the topics brought up.

As the ball is tossed and caught, in this process, there is something going on underneath the words. The ball helped to break the ice, the act of throwing the ball to a particular person involves making a choice and taking an action. The act of catching the ball involves acknowledgement of accomplishment (catching the ball) and a feeling of satisfaction, a little success. Near the beginning of group this exercise allows each person to have an easy win, a feeling of success, a sense of belonging. It is an invitation to a different way of discussing something that may have felt shameful or hidden. Group members eagerly wait hearing what the next person will say, and there is support for each person to speak. And even though we are all sitting safely around the table, this simple exercise is an experiential introduction to the creative process, free association, and improvisation. This exercise opens up what had been a shameful topic in a playful way, inviting flexibility. On the surface level, we are having a discussion. On another level we are building group cohesiveness, reducing anxiety, and sharing in the universality of having an eating disorder. On another level each person is being acknowledged and having a success and having their presence in the group noted.

Category Ball can also be used to brainstorm just about any topic. If someone has just identified that she hates when a boy who said he was going to call does not call, if the group doesn't naturally respond, I might take out the category ball and ask a few questions. "What are some of the feelings here?" "Embarrassment, he hates me, he doesn't care, I'm terrible, and it's because I'm fat." I might also ask, "What are some of the reasons he might not have called?" "He had a family emergency, he had to stay after school, he got arrested." Suddenly there are other possibilities.

Coping Skills with Category Ball

Another way we use category ball is to identify coping skills. When the group is reviewing the cognitive triangle or when someone is reporting that she doesn't know what to do with her food, I may take out the ball. "What are some coping skills that someone could use at this point?" The group may then come up with plenty, "take a bubble bath, write an angry letter, write in your journal, etc." It is a nice way to reduce the tension of the group by bringing a little levity into the room. It is also way to begin to gently begin to bend and break down rigidly–held thoughts and positions.

Write a Letter to your Eating Disorder

1. Group discussion about relationship with eating disorder. The group discusses how long they've had the eating disorder, ways it's helped their life, at least at the beginning.
2. Each group member is given three pieces of paper and instructed to write a letter to the eating disorder on the first page. "Dear Eating disorder. . . ." As if the eating disorder is an old friend, they are invited to discuss the relationship, benefits, and new feelings about the eating disorder.
3. Each group member is invited to read the letter and say how they feel.
4. Next they are asked to write a letter on the second page that is a letter from the eating disorder to the person. "Dear Suzie" This is where the eating disorder is able to speak to the person. "These are the reasons you need me. . . ."
5. These are then read in the group.
6. And then group members are asked to write a third letter, this is a letter back to the eating disorder saying that things are changing now, the person is invited to explore ways she wants to change her relationship with her eating disorder, i.e. "Even though you helped me get through difficult periods in my life, I'm wanting other things now, a relationship, a new job, etc. I am in charge of my eating, not you. I will no longer listen when you tell me I'm fa_. . . ."
7. This is read to the group as well and followed with discussion.

Finding your Wise Mind

1. Initially I would work introduce the DBT idea of "wise mind" and suggest that each patient recall a time when she was in a difficult situation and they were able to act. This might be an example of their wise mind.
2. Next patients are asked to turn to the person next to them and take turns with the following exercise. First, one partner tells the other a small issue they are coping with.
3. The partner is asked to imagine taking on the role of their partner's wise mind. They are directed to imagine this role able to acknowledge the emotional and reasonable minds and speak from this compassionate, kind, wise voice to give kind words or suggestions.
4. Partners were instructed to switch roles and were guided through the exercise again.

After the exercise members were asked to tell their partner how the partner was in the role of Wise Mind. Many were surprised to later get feedback from the partner that their compassionate advice was helpful, and that they were able to successfully able to play the role of each other's Wise Mind. This is a nice preliminary step of being able to access their own Wise Mind. This lead to expanded role repertoire, something that drama therapists value as an expansion of the range of roles a person allows themselves to play. While playing this role for their partner, they were able to access and speak from a compassionate place. Much, much later, I was able to call on this experience when leading them to play the role of their own Wise Mind, which of course 100 percent of the women in my groups assured me they couldn't access initially. Several follow–up exercises follow that can be used in the same group for a series of groups.

Wise Mind, Emotional Mind, and Rational Mind Role Play – Introduction

1. The group reviews the DBT concepts of Wise Mind, Emotional Mind, and Rational Mind.
2. Signs are handed out to each group member and they are asked to say something about the "mind" they see written on the sign.
3. Those who received a Emotional Mind sign are gently coached to take on the role of the emotional mind.
4. Those who received a "reasonable mind" sign are gently coached to take on the role of the reasonable mind.
5. Those who received a "wise mind" sign are gently coached to take on the role of the wise mind.
6. I would identify a possible situation dealing with an event that might trigger a binge, and ask each person playing one of the minds, to say how they felt about it in role.
7. Clients were directed to trade signs and roles, and try on a different "mind" as we did the exercise again with a new situation being offered.
8. We would discuss how it felt to "play" each of the minds, and discuss when they find themselves in each of the minds.

Once the group had warmed up to the idea of the different minds and was at least a little warmed up to the idea of taking a role, I would do the following exercise

Role Play Three Minds to Help With a Real Situation

1. One person would volunteer a dilemma she wanted to explore. For instance someone might bring in the problem of, "every time I go gro-

cery shopping, I try to buy healthy items, but when I pass the cup cakes and candy, I can't control the urge to buy them and then go home and binge for an hour or two."

2. I ask this person to choose one person to be their emotional mind, and give them a line to say, i.e. "I want those cup cakes, I worked hard, I deserve them!"

3. Choose one person to be the rational mind and give them a line, for instance, "You are going to stay on the strict diet and there are no exceptions, none."

4. Choose one person to be the wise mind and give them a line. Sometimes I would give a line to the wise mind if the person couldn't think of one. Something like, "I understand you worked so hard and you want a treat. We're going to buy everything on the healthy list and you can have a treat after dinner."

5. The three people playing the roles of the minds are seated on three chairs at one end of the room. I begin to conduct an orchestra that is made up of the three minds. Each one is to say their line. I model this for the person who's issue we are exploring.

6. The person working on this issue is given the conductor's baton and shown how to conduct the orchestra of her three minds by motioning for louder or softer, and choosing who to listen to for a solo. By now there is a cacophony of all the voices shouting at them at the same time, "I want those cup cakes," "You don't deserve any treats we're on a strict diet," and "I know that you really want those cupcakes AND you can have a treat after dinner tonight, and first we're going to shop with this list." I would support each client in conducting and directing the orchestra and then to gradually assume mastery by asking some of the voices to go silent. Emunah's (1999) emotional orchestra helped bring this usually hidden thoughts and behavior right out front in such an amusing way, shame was reduced and usually all or most members of the group were deeply engaged because everyone related to the issue. If the group is very warmed up I might take them into the next step. If they are not, I might end the exercise here and ask everyone to journal or make a collage about insights and realizations they had during the exercise and about any changes they might want to try.

7. At this point, if the group is warmed up, I would also use role play and psychodrama to guide the patient to take on each of the these roles for herself and have a conversation in roles that were appropriate for her to express what needed to be expressed, and then to claim her wise mind. In this process sometimes memories would be assessed of being teased in fourth grade, or of a boyfriend/husband telling them to loose weight. The understanding support of peers who were willing to play these parts was instrumental.

8. After this series of exercises, many patients reported that they were able, for the first time in years, to go to the grocery store with a list, and even though their emotional mind was shouting for binge food and their realistic mind was shouting for a strict diet, they were able to just buy the food on the list by tuning into the wise mind, and thereby avoiding the binge.

Interpersonal Effectiveness Drama Therapy Exercises

One member volunteers to work. She tells the group the situation she is trying to work on, i.e. being frustrated that her husband doesn't appreciate all the invisible things she does for him, or a boss that makes fun of her at meetings.

(1) *Talking to her three minds about the situation.* She is invited to choose group members to play roles in her role play: one person plays her wise mind, another plays her emotional mind, and a third plays her reasonable mind. They are gently led through a drama therapy process of listening to each of the minds and getting advice on how to deal with the situation presented.

(2) Role play the actual conflict. After the person has had a conversation with her three minds, she is then ready for the second part of the role–play. Another person is chosen to play her in the role play so that she can watch or direct the scene with my help. She then takes the advice of the wise mind to have a conversation with the person in conflict. The three minds, especially the wise mind can give advice to the person as she tries on new behavior setting boundaries, being effective, or speaking up for herself.

Game: Role–play to Explore Discussion Topics

1. Topics brought up during discussion are listed on the board. "What to do with a lot of food on your plate at the holidays." "What to do when you see someone else who has an eating disorder?" "How to talk to your eating disorder when it's trying to cause problems?
2. Roles and situation are written on index cards.
3. Group members are invited to choose a card
4. Cards identify the role and situation. One group does the role–play first.

Physical or Emotional Hunger

Clients are lead through a guided visualization, and asked to put their hand on their belly and notice the sensations and emotional reactions. This exercise leads the client in a journey of subtle sensations to tune into. Learning to be able to identify feelings fullness, and emptiness, hunger and fulfillment.

Emotional Regulation–Finding and Expressing The Forbidden Emotion of Anger

Many clients need help accessing feelings of anger that may be showing up in unconscious ways. Several exercises are: blowing bubbles and then clapping hard and loud to pop the bubbles, hitting balloons to push them away, drawing anger in a contained circle, and others.

Magic Weight

Often women with an eating disorder have a "magic weight" that they feel they are striving to get there through compulsive exercise, restricting, or purging. We discuss what they imagine will happen at this "magic weight." Others in the group often share that when they reached that weight, they were so busy doing all the compulsive behaviors to maintain it, they were not able to have the male attention or the perfect job and perfect life they had imagined. This can be further explored by writing a list or making a collage of the things the person wishes for at the magic weight. That can further be explored as to how to create these things in their life now, rather than striving for the weight, work toward the relationship or the job directly. This can then be taken into role–play.

Body Image

Draw 3 mirrors:
   1. The eating disorder mirror,
   2. The "reality check" mirror. Clients are asked how friends see them and we also may look at photographs.
   3. Future– this is a mirror without the distortion of eating disorder thinking.

Discuss: This exercise needs to be lead into gently with support and encouragement. Room for feelings is needed. Often group members are only able to draw the first mirror. We talk about the distortion of the way they see themselves, using support as they begin to challenge this. The next mirror usually benefits from group support and discussion. Often group members give feedback to each other that they are not "fat" or "ugly" but actually beautiful.

Talking to a Live Mirror–Role Reverse

After discussing the drawings, the next step may be to write positive affirmations.

A drama therapy prop that was used was large mirror frame without a mirror in it. Each person chose someone to play her middle mirror. Those who wanted to do this next part of the exercise would stand in front of the drama therapy mirror and the chosen partner would stand behind the mirror. The person would look into the mirror and say something positive to their reflection, who was actually the partner. The partner, in the role of reflection, would say positive things to the person peering into the mirror. This became a powerful exercise in which the person behind the mirror was often deeply affected by realizing how much her peer was putting herself down and would speak kind words. The rest of the group would applaud. All were learning how to say positive things to them. The exercise was deeply bonding for the partners doing the mirror work due to the eye contact and kind words. This mirror exercise is often referred to further along in treatment, "remember what your mirror said?" "Oh yeah, my mirror said I'm beautiful and she is proud of me." There can be a powerful moment when the voice in the mirror challenges the patient's distorted view of herself and models how she can say positive things to herself.

Self-forgiveness Exercise

Many women with eating disorders feel guilty for simply existing. The inner judge is vicious and can name every thing they didn't do perfectly. Some were not able to do the self–care and self–soothing exercises because they believed that they deserved to be punished, not comforted. This exercise helps with self–forgiveness to challenge this need to be punished. First identify what the person feels she is guilty for or needs to be punished for. Maybe it was for eating a whole dinner, or getting an A—instead of an A on a college paper,

1. Each person is invited write the "crime" on paper.
2. Neatly fold the paper into a small piece and then hold in her hands.
3. Close her eyes and follows the guided visualization into wise mind.
4. Visualize a wise or holy person.
5. Tell this wise person what your crime was.
6. Listen to the wise person's words of forgiveness.
7. Use this wise person's forgiving words to forgive yourself.

One client with severe anorexia held herself guilty for any comfort she offered herself—sitting on a soft chair was forbidden, eating anything more than starvation food was a "crime." When she did this mindfulness exercise she was amazed to see the Dali Lama in her meditation sit with her and tell her that she had done nothing wrong. This was a turning point in being able to coach her on taking small steps to let herself have little bits of comfort. The first change was to allow she to sit on the chair in the room that had a cushion.

We discussed having a sense of past and future in relationship to the eating disorder and life goals. Three chairs were set up in front of the room. Clients were directed to choose an object or symbol or group of objects to represent each of the three places in time. The first chair is the past, a life that was filled with the obsessions and hidden eating disorder behaviors. The middle chair represents the current self in relation to the eating disorder. The third chair is a place for an imagined future self. Clients can create a whole sculpture in each chair using the objects or symbols. After everyone is finished arranging their sculpture, the group comes back together. Each takes a turn sharing her journey with the group by sitting in or standing behind each chair and either embodying that they were in each position or telling about the symbolism they chose. The group can applaud each woman's story about living with her eating disorder and even imagine healing her eating disorder.

Drama Therapy Exercises to Use After Exploring a Cognitive Behavioral Triangle

Drama therapy techniques of role–play, line repletion, doubling, adding an internal nurturing parent, category ball, and storytelling were used to explore and challenge automatic thoughts and family dynamics beneath compulsive food or exercise related behaviors. I would first lead a psycho–education discussion about the cognitive behavioral triangle to help clients begin to understand triggers, thoughts, feelings, and behaviors that all happen in an instant and lead to unconscious compulsive eating disordered behaviors. We would slow down that process. What happened (triggering event), what did you think ("I'm no good"), what did you feel ("helpless"), what did you do ("start the binge"). We would identify coping skills that could be used instead of the eating disorder behavior. This could lead to a role–play about a current situation or a memory from the past about being teased in school or a boyfriend who said, "You have to loose weight." I would lead the person to identify what they story meant to them and what needed to be changed/healed. Sometimes I would take on the role of the wise adult and go into the scene and tell the mother or the brother not to tease them. Sometimes it would be a group member. Sometimes the whole group would be involved in telling off the boyfriend or talking to the angry boss in the scene. Sometimes the patient would at last be able to express long held anger after others in the group did, and say out loud, "You can't talk to me that way," or "It hurts when you say that." This could then lead to interpersonal effectiveness, learning how to set boundaries and how to present themselves so that they are heard, in current time in their life. I directed role plays to explore and challenge internalized family dynamics, automatic thoughts, and compulsive eating disordered behavior, as well as working with body image through a drama therapy mirror movement, and sensory awareness exercises.

References

Emunah, R. (1994). *Acting for real: Drama therapy process, technique, and performance.* New York: Brunner/Mazel, Inc.

Fairburn, C. (1995). *Overcoming binge eating.* New York, The Guilford Press.

Johnson, A. (1996). *Eating in the light of the moon.* Carlsbad, CA: Guize Books.

Linehan, Marcia.M. (1993). *Skills training manual for treating borderline personality disorder.* New York: Guilford Press.

Biography

Sheila Rubin, MA, LMFT, RDT/BCT is in private practice with offices in San Francisco and Berkeley, CA, as a licensed Marriage and Family Therapist and a Registered Drama Therapist and Board Certified Trainer. She developed this eating disorder program when she was the eating disorder specialist for five years at Mills Peninsula Hospital, Out–Patient Behavioral Health Services in Burlingame, CA. from 1998–2003, where she worked with adults and adolescents in the partial hospitalization program. She has since adapted this work into the "Women, Food and Feelings Groups" she offers in her private practice. She is an adjunct faculty and an alumni of CIIS, The California Institute of Integral Studies Psychology and Drama Therapy Dept., and also teaches at The JFK University Holistic Counseling Center supervising transpersonal and somatic psychology students. She is a past president of the San Francisco chapter of CAMFT, the California Association for Marriage and Family Therapists, and a past president of the Northern California chapter of NADT, the National Association for Drama Therapy. She has presented at numerous NADT conferences since 1997. To work with a wide range of client needs, her psychotherapy work combines drama therapy, expressive therapy, and somatic therapy (Haikomi, Focusing), with CBT, (Cognitive Behavioral Therapy), DBT (Dialectical Behavioral Therapy), mindfulness, transpersonal, attachment, object relations, family systems, and other theories. She also offers alternative track drama therapy training for therapists and workshops in embodiment, presence, and authenticity through improvisation and sacred witnessing in her Life Stories Self–Revelatory Performance Drama Therapy Workshops. Her website is www.TheHealingStory.com.

Chapter 12

THE SACRED AND THE PROFANE FOOD: RITUAL AND COMPULSION IN EATING DISORDERS – EXISTENTIAL DRAMA THERAPY WITH ADOLESCENTS AND THEIR FAMILIES

Cosmin Gheorghe

Anxiety: A Hundred Years of Solitude in Psychotherapy

The following chapter proposes Existential Drama Therapy, a *systemic* and *multidisciplinary* approach to eating disorders, which takes into consideration the interrelation and interaction between the *individual* and the *collective*, and between the *public* and the *private*. Psychology, mythology, theatre, physiology, biochemistry, sociology, politics and economics, are at the same time interwoven and transcended, with the intention to create an integral approach to the exploration and treatment of eating disorders.

It is important, from the author's point of view, to situate the patient in his/her familial, cultural, historical and socio–political context, in order to understand and adequately and efficiently treat any of the eating disorder syndromes. Therefore, creative arts therapists (CATs) find themselves in a privileged, although challenging, position, in comparison to any other mental health practitioner. Because of their intention and capability to make arts and science work together in a harmonious whole, CATs have the capacity and freedom to represent the point where several knowledge sources meet into a homeostatic mélange. Disciplines that appear to be unrelated or even in opposition, not only are able to coexist without confronting each other within CATs work, but they act in an elegant synergy, which produces treatment solutions that address simultaneously the individual and the collective, the mythos and the logos (in Greek *mythos = story*, and *logos = science*, or *rational knowledge*. Mythology could be therefore defined as the rational understanding of an imaginary story. For more information please see Mircea Eliade (1992), "The Sacred and the Profane"). Creative arts therapists, besides eliciting healing and health, have also the ability and duty to elicit social and sometimes political change, and therefore clients should always be approached only in the context of their familial, social, economical, political, and cultural environment. As James Hillman points out with his fine humor, "we've had a hundred years of psychotherapy and the world is getting worse" (Hillman & Ventura, 1993, p. 3). Locating and treating only "the psyche inside the skin" leaves out an entire world that is deteriorating. The author of this chapter believes that it is vital to recognize that "the soul of the world" has been ignored to the expense of the individual's soul, and "the buildings are sick, the institutions are sick, . . . the schools, the streets. . ." (Hillman & Ventura, 1993, pp. 3–4).

There is no one single cause that could fully explain the apparition and developments of eating disorders. Therefore, this chapter proposes that eating disorders are the result of the concurrence of several categories of factors, which feed each other back positively and negatively. Biological, psychological, and socio–relational factors, in a given family system, in the appropriate circumstances, elicit a psychosomatic syndrome (Minuchin, Rosman & Baker, 1979) related to food and the act of eating: the eating disorder.

Because of the limited space available within this chapter, I will focus my exploration on what I consider as one of the main issues associated with eating disorders: anxiety. "Anxiety is the reaction to the *threat to any pattern which the individual has developed upon which he feels his safety to depend,*" and "a reaction to a threat to some value which the individual holds essential to his existence as a personality" (May, 1977, pp. 162–163).

In the following paragraphs, I am going to demonstrate that *anxiety*, together with all its clinical manifestations (compulsion, obsession, social phobia, etc.), are at the core of the two best clinically described eating disorders: anorexia and bulimia nervosa. Then I will analyze, from a multidisciplinary perspective, the sources of and the role–played by anxiety, with direct reference to Family/Families of an Adolescent Diagnosed with Eating Disorder (FADED–see Definition of Terms at the end of the chapter). Next, I will show that *ritual* is one of the most efficient mechanisms to alleviate and conquer excessive anxiety; an analysis of the relationship between *ritual* and *compulsion* will follow. And finally, we will look into how Existential Drama Therapy can provide tools to explore and address the anxiety and fears which have been centered around eating and food in a FADED.

Although I am always mindful of the clinical diagnosis perspective, in my approach to counseling and psychotherapy, I am more interested in a multidisciplinary, holistic view of an illness or symptom. As Paul E. Garfinkel writes, "Awareness of psychological theory of development, unconscious conflict, or the therapeutic process is not needed to make a diagnosis. This absence of meaning must be addressed if we are to retain humanistic orientation, for it is impossible to treat suffering individuals if we are devoid of an awareness of history, symbolic meaning, conflict, ambivalence, social context and the primacy of existential concerns" (Garfinkel, 2002, p. 160). As we will see further on, in order to obtain therapeutic results that are stable and meaningful, eating disorders need to be examined within one's historical, developmental, and social context.

Eating Disorders and Anxiety

Clinical and epidemiological studies show that there is a substantial comorbidity between anorexia and anxiety disorders. In fact, "well over half of women with anorexia nervosa report the lifetime presence of an anxiety disorder—most commonly generalized anxiety disorder, obsessive–compulsive disorder, and social phobia" (Bulik, 2002, p. 194). In the acute phase of the illness, clients with anorexia experience a pervasive anxiety and obsessive preoccupation with any issue that relates to food, body shape, and weight. "Retrospective clinical information suggests that women with anorexia nervosa have premorbid obsessional traits, and they retain high scores on obsessionality indices" (Bulik, 2002, p. 194). Many studies indicate that the onset of anxiety disorder precedes the onset of anorexia nervosa. Also, early onset of an anxiety disorder is considered a serious risk for developing bulimia. More precise, "childhood anxiety represents one significant pathway towards the development of anorexia nervosa" (Bulik, 2002, p. 194).

Social phobia and generalized anxiety appear to be also the most common disorders that accompany bulimia nervosa. In fact, some treatment methods assume that bingeing and purging have anxiolytic effects (the anxiety reduction model), and that bulimic eating behaviors and attitudes are the result of a heightened social anxiety that fuels body dissatisfaction. Likewise in anorexia, early onset of an anxiety disorder is considered a serious risk for developing bulimia (Bulik, 2002).

Sources and Purpose of Anxiety in Eating Disorders

Existential Drama Therapy proposes that anxiety experienced by ADED has several sources: the developmental stage of the adolescent, where anxiety constitutes a normal ingredient; an unstructured, avoidant, ambivalent, family system (FADED); the social environment which, particularly in Western societies, is organized as a hyperreality (Baudrillard, 1985), and progresses towards more and more compartmentalization, ultra–specialization, alienation, disconnection from the natural rhythms and creation of virtual (pseudo) connections; and existential meaninglessness and loneliness (the experience of potentiality of freedom) (Kierkegaard, 1941). As I will show in the last part of this chapter, by placing the client at aesthetic distance, drama therapy allows for a deconstruction of automatic, destructive reactions generated by existential concerns.

The existential source of anxiety is related to four ultimate concerns: death, freedom, loneliness and meaninglessness (Yalom, 1980). It is very interesting to notice that the adolescent's individuation, seen as a cycle of separations/fusions, mirrors the existential cycle fear of life/fear of death described by Yalom (1980). Fear of life is a fear of separation, of existing as a separate entity, fear of not belonging and of not being connected. Fear of death is fear of fusion, of engulfment, of disappearing into an undifferentiated mass (Yalom, 1980). If we define anxiety as objectless fear (May, 1977), then we can assert that anxiety (objectified as fear of something) is the drive that pushes an individual to oscillate between states of separation and fusion (Gheorghe, 2001). These oscillations may lead to individuation and growth or to overwhelming anxiety (Gheorghe & Rojas, 2005), which will tend to be resolved through repetitive acts, like those related to food and eating.

In their paradoxical need and search for both individuality and belonging, adolescents are especially amenable by the social and cultural attitudes and behavior created around body image, success and failure, satisfaction and happiness. With some particularities from a country and culture to another, it is noticeable what Stice (2002, p. 103) calls *social reinforcement*, the process whereby people internalize attitudes and exhibit behaviors approved by respected others, and *modeling*, the process wherein individuals directly emulate behaviors they observe. As Stice (2002, p. 104) points out, "there is considerable correlational, prospective, and experimental evidence that mass media contribute to body image and eating disturbances," with "increased body dissatisfaction and negative affect." Also, "a natural experiment found that the rates of body image and eating disturbance increased following the introduction of Western media to Fiji, a culture initially devoid of thin–ideal images" (Stice, 2002, p. 104).

Many of us secretly hope or openly believe that our hair would look as great as Naomi Campbell's, if we only used the product she uses. That a cell phone, especially the thin one with camera, radio, and MP3 player, will instantly eliminate miscommunication, loneliness, and anxiety from our life. That we would be (more) liked, (more) popular and overall a much better person, only if we had Christina Aguilera's thin waist. Anxious, confused, aggressed or just bored, the adolescents make more and more space in their lives for the meaningless role of "voracious consumer" (Taffel, 2006, p. 36), hoping that by consuming the same products as the celebrities they will

become successful, powerful, and self–confident. "They're seduced into wor-
shipping physical perfection; to create at all costs, a flawless body 'to die for'"
(Taffel, 2006, p. 36). As we will see in the next part of this chapter, the modeling mechanism proposed by Stice (2002) is the twenty–first century substitute of what Eliade describes in the archaic societies as *ritual*: an imitation
(modeling! . .) of a divine prototype (Eliade, 1991).

It is important to note that the nature of social relationships has changed
significantly in the last half a century. The decrease of the individual's role
and identity as an active citizen in a democracy, and the expansion of the
consumer identity, have changed the way individuals interact within the society, community, and family. The audience has become *consumer of information and entertainment*; students have become *consumers of knowledge*; patients
have become *consumers of health*. In his critique and brilliant demonstration
on how business relationships tend to become the main way of social interaction, George Soros points out that there is an increased belief in Western
societies that "individuals and their interests are best expressed by their decisions as market participants. For instance, if they feel philanthropic they can
express it by giving money away" (Soros, 1998, p. xxv). Soros warns that in
this type of society genuine human interaction and all social activities are
being replaced more and more by "transactional, contract–based relationships, and valued in terms of a single common denominator, money.
Activities would be regulated, as far as possible, by nothing more intrusive
than the invisible hand of profit–maximizing competition" (Soros, 1998, p.
xxvii). As members of such a social structure, overwhelmed, and confused
parents and adolescents find refuge and comfort in a role and an environment that paradoxically expands their isolation, loneliness and alienation,
intensifying the overall anxiety. As we will see later on, the above mentioned
social mechanism (i.e., structuring an overwhelming and anxiogenic environment) is mirrored in the microcosm of the family system, where ADED
uses repetitive behaviors and thoughts related to eating and food, in order to
gain a sense of control. It is interesting that while life in the Western, "developed" countries goes towards an intense "globalization," the individuals living in these countries become in fact more and more isolated and lonely
(Beck, 2006). Additionally, the potentiality of freedom to have virtually
unlimited and instant mediated connection is accompanied by great anxiety
(Kierkegaard, 1977, p. 38). Written, audio and video connection with every
corner of the world is available, affordable, and, moreover, portable. Also, in
opposition with the apparent globalization, individuals' ways of understanding and approaching life tends to narrow. In an ultra competitive, global market there is a tendency at the individual level to ultra–specialize. One of the
most important consequences of ultra specialization, especially when that
happens in fields like mental health, medicine, art, and education, is the
decline of intimacy–sponsoring institutions (Yalom, 1980), which has dra-

matically increased social loneliness, meaninglessness, disconnection, and alienation

Another big source of anxiety in FADED is the family system itself, more precise, the way the family members relate to each other, which Salvador Minuchin calls the family dance (Minuchin, Rosman and Baker, 1979). The way FADED functions reproduces, at a smaller scale, the previously described societal functioning. Parental pressure to loose weight and family criticism regarding weight, modeling of abnormal eating behavior, parental body dissatisfaction, are significantly correlated with the appearance of eating disorders in adolescents (Stice, 2002). There is evidence that "general disturbances in family functioning are related to eating pathology, individuals with eating disorders reporting that their families are more conflicted, disorganized, critical and less cohesive compared to controls" (Stice, 2002, p. 105). However, although usually the family presents itself to the therapist divided in two confronting teams, i.e., parents on one side and the adolescent with eating disorder on the other side, I would like to emphasize that there is no specific family member to blame for the eating disorder. The anxiety that dominates ADED's life is the result of the family members' way of interacting and relating to each other. It is the family system, through its interpersonal transactions and feedback circularity which organizes the behavior of the family members in dysfunctional patterns, manifested as psychosomatic syndromes: anorexia and bulimia nervosa (Minuchin, Rosman & Baker, 1979). There are four characteristics of the family functioning, described by Minuchin and colleagues (1979), responsible for generating the intense anxiety in a family environment that is unpredictable, ambivalent, unstructured, and chaotic. They are (see Appendix of Terms at the end of the chapter): (1) *over involvement, enmeshment,* or *excessive togetherness;* (2) *overprotectivenes;* (3) *rigidity;* and (4) *a very low threshold for conflict,* combined with an intense *avoidance of conflict* and consequently a lack of conflict resolution (Minuchin, Rosman & Baker, 1979, pp. 30–31). It is the adolescent who reroutes, absorbs, and eventually expresses the family anxiety, by acting out (opposition, defiance, antisocial behavior) or, in FADED case, by acting in: self starvation, bingeing and purging, etc. As we will see in the next section, by mimicking an archaic structuring mechanism (ritual), ADED use destructive compulsive behavior as a "tool" to manage the intense and generalized anxiety s/he experiences.

Ritual and Compulsion: The Sacred and Destructiveness of Repetition

As previously discussed, unstructured, unpredictable, and chaotic environments are a great source of anxiety. In addition, anxiety itself *is* chaos, non–structure, dissolution, and non–being. As defined by Rollo May, anxiety is "the feeling of diffuseness and uncertainty and the experience of helplessness toward the threat," as opposed to fear, which May defines as "a reaction to a specific danger, to which the individual can make a specific adjustment" (May, 1977, p. 162). Whenever one perceives too much chaos/anxiety, one will push for *creation*, as a way of transforming unbearable anxiety into bearable structure. This is what happens in FADED: the anxious adolescent will precipitate into organizing the anxiety into something that makes sense, something that can be grasped, manipulated, and controlled. Although a structure, the solution found by ADED is a vicious structure, a vicious circle that leads to negative consequences and perpetuates the problem. As we will see in the last part of this chapter existential drama Therapy, besides creating awareness and connecting FADED with a meaningful existence, creates also a transitional space (Grainger, 1995; Johnson, 1998; Jones, 1996) where the deconstruction of the vicious circle and the *re–creation* of a meaningful spiral are possible.

In the following paragraphs, I am going to introduce and discuss the main hypothesis of this chapter: (1)ritual and compulsion are two different facets of the same behavior: *repetition;* (2) both are used by FADED to manage anxiety; (3) by understanding the structure and purpose of ritual, existential drama therapy allows the creative arts therapist to (a) deconstruct compulsion, (b) replace it with a meaningful structure, and hence (c) reduce intensity of and enhance tolerance for anxiety and non–structure, with a consequent submission of eating disorder symptoms.

In order to understand the connection between ritual and compulsion, and the way they relate to anxiety, I am going to analyze first the origin and purpose of ritual. *Webster's Dictionary* defines ritual as an established procedure for a ceremonious act, prescribed or customary in a solemn situation. In a broader sense, ritual is represented by any practice or pattern of behavior, regularly performed in a set manner (*Random House Webster's College Dictionary*, 2000). On another hand, according to the anthropologist Mircea Eliade, ritual represents a repetition of a primordial, archetypal act, which has been performed for the very first time by a god/goddess or a hero (Eliade, 1991). This archetypal act is considered *sacred*, because it happened in a mythical (sacred) time, which proceeded the actual, historical, and profane time. For that reason, Eliade calls it *illo tempore*, which translates from Latin as *that time*, the *once upon a time*, described in myths, fairy tales, and legends. The primordial act is sacred also because it happened in a sacred space, considered as a center of the world (in Latin: *Axis Mundi = the axis of the world*), around which communities gathered ever since. The most common examples of Axis Mundi are the churches and temples, and prayer is the ritual that is structured around the axis mundi that they represent.

Eliade (1991) argues that when one performs a ritual, one repeats and re–actualizes the quality of the act, gesture, or event performed originally in the sacred time and space, by a god (goddess), ancestor, or hero. That is, the performance of the ritual produces a consecration: the sacred contained by the archetypal act is invoked and re–actualized each time that act is performed. Through ritualization, an ordinary act is taken out of the present (profane) time and space, and projected in the mythical time and space becoming sacred. For the individual who performs it, the ritual provides structure and meaning, with alleviation of anxiety, which translates into peace, comfort, and healing.

Thus, ritual has three main qualities that are relevant for the creative arts therapist who wants to use existential drama therapy. First, ritual is a structured and predictable act, and consequently a tool that one uses to create meaning and structure in an unpredictable, insecure, chaotic environment. Second, it is organized around a core, a center, called Axis Mundi. And third, when performed, ritual lends the power, strength and sacred of the gods or heroes who originally performed it.

Looking closely to compulsion, we will notice that it has very similar qualities with ritual. First of all, likewise ritual, compulsion is a repetitive act. Also, compulsion manifests itself as a reaction to unstructured, out of control, anxiety producing environment. And finally, repeating something in a compulsive way offers anxiety relief. Observations that involved World War I veterans who had parts of their brain shot away showed that these patients had very limited capabilities to adjust to a dynamic environment. Changing the arrangement of their clothes and shoes, or placing the veterans in what they perceived as "catastrophic situations" (a space where objects were in disarray), elicited reactions of profound anxiety. As a way to protect themselves from the overwhelming anxiety generated by unstructured environments, these patients developed an acute sense of and need for order, which evolved into "compulsive patterns for orderliness" (May, 1977, pp. 57–58).

Compulsion is defined as "an irrational need to perform some action, often despite negative consequences" (online Wikipedia). Often, for parents of an ADED it does not make any sense: why does their adolescent keep doing the same harmful thing? If we look at compulsion as an altered version of ritual, a tool that ADED use to manage a diffuse uncertain threat to their core values, then things become more clear. ADED create their own rituals around food and eating in order to avoid or diminish the unbearable anxiety, and to gain a sense of control of an ambiguous and ambivalent environment, of a situation that they perceive as catastrophic, in which they cannot actualise their capacities, and with which they believe they cannot cope otherwise (May, 1977, p. 58). In anorexia nervosa for example, self–esteem becomes directly proportional with thinness: the thinner one becomes, the better one feels about oneself. "The patient holds on to her emaciation as a form of self–realization and identifies with her wasted body" (Beaumont, 2002, p.163). In bulimia, the anxiety is perceived as void, as *absence*, in its two major forms, *longing* and *loss*. As we will see later, Sysiphus and The Absent Angel are characters in FADED enactments, representing compulsion and respectively the internal void. Also, Thinness and Anxiety are Axis Mundi around which compulsion (and not ritual) is organized, and they are the main ingredients of the personification, externalization, and enactment techniques presented at the end of this chapter.

In conclusion, ritual is a structured, repetitive, and sacred act which provides self–empowerment, meaning, and comfort in anxiety producing situations. Compulsion is also a repetitive act, which manifests itself in similar situations and has the same purpose as ritual: to structure the chaotic, unpredictable environment (which initially created the compulsion) and to manage the accompanying anxiety. Thus, ritual and compulsion can be regarded as different facets of the same diamond: repetition. In fact, compulsion can be considered a *substitute* for ritual, hence a *pseudo–ritual*, employed in an environment that produces unbearable anxiety and which provides a harmful, pseudo–structure.

Rituals take place every moment in today's society and families, and they can play a key role in the way creative arts therapists approach the concepts of illness and healing. There are certainly differences between an archaic society and a twenty–first century society, mainly related to the continuous process that Eliade calls "desacralization" (Eliade, 1991, p. 28). However, there are two things that have persisted over the centuries. One of them is *anxiety* (with its existential and social component), although nowadays the quality of anxiety differs significantly. The second one is the way people cope with anxiety, which has remained essentially the same: (1) making sense of chaos and unknown through repetitive, structured behavior (ritual or compulsion), organized around an Axis Mundi, and (2) alleviating anxiety by infusing themselves with the power and the prestige of an archetypal–like being.

As it was shown in this chapter, the re–actualization through ritual is called by nowadays sociologists and psychologists *modeling* and *social reinforcement*. In order to achieve a sense of competency, security and belonging, the adolescent imitates the behavior and the look of a respected other (Stice, 2002), represented most likely in Western societies by celebrities: fashion models, musicians, criminals, politicians, financial managers, etc. In a social environment where progressive desacralization has been creating a chronic lack of meaning and a void of faith (May, 1977), celebrities are substitutes for the "old–fashioned" gods, goddesses and mythic heroes. Being thin, loosing weight, being fit, like the celebrities, is perceived by many adolescents (and often by their parents) as a condition sine qua non for being accepted, liked, and successful. Similarly, the adolescent in FADED attempts to eliminate the anxiety that s/he experiences by repeatedly performing specific acts, aimed at transforming the unknown and the unspoken within the family system into a somehow manageable experience: compulsions related to food and the act of eating. Physical exercise, calorie count, bingeing and purging, become compulsions, mere repetitive acts, aimed at structuring the undefined anxiety. But what differentiates in this case a ritual from a compulsion? First, the same act can be a ritual or a compulsion according to the circumstances and the frequency of the repetitive behavior.

Second, a compulsion lacks sacred. And third, the nature of the Axis Mundi is crucial in defining if a repetitive behavior will become a destructive compulsion or a meaningful, healing ritual. In fact, the meaningfulness of an act is given by the quality of the Axis Mundi. ADED structures their compulsion around a destructive Axis Mundi: the center of the specific world of the anorexic individual is the pursuit of thinness, and all of his/her life and actions revolve around that. The anorexic has as main purpose in life to be thin, and life ends up being perceived as meaningful only as long as it is in some way related to thinness. Around that are built activities related to food and eating, which eventually become compulsions, in the adolescent's relentless pursuit of structuring the anxiety, of gaining competency and control.

Treatment Techniques: A Mythical Model

> The imitation of the paradigmatic acts of the Gods, the Heroes, and the mythical Ancestors does not produce an "eternal repetition of the same thing," a total cultural immobility. . . . Though the myths, by presenting themselves as sacrosanct models, would seem to paralyze human initiative, actually they stimulate man to create, they are constantly opening new perspectives to his inventiveness. . . . The existence of an exemplary model does not fetter creative innovation. The possibilities for applying the mythical model are endless. (Mircea Eliade, "Myth and Reality," 1975, pp. 140–141)

With this we enter into the practical application of existential drama therapy. As we saw, for the archaic societies, connected to their environment physically and spiritually, this anxiety was resolved through ritual: "There is no reason to fear settling in an unknown territory," Eliade writes (p. 141). One, following the example of the Gods/Goddesses/Heroes, merely repeats "the cosmogonic ritual, whereupon the territory (= Chaos) is transformed into Cosmos. Therefore, repetition in a myth does not produce a vicious circle, but what in existential drama therapy is called a *meaningful spiral*. In this case, the therapeutic process has the function of the ritual: creates a transitional space (the equivalent of the mythical sacred space), and projects the FADED into illo tempore, the sacred time of the beginning. Also, existential drama therapy changes the quality of the ADED's Axis Mundi, from a destructive one that generates a vicious circles, to a meaningful axis, which opens new perspectives. By restoring the sacred, repetition does not manifest anymore as compulsion, but as meaningful creativity.

The main assertion of this chapter is that treatment efficiency of eating disorders increases significantly when the therapist uses a multidisciplinary approach. Gaining awareness of the deep and complex interconnections between one's behavior and the physical, social, and mythological reality creates a sense of belonging, and provides healing through the reduction of alienation and anxiety.

The techniques proposed by the existential drama therapy model are not complicated or never seen before. They are based on the assertion of this chapter that eating disorders (excluding organic deficiencies) are a psychosomatic syndrome and mainly an expression of the overwhelming anxiety the adolescent experiences. Therefore, working with and through anxiety at existential, social, and personal level, will reduce or eliminate the psychosomatic syndrome.

Mapping, Personification, Externalization, and Enactment

One of the main concepts I use frequently in my interventions is *Aesthetic Distance*. The term comes from theater and it is Robert Landy who introduced it in the drama therapy theory (Landy, 1994). For the purpose of this chapter, I will define Aesthetic Distance as *the optimal psychological distance or area at which one places oneself, so that one is not too close, and therefore invaded and engulfed by anxiety, but not too far, removed, denying the existence or the effect of anxiety.* The goal of the following techniques is to have the ADED become aware of and feel their aesthetically distanced area. This allows them to gain clarity and strength, needed to acknowledge the existence of the destructive Axis Mundi (thinness, bingeing and purging, anxiety, etc.) around which the eating disorder has been built, and to break the vicious circle.

As mentioned previously, Rollo May (1977) states that anxiety *"strikes at that basis of the psychological structure on which the perception of one' self as distinct from the world of objects occurs."* "One is afraid but uncertain of what one is afraid." "One cannot fight what one doesn't know" (May, 1977, pp. 206–207). It is the purpose of *Personification* technique to objectify, externalize, and make anxiety known. The client is asked to describe Anxiety in terms of a person. Would it be a woman or man? Is s/he a stranger or a known person? What is the age and the physical appearance of this person?

What is his/her name? Describe her/his clothes, behavior, voice, gestures, etc. Inspired by a book of Lewis Hyde (1983), I established that there are four ways of dealing with anxiety: to pretend it does not exist (denial), to permanently fight with it, to identify with it, and to invite it to a dialog. During the next few individual sessions, the client is asked to have imaginary dialogs with Anxiety, and processing time is allowed. During the family sessions, the description of Anxiety and the dialogs are discussed and the family is engaged in enacting them. Most of the time, the parents of ADED begin sharing about their anxiety and they way they deal with it. The therapeutic focus shifts from the adolescent and his or her disorder, to the way FADED deals with anxiety and in fact with each other. The compulsive and obsessive behavior is mentioned and situated within the specific environment (family, community, culture, etc.). As a result, the eating disorder and the anxiety are externalized, established as distinct from self, as the adolescent places himself or herself at aesthetic distance.

Mapping. Using sandtray figures (or pencil and paper), the adolescent is asked to choose or draw a representation of Thinness and place it in the middle. Next, the client is told to choose three people that are significant for his or her life and place them around thinness. Next, adding three emotions that are perceived as dominant in his/her life; then three meaningful smells/perfumes/fragrances; three sounds; and then three images or memories, or dreams, or a combination of these three categories. Various maps can be created, by placing Anxiety, Loss, Longing and then the client himself or herself in the middle. Stories that involve the map's elements are told, followed in the family sessions by sculptures and enactments with the participation of the family members (Emunah, 1994). The goal of mapping is to create awareness about the existence and the nature of Axis Mundi, and about the repetitive behavior organized around it: destructive (compulsion), or to constructive, meaningful and enriching (ritual). Also, an emphasis is put on the client's relationship with the environment, and the eating disorder is regarded as a result of systemic interactions.

The last technique involves mostly enactment. First, myths and stories involving the main characters are shared: Sisyphus (the personification and symbol of the vicious circle and being stuck); The Absent Angel (the personification of absence, nostalgia, loneliness, longing, etc.); Thinness; Anxiety. Using these characters and family members and/or scarves to represent them, the adolescent creates a sculpture, which moves towards enactment when each character is given a line. Old family and individual stories are explored, compared with and integrated in the world stories. New stories are developed and meaningful relationships with the world and with self are established.

CONCLUSION

Eating disorders are not merely illnesses that invade individuals. When a medical condition is not present, eating disorders are psychosomatic expressions of specific relationships established within the family, community, and society. Therefore, in order to properly understand and treat them, a systemic and multidisciplinary approach is needed. Patients need to be considered within the context of their social, economical and political environment. Anxiety is found at the core of eating disorders and it is the result of relationships established in "anorectic families" (Minuchin et al., 1978). The number of eating disorders cases is directly proportional to the levels of anxiety, isolation, and meaninglessness experienced by individuals, families and societies, which in turn are fostered by the replacement of social human interactions with contract–based relationships and market–based transactions (Soros, 1998).

Existential drama therapy uses Eliade's Mythical Model to explore the similarity between *ritual* and *compulsion*, as forms of the same act, *repetition*, which occurs in eating disorders as a way of providing structure to an unbearably chaotic and anxiety provoking environment. The repetition of a ritual, defined as the imitation of paradigmatic acts of Gods, Heroes and/or Ancestors, provides meaning and sense of belonging. On the same continuum with ritual, compulsion is a form of repetition that leads to even more anxiety, with possible negative consequences and destruction.

Using creative arts, as well as existential, systemic, and structural concepts, existential drama therapy proposes a few techniques, easy to use by any clinician. The author welcomes any questions, comments, or reports on the results of the concepts and techniques presented in this chapter (www.SynergisCounseling.com, cosmin@SynergisCounseling.com)

Appendix–Terms

FADED–Family/Families with Adolescent Diagnosed with Eating Disorder.

ADED–Adolescent(s) Diagnosed with Eating Disorder.

Over involvement/enmeshment/excessive togetherness–"an extreme form of proximity and intensity in family interactions," which "brings about a lack of privacy" and intrusion "on each others' thoughts and feelings" (Minuchin, Rosman & Baker, 1979, pp. 30–31).

Overprotectivenes (or hypersensitivity)–"high degree of concern of family members for each others' welfare" (Minuchin, Rosman & Baker, 1979, pp. 30–31).

Rigidity–an intense commitment for maintaining the status quo of a given family (Minuchin, Rosman & Baker, 1979, pp. 30–31).

References

Baudrillard, J. (1985). *Simulacres et simulation.* Paris, France: Galilee.

Beck, A. (2006). *Americans are more socially isolated than 20 years ago.* Retrieved June 23rd, 2006 from www.yahoo.com/news.

Bulik, C. M. (2002). Anxiety, depression and eating disorders. In C. G. Fairburn & K. D. Brownell (Eds.), *Eating disorder and obesity: A comprehensive handbook* (pp. 193–1998). New York: Guilford Press.

Eliade, M. (1991). *Eseuri: Mitul eternei reintoarceri. Mituri, vise si mistere.* Bucuresti, Romania: Editura Stiintifica.

Eliade, M. (1992) Sacrul si profanul. Bucuresti, Romania : Humanitas.

Emunah, R. (1994). *Acting for real: Drama therapy process, technique and performance.* Levittown: Brunner/Mazel.

Garfinkel, P. E. (2002). Classification and diagnosis of eating disorders. In C. G. Fairburn & K. D. Brownell (Eds.), *Eating disorder and obesity: A comprehensive handbook* (pp. 155–161). New York: Guilford Press.

Gheorghe, C. (2001). *The retrieval of the lost time: My three steps toward aesthetic distance.* Unpublished manuscript.

Gheorghe, C., & Rojas, P. (2005). *Individuality, individualism, individuation: The therapy and politics of separation.* Paper presented at the International Conference of Family Therapy, organized by American Association of Family Therapy (AFTA).

Grainger, R. (1995). *Drama and healing: The Roots of drama therapy.* London, U.K.: Jessica Kingsley Publishers.

Hillman, J., & Ventura, M. (1993). *We've had a hundred years of therapy–and the world is getting worse.* San Francisco: HarperCollins.

Hyde, L. (1983). *The gift: Imagination and erotic life of property.* New York: Vintage Books, Random House.

Johnson, D. (1998). On the therapeutic action of the creative art therapies: The psychodynamic model. *The Arts in Psychotherapy, 25,* 85–99.

Jones, P. (1996). *Drama as therapy, theatre as living.* London, U.K.: Routledge.

Kierkegaard, S. (1941). *The sickness unto death.* New York: Doubleday.

May, R. (1977). *The meaning of anxiety.* New York: W.W. Norton & Company, Inc.

Minuchin, S., Rosman, B.L., & Baker, L. (1978). *Psychosomatic families: Anorexia nervosa in context.* Cambridge, Massachusetts: Harvard University Press.

Random House Webster's College Dictionary. (2000). New York: Random House.

Soros, G. (1998). *The crisis of global capitalism: Open society endangered.* New York: Public Affairs.

Stice, E. (2002). Sociocultural influences on body image and eating disturbance. In C. G. Fairburn & K.D. Brownell (Eds.), *Eating disorder and obesity: A comprehensive handbook* (pp. 103–107). New York: Guilford Press.

Taffel, R. (2006). The divided self. *Psychotherapy Networker, July/August,* 32–39.

Yalom, I. D. (1980). *Existential psychotherapy.* San Francisco: HarperCollins.

Biography

Cosmin Gheorghe is a graduate of the Counseling Psychology program, concentration in Drama Therapy, from California Institute of Integral Studies in San Francisco, CA. He also holds a Medical Degree in General Medicine, obtained at the University of Medicine and Pharmacy Timisoara, Romania. He is a Licensed Marriage and Family Therapist in California and New York. Cosmin's knowledge and experience have been enriched by his participation in numerous international workshops and conferences in France, Netherlands, Czech Republic, Romania and the U.S. His presentations include *Reorganizing Vicious Circles into Meaningful Spirals: Aesthetic Distance and Existential Drama Therapy* and *Individuality, Individualism, Individuation: The Politics and Psychotherapy of Separation.* Together with Patricia Rojas, MFT, he founded in San Francisco *Synergis Counseling, Psychotherapy and Consulting,* a private practice that reflects the idea of a synergic, multidisciplinary and meaningful approach to psychotherapy and life.

Chapter 13

NOURISHING THE INNER CHILD: THE SESAME APPROACH OF DRAMA AND MOVEMENT THERAPY WITH TEENS RECOVERING FROM DISORDERED EATING

PRIYADARSHINI SENROY

Abstract

The chapter begins with a very brief statistics of teens with disordered eating in Ontario, Canada. It then gives information about the day treatment program where this research takes place and the challenges faced by the author while facilitating the group sessions. The chapter continues by explaining the *Sesame Approach* that formed the basis of the therapeutic work, on the theme chosen, nourishing the inner child. Three session vignettes explain the process work and the approaches which were chosen to explore the areas of rediscovering and nourishing the feeling, intuitive, spontaneous, and creative inner child. The chapter finishes with a conclusion followed by bibliography.

Introduction

In a 2001 school–based study published by the Canadian Paediatric Society, 27 percent Ontario girls, aged 12–18 years old were reported to be engaged in severely problematic food and weight behaviour (Jones et al., 2001). It lists eating disorders to be the third most common chronic illness in adolescent girls. While the most common age of onset is between 14 and 25 years of age, eating disorders occur in a wide range of ages and are increasingly seen in children as young as 10. With such high numbers, teens exhibiting symptoms of eating disorders often require evaluation and treatment focused on biological, psychological, and social features of these complex chronic health conditions. Assessment and ongoing management are usually interdisciplinary and is best accomplished by a team consisting of medical, nursing, nutritional, and mental health professionals. Hospitalization of an adolescent with an eating disorder is necessary in the presence of malnutrition, clinical evidence of medical or psychiatric manifestations, or failure of outpatient treatment. In this case, ongoing treatment is usually delivered with appropriate frequency, intensity, and duration. In the province of Ontario, Canada, there are several day treatment programs as well as hospitals where teens are referred to undergo various kinds of treatments according to the severity of their disorder (Adolescent Medicine Committee, Canadian Paediatric Society, 2001).

The Setting

The research took place in one of the many Eating Disorders Programs based in a children's hospital in Ontario, Canada. This program is an intensive treatment option for adolescents suffering from Anorexia Nervosa, Bulimia Nervosa, and Eating Disorders Not Otherwise Specified. Key components of the program include Outpatient Services, Day Treatment Program, Inpatient Services, and Parent Support Group. The Day Treatment Program is for adolescents with serious eating disorders who are medically stable but who require intensive treatment and support due to the severity and complexity of their disorder. The program operates 8–10 hours per day, five days per week. This program can accommodate up to 12 patients at any one time and the expected average length of stay is three months.

The Approach

There are many creative therapeutic modalities, which were used successfully to work with the eating disordered population. Many are direct approaches and some are indirect. One of the key components of the treatment program used as an alternate and indirect therapeutic intervention technique was drama and movement therapy based on the *Sesame Approach*. This approach is unique as it combines dramatherapy and movement therapy in one experiential process oriented methodology. The Sesame Approach works obliquely, based in the knowledge that most of us reveal the nature of our difficulties through metaphor and symbol. Exploring drama and movement in a safe and structured environment enable people to find ways of expressing their needs, fears, anxieties, and frustrations spontaneously and naturally. Having established the difficulty, the Sesame Approach uses drama and movement to promote healing and change through an indirect rather than direct approach to them. The Sesame Approach shares the holistic approaches found within drama and movement therapy, but it also has its own individual method and practice. This incorporates the therapeutic use of movement observation developed by Rudolf Laban, child drama discovered by Peter Slade, and the enactment of symbolic stories based on Carl Jung's concept of the psyche (Pearson 1996). The client is never judged by the quality of their contribution, as the work is not geared towards performance. All the work of the session is done within the art form, with no attempt at interpretation of personal material (Pearson 1996).

Rationale of Using the Sesame Approach

Carl Jung, the analyst, whose system of thought informs the basic theory of the Sesame Approach, saw the psyche as a self–regulating system with a natural tendency towards balance, growth, and consciousness (Pearson, 1996). It is in the nature of unconscious material to seek expression and psychological health depends on the integration of this material into consciousness, which is a vital aspect of the creative process. The psyche has a way of reasserting its lost meaning through symbols. These arise naturally in art, story, dance, music, dreams, and play (Pearson, 1996). All these qualities of the Sesame Approach made the process work accessible to the teens who undertook the therapeutic journey to explore and express a variety of emotions. The emphasis was working with inner child. The inner child is the original, often forgotten, authentic part of us which experiences life in a spontaneous, creative, intuitive, and innocent manner. The inner child is a reflection of our emotional makeup. Through inner child healing, one comes to understand their emotional child, their sabotaging and self–esteem issues, and eventually empowers themselves into freedom of body, mind, and soul.

During the experiential process, the teens found ways to communicate with their feelings, spontaneity, creativity, and intuition of their inner child in a non–judgmental atmosphere created by the playful and spontaneous structure. The drama and movement therapy, through their ability to access the unconscious easily, was able to quickly bring out information and lead to insights that were new to the teens, individually as well as a group. The teens found that the process of making images in therapy allowed them to see, sometimes for the first time, aspects of their inner world that they were previously unaware of, or perhaps unable to explain. Teens with eating disorders often have opposing thoughts about body image, about how to feel good about themselves, about how to deal with their needs. The creative modalities exposed those puzzles that were then worked on therapeutically in with their psychotherapists. The sessions were lively and invigorating. Much of it was participative and experiential. Popular music, myths and legends, creative writing, free movement. and verbal discussions were used to explore and respond to the individual needs of participants. All the activities chosen were used to explore emotional responses, dispel myths, and discuss current concerns.

Sessions

The sessions happened over a period of two years. The group of teens met twice a week for two one–hour sessions. Participation in the sessions was part of their overall commitment to the program. The sessions were co–facilitated by a Child and Youth Worker attached to the program. Further, the sessions were recorded at the end of every week. A senior staff provided regular supervision. As the turnover of the group was short, all interventions were short term in nature and needed to be comprehensive and compact. As a result, there was always an overlap between new and old clients. Some of the teens were there only for three or four sessions while the others were there for a longer period. As a result, the groups had to be catered and planned according to themes and self contained in one sessions. Continuity was difficult during transition times. The working contract of the sessions had to be clarified and the boundaries clearly defined to accommodate new members joining the group. At the same time, sessions had to incorporate therapeutic endings to facilitate smooth transition for members leaving the group.

The session vignettes which are being shared are some of the *golden moments* that took place with respect to the Sesame sessions. A golden moment, when it happens in a Sesame Session, is described as when the participant finds release and growth through touching on a symbol of the self. Such moments can arise when involuntary connection is made to an image in the session, which may come about because of an unconscious choice of role and movement pattern (Pearson, 1996). The scope of the chapter was not able to include the many such sessions, which took place, but never the less had psychological impacts on the teens. The degree of participation and expression varied in the group depending on their level of comfort and knowledge of the Sesame Approach. Each session was structured through a warm–up, main event, and grounding. The Sesame toolkit included enactment, spontaneous dramatic play, and non–verbal expressions using movement, and music. Verbal feedback was also encouraged to emphasise the importance of expressive language.

Session Vignettes

The first vignette focuses on rediscovering and nourishing the intuitive inner child. Intuition is a different kind of knowing (Johnston, 1996). It is composed of inner hearing, seeing, feeling, and knowing. It acts like an inner lighthouse that guides one's senses and helps one to trust one's instincts and insights while navigating through un–chartered waters of the unconscious. In eating disorders, one's intuition gets lost, is buried and loses its value through self–doubt, negative self–image and low self–esteem. Recovery from disordered eating involves reclaiming one's intuition, that inner authority that provides knowledge and compassionate guidance to develop an appreciation of the inner wise self. According to Johnson, the intuitive mind has access to a broader and deeper supply of knowledge (Johnston 1996).

One of the many therapeutic vehicles that the psyche uses to tap into this broader, richer and deeper supply is the art of storytelling and enactment. In this way, the individual is able to draw on the collective range of experiences and possible solutions, which are beyond their own experience and re-sources. Stories can therefore aid the individual's mastery over internal processes and external reality (Harper & Gray, 1997).

The Sesame Approach

The Sesame Approach uses myths, fairytales and stories from different cultures, roots and ages to connect the inner world of the child with the external reality of the society. These stories, as Jung Joseph Campbell, Marie Louise von Franz and Bruno Bettelheim have variously pointed out, originate and resonate in a very deep part of the psyche, calling up energies and feelings that seem to be universal and straight from the heart (Pearson, 1996).

Bruno Bettelheim in his work with children found why fairy tales were successful in enriching the inner life of the child. He realised that these tales appeal to the here and now of the psychological and emotional being of the child. He continues by explaining that the fairy tales speak about the severe inner pressures in a way that the child unconsciously understands, and without belittling the most serious inner struggles which growing up entails—offer examples of both temporary and permanent solutions to pressing difficulties (Bettelheim, 1976).

One such popular Russian fairy tale was chosen to explore the inner intuitive nature of the teens. This tale is a woman's initiation story. The feminine calls upon one's intuition and instincts in order to "sniff things out," use all the senses to wring the truth from things, and to extract nourishment from ideas. In the tale, Vasalisa the Wise is given a doll by her dying mother with these words of advice: "Should you lose your way or may be in need of help, ask this doll what to do, you will be assisted. Keep the doll with you always" (Estes, 1992). Vasalisa carries the doll during her journey to get the adventures in the forest to earn what she needs from Baba Yaga. From time to time, her doll gives her advice, and in the end, Vasalisa is able to bring the "fire" and in the process learn to trust her own intuition. The doll symbolises the inner intuitive child of Vasalisa, and by having it with her physically, helped her to readily access her unconscious instinctual self.

The group of teens first enacted the fairy tale with setting the different stages of the tale in different parts of the lounge where the sessions would take place. The sofas and coffee table became the symbolic forest of the unconscious, the unknown, and dark part of the psyche, which must be traversed during the heroine's journey to reach her goal. A revolving chair with three legs became Baba Yaga's chicken legs house. Orange, red, and yellow crepe papers were taped to a stick to resemble the fire.

Beginning from a point of silence, with predetermined roles voluntarily chosen by the group members, the enactment began. The tale unfolded as the characters came into the scene, did their part, and departed to form other parts of the story. Two members who went through the forest played Vasalisa and her doll as they clutched and talked to each other as the background of scary, eerie noises threatened their journey from time to time.

Upon reaching Baba Yaga's house, members who were part of the forest joined voices to portray Baba Yaga. It needs to be mentioned at this point that none of the members chose Baba Yaga's role and so the group and the therapist mutually decided to use voice and props to represent her. What followed next were the various tasks that Vasalisa had to accomplish with the help of her doll in order to get the "fire." Every time Vasalisa became frightened, her doll would say the right words to encourage her and every time Vasalisa would begin to lose faith in her self, the doll would say the right words to keep up her hope. The dialogues were improvised as the enactment was in process and the other group members would throw in encouraging words to Vasalisa. Once Vasalisa completed the impossible tasks just by listening to the guidance of her wise doll, Baba Yaga gave her the fire. Vasalisa returned with the fire and in the end, the same fire destroyed the stepmother and stepsisters.

As the enactment ended, the members were completely silent and on their own began to take down the props, bring a natural derole to the whole process. What followed was a verbal feedback. As the group deconstructed each phase, the therapist echoed back some of the scenes that were seemed to be powerful and thought provoking. The group first gave a feedback on the character roles that they had chosen. When mentioned that no one wanted to be Baba Yaga, one of them replied that she personally found it difficult to be a character which she thought was powerful and mean, yet provided the solution of the tale. The other members echoed and mentioned that no one wants to carry the archetype of the "shadow" even though there was gold in this "shadow" in the form of the fire. By getting the fire, Vasalisa was able to conquer not only her fear but also begin to listen to her own instincts represented by the doll. All the group members agreed that the doll represented Vasalisa's inner child, in a way their inner child. By going through the dialogues, the members who portrayed the roles of Vasalisa and the doll mentioned that now that she was thinking about her role, as she realizes that after some time in the enactment process, Vasalisa was talking to herself with encouraging words. And the member who played the role of the "doll" said that maybe that was the moment of truth, the moment of learning, the moment of healing, when Vasalissa did not need the doll physically to reconnect with her inner child. That was the time when Vasalisa looked into herself and found the inner strength by listening to herself. At this point, the therapist invited the group to reflect about any part of the story that they could personally relate to their disordered eating. What followed was a sharing of the different feelings the teens felt during many times when faced with relapses during their process of recovery. Some mentioned that even though a tiny voice inside themselves said that they could do it, that they could follow through with their plans and strategies, the external factors were too big and they often gave up on their "inner child"–they did not listen to their instincts, they did not nourish their inner child, their intuitive doll, with words of encouragement. They were not strong enough to defend their inner voice. The therapist mentioned that maybe by taking part in such narratives the teens were given important opportunities to gain insight into the way they arrange their life experiences and to develop intervention strategies, which will a provide greater understanding and coherence for growing up in an often complex and bewildering world (Gardner & Harper, 1997). They knew that they had the inner strength to overcome such forces, and no matter how fearful the shadow was, there was gold in it. No matter how impossible the tasks were, no matter how intimidating the jungle was, the main thing was to get the fire, and no matter how demoralizing the external factors were, they always had the intuitive doll within them. During her journey through the dark woods as she became more frightened, Vasalisa would pat her doll in her pocket and say: "Just touching the doll, yes I feel better." The same way whenever the teens would feel overwhelmed by their disordered eating, they would close their eyes and touch their inner child and say, yes, I feel better, yes, I can do this.

The second session vignette focuses on rediscovering and nourishing the feeling inner child. Research shows that many patients with eating problems struggle with alexithymia, which is defined as difficulty in putting feelings and fantasies into words (Zerbe, 2006). Eating disorders are incredibly complex and one of the ways the problem manifests is because of an individual's best attempt to cope in some way with internal or external stress. Feeling states manifest in the body, and the "site" of the eating disorder is the body itself, making body–based therapies ideal in helping those with eating problems.

Dance/movement therapy is effective as a technique to help those with eating and body image problems. In the eating disorders program, one of the areas to be addressed by the professional team was the area of dealing with alexithymia and how the movement therapy sessions would serve as an indirect approach for the clients to give a voice to their inner feelings via the non-verbal modality of using the body as a communication tool. The basic task in this area of work was to find the appropriate dramatic vehicle, which would enable the client to explore their experience, shift in behaviour, and relationship to body self and others (Dekker, 1996).

The human body in movement, however minimal that movement may be, speaks. The person moving feels freer and less self–conscious if movement is given motive – so a drama builds up with moods, inner states or characters being given living form. Movement may be the language that can become a spontaneous improvisation or it may be given a framework, using only key words that help to carry the heightened moments that are being experienced bodily. Such imaginative creativity opens doors of possibility, which may have been locked for years. The Sesame Approach of Movement Therapy sees itself as offering a key (Dekker, 1996).

When the movement therapy sessions were first introduced, almost all the members of the group showed certain degrees of confusion, fear, anxiety and apprehension. Some of the mentioned that they did not like moving or working with their bodies, some said they did not know how to dance, while one mentioned that they did not know how this would help them The therapist affirmed that them acknowledging their feelings was the first step in the right direction. Being aware of how they felt meant that they were beginning to feel again. They were beginning to get in touch with who they really were, their child within, their real self (Whitfield, 1990). Like any Sesame sessions, the therapist invited them to participate voluntarily and try not to think so much while doing. The group started by passing a hand squeeze in a circle to acknowledge, greet, and become one. The facilitator started a simple series of physical warm–ups and then opened it to the group to continue with their inputs. As the members began to tune up and started to listen to what and how their bodies wanted to move, their movements begin to evolve in a progressive manner. Initially, some of them were keeping themselves to their personal space and all the movements were close to their bodies, smaller in moving and did not use up the whole space. Their movements were also disjointed and the body did not move in unison. The movements were heavy and every step seemed to take a lot of effort. Applying Laban's terminology, we might suggest that in the early stages of the group experience the movements were firm, sudden, direct, and bound which seemed to reflect their disjointed and feelings of being split (Wethered, 1993). For many weeks through repeated music and movement activities, the patterns of movement began to change and the bodies started to move and explore the qualities of fine touch, flexibility, sustain, and flow. The sessions always had movement–based activities in conjunction with using props, visuals, artwork and music to facilitate the member's participation. In addition, this is what helped the members to see for themselves and others how their feelings effected their movement.

Such a session is described below giving individual responses and golden moments where a shift in physical, psychological, and emotional state was seen.

T changed into her pants when she found out that the session would involve movement.

S was coming to the group for the first time, so T refreshed on what we did last time and said that it was fun. Unlike the others she was not feeling lethargic and while doing a improvisation of walking in the park; while the rest of the group had a slow pace to their movement, she had a cheerful "skip" in her steps. She wanted to know if we would do masks in the end. She used paper to make waves like features and wrote her name on them. She then wore the masks and did a small "dance" using the waves as movement patterns and her name as the key word. In the feedback, she said that she enjoyed the name making activity, and she liked the movement part.

W was very sleepy and initially her movements were slow and sluggish, but picked up in the middle. Her name making involved using negative words of confusion, and she chose to use voice variations to spell out her name. She used angry voice, surprised voice, shaky voice, and dejected voice to spell her name. She showed creativity and imagination.

D was feeling sluggish too but managed to come out of it and worked well with the materials. Her name had a kind of zigzag pattern beneath the name print. I commented that it looked like heartbeat to me – a very dynamic one.

S came in with her hood on, saying she was feeling cold and her body was all hunched up. As the session progressed and came to moving in different ways her movement patterns changed and she was making her figure skating movements. She "opened" up both in her movements and in her contributions as the session progressed. While doing the name activity, she commented on W's work, saying that she liked it. Her name was made out of a picture representing the seaside with dolphins, boat, sun, tree, and so forth. By the end, the hood was gone and her inhibitions. What the group displayed was laughter, movement work incorporating touch, exploring, and experiencing the body in relation to space, time and directions, using voice work, and the art activity in a creative and imaginative way.

As the sessions progressed, the members began to use all categories in various ways and began to expand the repertoire of their movement vocabulary. Every session had a main theme based around feelings. Over a period of sessions, they used music, props, and voice as well as movement games to become less inhibited and more cohesive in their movement. In another session, the group developed body movement patterns through drawing lines, used words, and then associated them with feelings. For example: horizontal lines expressed restful and calm feelings, short vertical lines expressed rigidity, and crisscross line depicted conflict. They made a conscious effort to give words, images and expressions to how they were actually feeling. This seemed to have given them nonverbal vocabulary and helped them to be aware how feelings affected their body movement and how their movements expressed their feelings without them being aware of it. By entering into this dramatic act or space, a change in the way the individual experiences their body and the relationship between their body and identity can occur. Being in this special state, involves an alteration of perception, a change of focus and responses, and the sharpening of senses (Jones, 1996).

The third session vignette focuses on Rediscovering and nourishing the spontaneous and creative inner child. Spontaneity is closely linked to creativity. It acts a as catalyst or a companion to the creative process. Our spontaneity warms up our creativity. According to Moreno, the founder of psychodrama, spontaneity meant that we are ready to respond as is required by the situation (Dayton, 2005) and not by predetermined factors or behaviour patterns like perfectionism as is often found in clients, which are suffering from eating disorders. By being spontaneous, the clients get a chance not to think about the preconceived notions or behaviour patterns, thus plying out emotions with out the loss of face. By taking part in a variety of make believe play, the child in us is given the opportunity to grow and find itself, where we can relate to this child in ourselves and lead it gently by the hand to join up with our mature selves. According to Peter Slade, spontaneity may be guided by only suggesting what to do without showing how to do it (Wethered, 1993).

Sesame's method is to engage the body creatively and allow the emotions spontaneous expression within the freedom and protection of role and metaphor (Dekker, 1996). Through the art forms of drama and movement in a Sesame session, it is possible to make a reconnection with the ability to play. This can in turn serve the function of recreating the way reality is perceived, which over time can lead to the recovery of that spontaneity we think of as childlike (Deane, 1996). Jung recognized that the psyche could be best heard attended to and befriended by our engaging in some form of creative and imaginative play. Play, as a structured form, acts as a vessel, wherein many healing transformations can occur. Jung always recommended the practice of an art form to an analysand. The Sesame approach is just such a vessel, in which imagination is liberated. By imagining these, we discover, and come into relationship with, the many aspects of ourselves and of the human condition (Dekker, 1996).

Play would form the basis of one such session that features guided active imagination to set the stage for spontaneity and creativity. In this session, where there was a golden moment, the clients were taken through a guided imagination of exploring and playing like kittens. The activity started after an initial warm up lying down, relaxing the body, and inviting the members to imagine that they are going to sleep and is now dreaming. The dream starts with them finding themselves as kittens and lying in a curl of ball. As the exercise progresses, they were then encouraged to start uncurling, stretching their body parts, rubbing their backs just like a kitten. As the members began to become aware of their surroundings and notice other kittens, they were then encouraged to start to play with the other kitten. Balls of yard, and other kitten related toys were introduced to facilitate and stimulate the imagination. Almost all the members continued into this imaginary world, one member which all be referred as Lucy here, stayed curled up longer than the others did. The therapist sensing that Lucy might need assistance in moving on entered into the dramatic space in the role of adult kitten owner. This therapeutic interaction occurring within the art form is part of the Sesame Approach. In this dramatic space, the therapist engaged in role according to the observed need of the participant within the dramatic context. This intervention helped to support, mirror, validate and was made more real by the way it was received and developed by the therapist in role (Dekker, 1996) She acknowledged the kitten and said may be the kitten needs help to move on, the kitten replied with a soft meow. The therapist gently started to stroke the kitten's back, massaged its paws and after a little while Lucy the kitten began to slowly uncurl, keeping her eyes closed. She then turned on her back and the therapist approached with caution, gently rubbed her tummy making slow gentle strokes. As Lucy accepted the strokes and gradually opens her eyes, the therapist encouraged her to sit on her paws, stretch a little and then introduced her to the others. The other group members still in role, accepted Lucy in their group and slowly but with repeated engagement invited her to join them in different kinds of play. The therapist still in role, introduced more objects to stimulate different movement styles to make the body respond to moving in different ways, using the space and direction of the movement, the heights, and levels.

The active imagination was gradually brought to an end, with the therapist coming out of role and inviting the group to find a resting space where the kittens needed to rest after the play. As the kittens found a space and started to curl up into a ball again, the therapist invited them to imagine that they were going to sleep and hearing the alarm clock, they would get up and return to the reality. The deroling took some time as Lucy again found it challenging to come back to the here and now. The others who had already deroled and the therapist acknowledged that the person lying down was Lucy and asked her how they might help her to derole. She suggested that maybe they can all call her name out gently and then tell her things about Lucy, like how old she is, where she lives etc. The therapist also acknowledged Lucy asking that while in role Lucy seemed to have found a place of comfort and safety where she was able to explore her spontaneity and creativity. Maybe she should remember that and bring it back to the here and now and find opportunities to explore these qualities in other areas of drama therapy. The session took longer to derole but it was important to let all the members return to the here and now. In Sesame, deroling followed by grounding is an important part of the grounding process. The process was then talked about in the feedback session, where the space was left open with the members invited to share their thoughts. While one member said that she had never moved like a kitten before, another said that it was fun and playful to move in different ways and to move with the others in spontaneous fashion. Lucy mentioned that she found it difficult to move on from the space of comfort into the space of action, but acknowledged that she appreciated the help from the therapist and the others in role to encourage her to move on. She shared that in real life she often finds it difficult to move on and in the process miss out on many actions. As hard it was to get in to action, it was difficult to come out of it. The reason being that she had discovered a different way of feeling – the feeling of being free, spontaneous and creative– and feared that all of those would be taken away from her once she came back to reality.

At this point most of the group members shared that while at times they were afraid to let go during the enactment, wanting to keep all their movements perfect and controlled, the urge to let go was immense and while some gave themselves the permission to letting go, others did control certain aspects of their movements. The therapist acknowledged that maybe all the movements and the feelings of spontaneity and creativity have always been there and now that they had experienced it, maybe over a period of time they might think about their needing to be perfect and controlling how their bodies moved or looked like. The therapist acknowledged that the in being spontaneous and child like, the group was able to recapture the expressive use of the body as a means of communicating. The group was able to enjoy the sheer fun of creative physical play, the movement spontaneity of their inner child seemed to have reappeared and she encouraged the group to give themselves the permission to be spontaneous and playful. While it is impossible to create spontaneity, it is possible to create a situation in which spontaneity can emerge. This can only happen when somebody does not feel self–conscious. The paradox of letting go of the self–conscious ego results in becoming more dynamic and flexible. In the same way, it is by expressing and integrating uncounsious material that the ego becomes stronger and more able to manage what may previously have been felt as overwhelming emotions ands experiences (Syz, 1996).

Conclusion

"I come upon memories of Sesame Dramatherapy and a smile spreads itself across my face. Who ever knew that in my imagination, the Little Red riding Hood lived in Finland? Or that doodles could tell a story? Or that a hat could create such a character? Or that a story could be told in so many different ways? Or I could move without boundaries and enjoy my body for moving? I look back and I see the important lessons of team work, of acceptance and of leadership that I have learned. The freedom and creativity that I felt in each Sesame session will never be forgotten."
(Teen recovering from Disordered Eating, Eating Disorders Program, Ontario, Canada)

As seen in this feedback, the Sesame Approach has been found to be very innovative with teens dealing with the different kinds of issues around recovery from disordered eating. The drama and movement therapy sessions provided a space to find out how the group used the various modalities to explore and express their emotions and in their own way nourish themselves. The non–threatening and secure environment provided in these sessions were needed to give an opportunity to the teens to reclaim their lost childhood in a playful and spontaneous structure. They also learned to regain and redevelop healthy and trusting relationships with their inner child.

Appendix–Terms

The Sesame Approach–At the heart of the Sesame Approach is a metaphor. Just like the ancient story that uses the phrase "Open Sesame" to open the cave door and reveal treasure, the Sesame Approach uses drama and movement as powerful resources to promote healing and change in people.
Jungian psychology in Sesame Approach–Sesame sessions offer the opportuni-

ty for people to work safely with the fundamental experiences of being human and alive. For example, when we enact the Myth of Parcival's Quest for the Holy Grail, we open ourselves to the possibility of being brave, lost, alone, and finally saved. These are the archetypal states of being that are held within the Jungian Psychology that is the theory underpinning the Sesame Approach.

Storytelling in Sesame Approach—Here Sesame sessions offer the possibility of connection with archetypal qualities through the enactment of mythology and fairy tale. Therapeutically the experience offers the participant a real validation of their creative expression through the ritual of performance and being witnessed by others. This involves the sustained immersion in a character and the subsequent devising of a scene that can be presented and witnessed. This stage can also be the enactment of a told story or myth and the selection of an existing role from within the story.

Improvisation and the setting in Sesame Approach—Improvisation, within the dramatic context, is the ability to respond in the moment and to spontaneously create enacted narrative. Therapeutically Sesame sessions offer participants the opportunity to transfer these skills and experiences to their real lives.

Reflection in Sesame Approach—Sesame sessions help people to develop a capacity to contemplate personal meaning from their experience. In short, to notice what they noticed about their experience of being in this session. This stage involves coming out of character or experience and reflection on the return to the here and now.

Ritual in Sesame Approach—There is an established sequence of events in a Sesame session. This sequence forms the ritual of beginning, middle, and end and acts as a container for whatever therapeutic work takes place.

Movement in the Sesame Approach—The focus on opportunities for movement in a Sesame session is informed by the work of Rudolph Laban. Laban worked in the early twentieth century as a dancer and choreographer, and developed a language of movement observation and analysis in order to find the connections between motion and emotion. Laban identified the four movement qualities as being: Flow, Weight, Space, and Time. He observed the outer use of these four elements and used them as tools to work with the inner world.

Flow is linked to feeling—it can be free or bound. Free flow moves endlessly on and on and can be difficult to end. Bound flow starts and stops, it has a pizzicato feel to it and is much less spontaneous and more rigid.

Weight is linked to intention—it can be firm or fine. The energy or force which is used to do things may relate to firm or fine purpose.

Space is linked to thinking or attention–it can be direct or indirect and relates to the way a person inhabits and learns about the world.

Time is linked to decision–making–it can be sudden or sustained and relates to the speed at which choices are made.

Touch in Sesame Approach–Sesame sessions use the possibility of physical contact between participants and therapists to work safely with touch, which is often regarded as taboo in therapy.

Play, Peter Slade and Human Development in Sesame Approach–Sesame sessions offer participants the chance to re–experience the spontaneous, creative qualities that can be seen when children instinctively play. Our assertion that plays is a vital part of therapy comes from the work of Peter Slade. The research of Peter Slade's work on how children play spontaneously and his influence can be found within the art forms of Sesame session work. His central contribution was to draw from observing that children spontaneously enact scenes from their imagination when left to themselves to play freely and dramatically.

References

Adolescent Medicine Committee, Canadian Pediatric Society. (1998). Eating disorders in adolescents. *Principles of Diagnosis and Treatment, 3*(3), 189–92.

Bettelheim, B. (1976). *The uses of enchantment: The meaning and importance of fairy tales* (pp. 6). London: Penguin Books.

Dayton. T. (2005). *The Living Stage* (pp. 61). Florida: Health Communications, Inc.

Deane, M. (1996). *Self through drama and movement: The Sesame Approach* (pp. 117). London: Jessica Kingsley Publishers.

Dekker, K. (1996). Why oblique and why Jung. In J. Pearson (Ed.), *Discovering the self through drama and movement: The Sesame Approach* (pp. 40–42). London: Jessica Kingsley Publishers.

Estes, C.P. (1992). *Women who run with the wolves* (pp. 75). London: Rider.

Gardner, D., & Harper, P. (1997).Using metaphor and imagery: An illustrative case study of childhood anxiety. In K. N. Dwivedi (Ed.), *The therapeutic use of stories* (pp. 100). London: Routledge.

Harper, P. & Gray, M. (1997).Maps and meaning in life and healing. In K. N. Dwivedi (Ed.), *The therapeutic use of stories* (pp. 42–43). London: Routledge.

Johnston, A. (1996). *Eating in the light of the moon* (pp. 86). California: Gurze Books.

Jones, J. M., Bennett, S., Olmsted, M. P., Lawson, M. L., & Rodin, G. (2001). Disordered eating attitudes and behaviours in teenaged girls: a school based study. *Canadian Medical Association Journal 2001; 165*(5) 547–552.

Jones, P. (1996). *Drama as therapy, theatre as living* (pp. 164–165). London: Routledge

Pearson, J. (1996). (Ed.), *Discovering the self through drama and movement—The Sesame Approach* (pp. 2, 16, 187). London: Jessica Kingsley Publishers.

Syz, J. (1996). Working with symbol in the Mental Health Centre. In J. Pearson (Ed.), *Discovering the self through drama and movement—The Sesame Approach* (pp. 150, 152). London: Jessica Kingsley Publishers.

Wethered, A. G. (1993). *Movement and drama in therapy: A holistic approach* (pp. 45, 82). London: Jessica Kingsley Publishers.

Whitfield, C. L. (1990). How can we heal our child within. In J. Abrams, *Reclaiming the inner child* (pp. 173). Los Angeles, CA: Jeremy P. Tarcher, Inc.

Biography

Priyadarshini Senroy (MA, DMT, CCC) is a Drama and Movement Therapist residing in Toronto, Canada. She works with children and adults with special needs and mental health issues. She is also on the board of the Creative Arts in Counseling Chapter of the Canadian Counseling Association. She has taught at various training programs in India, Thailand, and Singapore. Also, Ms. Senroy has international experience in facilitating workshops in the UK, USA, and Canada. She has presented her multicultural work using Drama and Movement Therapy at conferences and has contributed to newsletters and journals all over the world.

Chapter 14

TALKING TO THE SOCIAL ANIMAL: AN EVOLUTIONARY APPROACH TO WORKING WITH ANOREXIC AND BULIMIC CLIENTS

SHINTA HERMANNS

Introduction

The study of the psyche has largely focused on developmental issues within the human lifespan, especially the early formative years of childhood. But if we universally acknowledge the influence that early childhood experiences have on future psychological and behavioural development, how can we afford to overlook the developmental childhood of our species and its likely impact on modern man and woman? The field of biology has proven this through the discovery of DNA and the mapping of the human genome. Many psychiatric illnesses are now being linked to genetic predispositions for developing them, including eating disorders (Kaye & Strober, 1999). The finding of a genetic connection is an indication for the biological evolution of the psychological and behavioural pattern that we diagnose as anorexia or bulimia today. In terms of natural selection, eating disorder symptoms may be interpreted as archaic blueprints for behaviour that must have been adaptive for our far distant ancestors' survival fitness, even if they lead perversely in our modern environment to the most lethal of all psychiatric illnesses. So in order to really understand the modern phenomenon of eating disorders, I contend that we have to look back to the developmental environment of our species and try and find out what natural selection benefits certain psychological and behavioural mechanisms could have had. This may give us valuable insights into eating disorders, help us interpret modern environmental triggers and aid us in devising more successful interventions.

Adaptation to Starvation of a Social Animal

During World War II, A. Keys conducted the so-called "starvation study" at the University of Minnesota (Keys, 1950). Thirty-six physically and mentally healthy male adults were put on a semi-starvation diet for half a year and their behaviour was recorded prior to, during, and after the experiment. The researchers soon witnessed progressively severe psychological and behavioural changes in the men. The subjects became increasingly self-centered and aggressive. They started to hoard food, as well as unrelated items, and increasingly withdrew from social contact. These are starvation-related observations that can also be made in societies affected by famine (Dirks, 1980). While at first people tend to help each other out, the longer and more severe the food shortage, the more we can witness the breakdown of society and even close family relations. Subjects also suffered from depression, sleep disturbances, and increasingly neurotic traits like anxiety and obsessions. They showed low self-esteem, developing intense feelings of inadequacy, and self-criticism. Some subjects reported instances of uncontrolled binge eating after which vomiting occurred, which in turn caused immense guilt and self-disgust. Other subjects started to exercise excessively to loose more weight in order to be allowed more rations or avoid having rations shortened. After the starvation period of the experiment ended, subjects reported problems like confusion, anxiety, and stress with returning to normal eating habits for several months. Two subjects had to leave the experiment prematurely due to the severity of the psychological changes they underwent. Anorexics and bulimics self-induce a state of semi-starvation. The motivation behind food deprivation may differ from the subjects in Keys' experiment; however, the physical and psychological pattern that sufferers display are akin to those observed in the study. We may infer from this that a lot of the psychological and behavioural symptoms that we associate with anorexia and bulimia appear to be due to the biological changes that semi-starvation activates in our species, male or female.

During the experiment, the subjects were not kept in total isolation with other starving people, as in a famine situation. They remained part of a wider social group that maintained normal eating habits. This experimental setup recreated a developmental environment in which food resources were available, but where access to them was restricted. This seems to me a pivotal, though slightly overlooked, point of the study. A selective group of people was deprived of food, the subjects, whereas another, the researchers, retained access to food. Moreover, the researchers were with regard to food regulation in a position of power, i.e., dominant, whereas the subjects were by the very rules of the experiment accountable for their food intake to the researchers' judgment, i.e., submissive. Thus, the observed symptoms associated with eating disorders may not be reactions to starvation exclusively but, more accurately, adaptive strategies to starvation within a social context where access to food is restricted and dependent on an individual's dominant or submissive status. Exploring this hypothesis, I will now move on to show the relationship between food and rank in our ancestral environment and explain how eating disorder symptoms may be interpreted in this context.

"Three hundred million years ago our ancestors competed for resources (food, territory, mates) on an individual basis . . . then, as group living became established and territory began to be shared, individuals ceased competing directly for territory and instead started to compete for rank. Once acquired, high rank brought with it access to the resources that were desired" (Stevens & Price, 1996, p. 47). The close relationship between high rank and access to vital resources like food is clearly visible by observing our closest hominid relatives: chimpanzees, bonobos, and gorillas (de Waal, 1988). Food resources are distributed according to social ranking, i.e. dominant group members usually have first choice of food resources, the weaker or lower group members eat after; whatever is left or given to them. It is highly likely then that access to food resources within early human societies was also based on a social ranking system. But how does a social animal attain rank and status? Looking at primates and their behaviour again, Michael Chance (1970) found that there were two different social systems at work: the agonic and hedonic mode.

The hedonic mode evolved sometime in the last ten million years with the development of the limbic system, or mammalian brain. The limbic system allowed our mammalian ancestors to form emotional connections and develop social groupings based on attachment. Rank in such a hedonic environment is based on how much emotional involvement and care an individual can elicit from others, preferably higher ranking individuals, within the social grouping. If an individual has what Gilbert (1989) terms a high social attention holding potential or SAHP, then the social status rises; if the individual cannot gain social attention then, consequently, that social animal's rank will decline. In a hedonic society, access to essential resources such as food and mating partners are intrinsically linked to competition for social attractiveness. The hedonic mode is at the heart of the human family unit, which is the root of human society. However, we have already mentioned how societal structures and familial relations break down during times of famine. It appears that in a fight for limited food resources human beings fall down the evolutionary ladder and a much older mode of interaction and social competition is activated: the agonic mode.

Out of the antagonistic fight for resources between individuals evolved at first the agonic mode of social living (Chance, 1970). In order for any communal living to be possible, continuous violent contests between individuals need to be inhibited. In the agonic mode actual violence is therefore mostly substituted with intimidation and the threat of violence. Most animal species have evolved a very specific or ritualised behaviour pattern regarding agonic contests for supremacy, e.g., dogs growl and show their ready–to–bite teeth. Ritualistic pre–attack posturing allows each combatant to assess their own chances in a potential fight to hold the desired resource against the opponent and take appropriate action, i.e., fight, submit or flee. To win such a ritualised conflict transfers resource holding power (Parker, 1974) or RHP and high rank onto the victor and they emerge as dominant. The looser displays after such a ritualised contest what Price (1987) calls involuntary subordinate strategies, innate behaviour that signals defeat, thus preventing attack. With regard to the effect of winning or loosing RHP on human beings, I quote Stevens and Price again (1996, p. 47):

> The human equivalent of RHP is self–esteem, and defeat can have similar effects on both the behaviour and self–esteem of human beings as it has on the behaviour and RHP of reptiles, mammals and primates. . . . An essential aspect of high self–esteem is the subjective awareness of being able to control desired social outcomes, while low self–esteem is the awareness of not being able to control such desirable assets, and it is associated with submissive forms of behaviour, as well as with a liability to anxiety, depression, or social withdrawal.

These are all symptoms which the starvation study revealed and which are common in both anorexic as well as bulimic patients. From an evolutionary point of view we can now interpreted them as signs of defeat in an agonistic conflict for resources. In all social animals, we can observe two mayor self–protective strategies when faced with an opponent that is perceived to have superior RHP: the self–assessed loser will either *flee* or *yield.* I propose to view anorexia as essentially a strategy of flight and bulimia as a strategy of submission.

Hyperactivity, the excessive will to control weight and the total denial of starvation are all features of anorexia. Shan Guisinger (2003) put forward an evolutionary perspective of anorexia nervosa as an adaptation to flee depleted territories. The overriding drive to move or flee may have been of adaptive benefit, allowing our ancestors to forage further and longer. Those individuals that had the strongest motivation to move on would have been the most likely to survive. The possession of a strong will or motivation should make a person a prime candidate for a dominant role, because strong–willed individuals would not easily back down in an agonic ritualistic conflict scenario. Instead, anorexics have low self–esteem and are prone to depression and anxiety, which are all submissive features. This seeming contradiction may be explained if we think again in terms of a group context. Anorexic behaviour pattern may be related to the behaviour of group members that are striving for group dominance, but do not have sufficient RHP to top the highest ranking group members. Such individuals would be in constant physical or mental competition with the ruling dominants for status and resources and thus live continuously poised between fight and flight. Especially illuminating is a phenomenon that Chance (1970) observed as typical within agonic social groupings, the so–called "reverted escape." A subdominant animal strays to the boundary of the group's territory, presumably getting ready to escape, but is prevented from actually fleeing by the dominant group member's threat of attack. Each defeated or reverted escape lowers the subdominant's RHP, which would sooner or later lead to a display of more submissive and harm avoiding behaviour. In other words, the reverted escape mechanism is a social downgrading process during which the subdominant animal is forced to come to associate challenging behaviour with instant retribution on the one hand, as well as self–control and perfectly submissive behaviour with harm avoidance on the other. I propose that the symptoms associated with anorexia are in fact psychological and behavioural patterns that have their origin in such an agonic inverted escape mechanism. To look for possible supporting evidence for this hypothesis I turn to biological research into the nature of eating disorders. Recent studies have found a link between the neurotransmitter serotonin and anorexia. Serotonin is linked to food, mood and impulse regulation, which are all the "ingredients" necessary for an agonic power struggle. Walter Kaye's research has shown that serotonin imbalances appear to persist even after recovery. His findings seem to support the hypothesis that the increased concentrations in AN and BN may be associated with exaggerated anticipatory over concern with negative consequences (i.e., "harm avoidance") (Kaye et al., 1999). Natural selection may have evolved these lasting changes to the chemical makeup of the brain, because it adapted the outranked submissive animal to continue displaying the correct harm–avoiding behaviour, thus increasing its chances of survival within the agonic social group.

Bulimics on the other hand appear to follow a yielding subroutine of submission to avoid harm. As a psychological profile, bulimics tend to be anger and conflict avoidant and may be overly preoccupied with pleasing others. This kind of behaviour is consistent with a fully submissive group member. Eating according to the group's RHP or SAHP hierarchy is adaptive, because in this way vital resources are safeguarded for those specimens that have the highest level of survival fitness within the group. This means, however, that lesser group members are seriously disadvantaged with regard to food distribution and may be more tempted to cheat and eat more than "their due." The feelings of disgust, shame, and self–hate that are experienced after binging by bulimics may well be part of a subordinate strategy that evolved because it helped to reinforce avoidance of such "cheating" behaviour. Binge eating in general can be interpreted as an adaptive strategy to an ancestral environment of unstable food supply. If one could never be sure of encountering sufficient food the next day, then reacting to food abundance by binging on it as and when it was available made sense. This ensured that valuable resources would be stored as body fat and could be lived off in leaner times (Stevens & Price, 1996). The only time this would not be beneficial is when an individual is extremely malnourished and the body has adapted to this deprivation by starting to use up internal fat resources. To start eating again, facilitating the shift from fat to carbohydrate metabolism, food intake needs to be increased slowly, because overindulgence could well have lethal consequences (Hearing, 2004). In order to avoid such potentially fatal foodbinges, we can assume again that adaptive strategies have evolved that helped to discourage or deal with such instances of overindulgence, e.g., nausea, vomiting. Bulimics may be sliding into binge–purge cycles, because the purging activates starvation level deficiencies, which in turn may activate mechanisms that encourage the body to void itself of "dangerous" binge amounts of food. As for the motivation to start binge eating, in the hedonic mode access to food denotes a high amount of social attention holding potential. Being given food is the primeval sign for care in the hedonic mode, and binge eating can then be interpreted as the attempt to self–inject the feeling of being cared for and equally fuel the make–believe of higher SAHP. Of course, if the reality of the submissive social animal does not mirror such high SAHP, then eating can spin out of control as such an individual can never eat enough.

This chapter explained how social rank was linked to access to vital food resources in our ancestral environment and introduced the hypothesis that anorexic and bulimic symptoms may have their origin in subordinate strategies within an agonic or hedonic mode of group structure. In the following chapter, I will look at our modern environment and interpret triggers on the basis of this evolutionary insight.

The Modern Phenomenon of Eating Disorders

Anorexia and bulimia are prevalent in societies where starvation due to natural causes has essentially been eradicated. Instead, degrees of starvation have become a modern life–style choice. At the same time obesity has become a problem of epidemic proportions throughout the industrialized world. According to the American Obesity Association, 65 percent of American adults are overweight and half of these adults fall into the obese category. Interestingly, in our contemporary environment of a generally overweight population, the current aesthetic ideal of beauty is one of carefully cultivated emaciation. Looking back at statistics for the increasing obesity problem since the 1980s, and comparing that to the way in which model sizes in the media decreased over the same period, we can make the following layman's observation: the fatter we become, the thinner the ideal figure seems to be getting. The "cult of thinness" (Hesse–Biber, 1996) is usually blamed on the media, the fashion industry, female exploitation, and so forth rarely on nature herself. After all, it seems such an unnatural phenomenon. But it could well be interpreted as nature's way to strike a homeostatic balance by letting us perceive such a physical condition as beautiful, which may be valuable to the reproductive fitness of our species. In a climate of food overindulgence reproductive fitness may very well favour those individuals that resist indiscriminate food intake, those that can exert self–control and stick to a proper diet–in other words, those that look thin. Thinness, as a sign signal for reproductive fitness (Abed, 1998), would become a social asset to be desired; a new naturally selective, social attention–holding device. If we stay with this hypothesis, dieting can be understood as a way of determining rank within gender specific social groupings, i.e., females comparing themselves to other females and competing for the thinnest figure, because this would result in sign signals that increase one's SAHP or mate value (Symons, 1987). It is important here to note that SAHP is a subjective assessment tool. The perception or feeling to be bigger than everybody else, i.e., have lower status than everybody else, activates the same submissive psychological and behavioural pattern, as if that self–judgment was based on fact. This may account for a body image gap that grows totally out of proportion with eating disorder sufferers. When people look into the mirror they judge and compare their own SAHP with that of others. If people start to diet who possess a critically low level of SAHP and do not, despite their best effort to control their weight, attain higher SAHP, i.e., reap the promised social recognition, then it stands to reason that they will never perceive themselves to be thin or good enough. To summarize, extreme dieting as seen in anorexics and bulimics, can be understood as a desperate and competitive bid for self–improvement on the social ranking scale in a contemporary hedonic setting.

Marya Hornbacher, talking about her own struggle with anorexia and bulimia in *Wasted* (1999, p. 68), says: "Too often the shrinks assume an eating disorder is a way of avoiding womanhood, sexuality, responsibility, by arresting your physical growth at a prepubescent state. . . . Some of us may be after something quite different, like breathing room, or crazy as it sounds, less attention, or a different kind of attention. Something like power." To go on a hunger strike is an extremely powerful political tool in a society in which the hedonic mode is at the heart of social interaction. "The efficacy of food refusal as an emotional tactic within the family depends on food being plentiful, pleasing and connected to love," according to Brumberg (1988, p. 139). In a hedonic society, based on caregiving and receiving, the feeding of loved ones is one of the most fundamental of social behaviour patterns. This whole archetypal system depends on two powerful innate mechanisms that are reciprocally activated: one on the part of the dominant—to give care and food, and the other on the part of the lower ranking individual—to solicit care and food. The most primal example of this would be the emotion of love between mother and infant (Bowlby, 1979). A lower ranking group member, who refuses food in order to protest against their own powerlessness, will activate compelling feelings of guilt and responsibility associated with neglect of care in the dominant group members, e.g., the family or society. This high psychological tension would prompt an immediate increase in caring behaviour towards the starving person in order to alleviate such stressful psychological tension. So a hunger strike empowers an individual, because it raises the level of social attention invested in that person by the dominants and thus elevates the perception of one's own SAHP. This is the evolutionary explanation behind feminist approaches, such as Susie Orbach's (1986) theories. The hedonic explanation model can help us understand the initial motivation behind restricting one's food intake which can lead to anorexia and bulimia by explaining what confers SAHP on an individual in our contemporary social environment and by explaining the relationship between care giving and attention holding potential with relation to food refusal by a low ranking individual. However, we have said earlier how the very act of starvation can put in motion behaviour mechanisms that have less to do with the hedonic but with the more primitive agonic mode of social interaction.

In contemporary society, where food is readily available, rank is no longer conferred on the one *holding* the resource, but on the one *withholding* the resource. In a complete reversal to our adaptive environment, power no longer resides with the one who eats but with the one who does not. Unfortunately, only because modern society has changed the rules for what gives an individual high SAHP, this does not mean that the rules for innate behaviour belonging to RHP will be negated. The more modern part of our brain says, if you are thin you are a success, whereas the archaic part of our brain says, if you are thin you are a failure. This is in my opinion the evolutionary trap that eating disorder sufferers fall into. The social rules of the hedonic setting motivate anorexia and bulimia sufferers to diet in order to raise their sense of self–esteem. What they activate through their self–starvation, however, is the psychological and behavioural profile of the submissive group member in the agonic mode. This creates a vicious circle in which any original sense of powerlessness only gets reinforced and amplified, in some cases with tragic consequences. C. G. Jung (1998, pars. 200–203) based his analytical psychology on the activation of such archetypal patterns within the individual's psyche and wisely pointed out that "everyone knows nowadays that people 'have complexes'; what is not so well–known is that complexes can have us." It is not so much the anorexic or bulimic person that has an eating disorder, it is the eating disorder that has them.

Talking to the Social Animal through Drama and Movement Therapy

Traditional forms of therapy offer the "talking cure." Verbal communication is indubitably the most evolved natural form of human communication and is a testimony to our species' cognitive abilities. However, eating disorders are for the most part completely "unreasonable" phenomena and highly resistant to traditional methods of therapy. This could be because the mechanisms they may be related to pre–date the further evolution of the brain and are animalistic and pre–verbal in nature. It stands to reason, then, that in order to reach the part that fuels anorexia and bulimia, the social animal, we need to attempt to "talk" to the more primitive parts of the human brain, i.e., the mammalian and reptilian brain. The communication signals that will be accessible to us to do so are not words but body language and sound. According to Bernie Spivak (1996, p. 165): "There are so many ways the voice can be used to good effect. For instance, you can suddenly whisper and people will stop and listen. . . . To be able to firm up your voice and make it a little louder or vary its tone is a great asset." The ability to consciously vary volume or pitch of voice and stance of body posture in attunement with clients' needs is a great instrument to have in any therapist's toolbox. Non–verbal communication has traditionally been less investigated as a therapeutic tool, but has been proven to be much more powerful than any linguistics by Mehrabian (1972). He found that in order to evaluate communication we rely only 7 percent on the actual meaning of the word; the majority of communication happens through body language and voice. It seems imperative, therefore, that therapists become as well trained in communicating and interpreting non–verbal signs as they are in dealing with verbal ones. The first conversational tip for working with the social animal, then, is to use its language and become very aware of body language and vocal quality in interaction with eating disorder clients.

My second conversational tip deals with the therapeutic relationship. Most research into the effectiveness of psychotherapy stress the quality of the relationship between client and therapist as the single most important factor for effective therapy, including Howe (1993). So we need to ask whether there may be a kind of quality that could be looked for in a therapist by eating dis-order clients in general; a quality that would be developmentally needed on an evolutionary level by our clients, not as individuals, but as sufferers from a collective archaic behaviour pattern. I spoke at length about submission and dominance in earlier sections, and that raises the question of power with-in the therapeutic relationship, a distinct "taboo" subject. During my Sesame training, the emphasis was on non–directive and client–led therapy to avoid overpowering vulnerable clients. This created a therapeutic attitude that has been tremendously valuable to me over the years. However, the effect of my repudiation of power and superior status on my first eating disorder clients was not empowering at all, on the contrary. The social grouping collapsed, as if I as the dominant group member had failed by not asserting myself enough to maintain group stability. Through this unsettling experience, it became clear to me that in order to work with this client group, I needed to regain a positive sense of power within the therapeutic relationship. Stevens and Price (1996) view eating disorders as rank and attachment related ill-nesses. What kind of rank should I as the therapist hold? The attitude that appeared to be demanded by my clients was not so much one of equality, but of the therapist as the dominant group member. It should be stressed here that I am not talking about feeling personally superior to clients, but about the need for therapists to play the part of group leader with conviction and acceptance of the dominant status that this role, at least initially, entails. To draw on the social animal scenario, an animal that is desperate to ascend the social ladder will not gain status by winning agonic or hedonic contests against individuals that are already more submissive than they are. They can only rise up and gain a sense of empowerment and self–esteem by either defeating or soliciting attention from higher ranking individuals. The thera-pist therefore needs to cooperate by providing the strong and supportive sur-face against which the client can lean the metaphorical social ladder and climb up. Climbing steps that are "artificially" lowered by the therapist will not get the client any further, but having to reach up and being supported through that struggle by the higher ranking group member will. The ultimate aim for working from a secure base of benevolent power, then, is to allow more and more control and assertiveness to reside with the client; for the client to become in fact the "good enough" (Winnicott, 1958) leader of their own life. As far as the therapeutic relationship is concerned with eating dis-order clients, my second conversational and maybe controversial tip for talk-ing to the social animal is to do so from a point of acceptance and care with regard to one's own powerful role within the therapeutic relationship.

My third tip is with regard to starting a dramatherapeutic conversation. In my experience, the least likely scenario to engage clients and liberate their innate creativity is what we could call an "empty stage" scenario. I once worked with a director who would leave the improvisational process completely to us actors (in the name of communal artistic expression) and whose ominous presence waited, quietly watching in the darkened auditorium. Instead of enjoying this freedom of expression the whole cast would stand around the expectation–laden empty stage and furtively look at one another to start somewhere, somehow. To stay with the theatre analogy: if the therapist is playing the audience by, for example, not taking an active part in a proposed activity, and the clients are unwilling or unable to engage with the material and step up onto the stage to be the actors, then this may create a vacuum of expectation within the play space that will paralyze the dramatic and with it the therapeutic process. I have found the most effective method of interaction with this client group is to first lead actively from the front or the middle, being the group leader, guiding director, or a supporting actor. Only when clients are comfortable enough to fill the space on their own will I take a more passive role and be their witnessing audience. An actively engaged therapist is also not as likely to be perceived by clients as "judging" their performance at all times. Eating disorder clients in particular are constantly preoccupied with doing things right, trying to stay in control and not taking up too much space (Jacobse, 1994). Being watched can be unbearable for these clients, as it heightens the psychological tension between needing to do everything in a correct manner and the fear of being judged a failure and inadequate. Psychological tension within the submissive social animal can only be alleviated by displaying appropriate submissive behaviour. This being the case, expressive arts therapies can be experienced as an ordeal for anorexic and bulimic clients. At the heart of most arts therapy approaches is the concept of creativity, the very absence of ground rules and right and wrong behaviour. But if no guidelines are given about what may constitute "right" behaviour by the group leader, e.g., by using the routine saying "do what feels right to you," then we may, in fact, be putting our clients under an oppressive amount of stress because they will not be able to identify the correct harm–avoiding behaviour. This is why, when I now begin working with a group, I teach clients physical and vocal techniques, always making sure that the exercises I ask the group to follow are clearly defined. I do not, at such an early stage of therapeutic work, want to confront clients with a potentially overwhelming and paralyzing choice of options. Admittedly, a more directive approach carries with it the expectation to engage in a certain way, which some therapists may find objectionable and stifling to the clients' creativity and self–worth. I have found the opposite to be true. The social animal will instinctively look for strong behavioural boundaries and associate non–submissive behaviour with laying oneself open to dire social consequences. It can only learn more creative self–expression by practice. Practicing needs to consist first of engagement in a shared social activity; secondly, of achieving a sense of capability through being able to engage according to the rules of the group; and thirdly, by not being punished but rewarded through positive social attention for beginning to show a higher degree of assertiveness or self–expression. Spontaneous improvisation with an anorexic or bulimic client group is, in acting terms, the height of achievement for the social animal. In psychological terms, it means that the clients have reached a level of self–esteem through the dramatic training and guided support, which allows them to express themselves openly, liberated from the submissive yoke of harm–avoiding "über"–controlled and planned behaviour patterns. It is a sign that their perception of SAHP has been upgraded and they can consequently afford to present themselves without excessive self–restrictions.

My fourth and final conversational tip is to share some of the exercises that I found useful in raising an eating disorder client's SAHP or RHP. In order to design suitable exercises, I researched how our hominid relatives behave when they compete for social attractiveness or resources, and tried to "ape" their strategies. Grooming is an activity that is enjoyed by all primates and another way to show care that is not food related. Being good at grooming, as well as continuously offering to groom a dominant group member, can give a submissive animal higher status (Attenborough, 2003). This may be the reason why people suffering from eating disorders find it much easier to give than receive care. For this reason it is also important to design exercises involving the offer of care, where care is returned in kind. Reciprocity allows the submissive animal to be coaxed into being cared for and thus experiencing themselves as "worthy" of care and attention. Touching and being touched is especially difficult for this client group. As Marya Hornbacher (1999, p. 14) explains: "I did not like to be touched, but it was a strange dislike. I did not like to be touched because I craved it too much." A central aim of my work with eating disorder clients is therefore to make appropriate touch a more normal experience and part of social interaction.

> Touch can be an integral aspect of group drama and movement. I encourage the development of confidence in this area through many different activities including games, massage and relaxation. . . . It can be a valuable and direct route to enhancing the quality of relationship and communication. . . . Within the context of therapeutic work it (touch) can be a source of reassurance and comfort, a demonstration of unity, care and support, where words are inadequate. Touch was always a healing art in its own right. Jocelyn James' (1996, p. 214)

Using touch in the socially acceptable, ritualistic form of massage has been a very good tool to develop hedonic trust with eating disorder groups, e.g. massaging a partner's hands or shoulders and having one's own massaged in turn. Touch and allowing to be touched can evoke powerful emotions as it speaks straight to the social animal within and may bypass our clients' conscious and verbal defenses. The therapist working with this nonverbal means of communication needs to be sensitive to this.

Raising an individual's RHP has all to do with winning agonic contests by getting better at displaying the physical signs of dominance. Real conviction will come with being more able to stand one's ground, but in order to do so anorexic, and especially bulimic clients, will first have to practice sending higher RHP signals, rather than their familiar submissive ones. To quote Phil Jones (1996, p. 165): "The sense of identity of an individual can be altered by physically changing appearance and body language in dramatic activity." If an actor needs to be in an agitated mood, then bringing the body into a state of agitation by running as quick as possible around the space can arouse corresponding emotions. What we want to arouse in our clients is a sense of high RHP self–esteem. A low level of self–esteem is visually represented by a person through defensive or submissive body language, e.g., through lack of eye contact, protective arm bracing or hunched–over posture. The aural signals through voice include very soft volume or artificially high and defenceless pitch. In order to activate an emotional state of feeling more dominant then, we need to offer clients the experience to embody more dominant positions, physically as well as vocally. Physically, this can be done through small improvisations in which clients are asked to walk a certain way, i.e. with high–heels to a movie premier, or as if they have a chip on their shoulder, etc. It may be helpful to lead such an exercise from the middle and exaggerate high status postures, so that clients have the possibility to see and copy a role model. Mixing low status and high status walks can also help to explore the physical differences between the usual posture clients may habitually display and higher status postures. Another training aspect is raising the clients' ritualistic agonic behaviour. This can be done within the dramatic art form by enacting ritualised or choreographed fights in which avoidance of actual physical contact is stipulated as a safety boundary. Such ritualised fights mimic the agonic conflict scenario and can be played out either as a partner exercises or as a whole group "battle." As for the vocal work, eating disorder clients often speak very quietly, minimalising the amount of space even their words take up. Voice training can help clients explore more powerful volumes and pitches, but is often experienced by eating disorder clients as more difficult than other body work. An exercise I often use, and which combines aggressive behaviour and vocal expression, is to teach a group of clients how to shout out loud without injuring the voice. I ask the clients to hold a pillow and shake it whilst saying "Aah" and trying to make that sound as loud as possible. When it is as loud as possible, they are asked to throw the sound against the wall at the same time as letting the pillow fly. The aim is to keep the throat as open as possible and let sound out at the same time as coordinating a volatile movement without self–restriction. These are just a few examples of exercises that I found particularly useful in talking to the social animal and teaching it to raise its RHP, SAHP, or self–esteem.

My personal conversational tips for speaking to the social animal were:

1. Become more aware of and attuned to using non–verbal communication as a therapeutic tool.
2. Own the power the role of group leader entails in a positive way with assurance and care.
3. Avoid the "empty stage" scenario by engaging in the action and do not give too many options initially. Creativity and freedom of self–expression may need practice.
4. Devise exercises that help raise self–esteem by raising social attention holding potential (SAHP) and resource holding potential (RHP) through body language and voice work.

In this chapter, I have laid out my hypothesis about the evolutionary nature of eating disorders and introduced the reader to a psychosocial approach to working with eating disorder clients based on this evolutionary insight. I hope this new approach of looking at eating disorders will be of interest to all clinicians working with this client group and that the experiences I have made in my practice will be of use to other creative therapists.

References

Abed, R. (1988). The sexual competition hypothesis for eating disorders. *British Journal of Medical Psychology, 71*(4), 525–547.

American Obesity Association. (2006). *Obesity statistic,* retrieved August 20, 2006, from http://www.obesity.org/subs/fastfacts/aoafactsheets.shtml

Attenborough, D. (2003). *The life of mammals.* London: BBC.

Bowlby, J. (1979). An ethological approach to research in child development. In *The making and breaking of affectional bonds.* London: Tavistock Publications Limited.

Brumberg, J. (1988). *Fasting girls: The emergence of anorexia nervosa as a modern disease.* Boston: Harvard University Press.

Chance, M. (1970). *Social groups of monkeys, apes and men.* New York: Johnathan Cape/EP Dutton.

de Waal, F., (1998). *Chimpanzee politics.* Baltimore, MD: Johns Hopkins University Press.

Dirks, R. (1980, February). Social responses during severe food shortages and famine. *Current Anthropology, 21*(1), 21–44.

Gilbert, P. (1989). *Human nature and suffering.* London: Lawrence Erlbaum Associates.

Guisinger, S. (2003, October). Adapted to flee famine: Adding an evolutionary perspective on anorexia nervosa. *Psychological Review, 110*(4), 745–61.

Hearing, S. D. (2004, April). Re–feeding Syndrome. *British Medical Journal, 17*(328), 908–9.

Hornbacher, M., (1999). *Wasted–Coming back from an addiction to starvation.* London: Harper Collins Publishers.

Howe, D. (1993). *On being a client.* London: Sage Publications.

Jacobse, A. (1994). The use of dramatherapy in the treatment of eating disorders. In D. Dokter (Ed.), *Arts therapies and clients with eating disorders.* London: Jessica Kingsley Publishers.

James, J. (1996). Poetry in motion. In *Discovering the self through drama and movement.* London: Jessica Kingsley Publishers.

Jung, C.G. (1998). *CW6–The essential Jung.* London: Fontana Press.

Jones. P (1996). *Drama as therapy–Theatre as living.* London: Routledge.

Kaye, W., & Strober, M. (1999, May/June). Serotonin: Implications for the etiology and treatment of eating disorders. *Eating Disorder Review, 10*(3), Retrieved July 20, 2006, from http://www.gurze.com/client/client_pages/newsletter22.cfm

Kaye, W., Strober, M., & Stein, M. (1999, May). New directions in treatment research of anorexia and bulimia nervosa. *Biological Psychiatry, 45*, 1285–1292.

Keys, A. (1950). *The biology of human starvation.* Minneapolis: Univ. of Minnesota Press.

Mehrabian, A. (1971). *Silent messages.* Belmont, CA: Wadsworth.

Orbach, S. (1986). *Hunger strike.* London: Faber and Faber.

Parker, G. A. (1974). Assessment strategy and the evolution of animal conflicts. *Journal of Theoretical Biology, 47*, 223–243.

Price, J. (1987). Depression as yielding behaviour. *Ethology and Sociobiology, 8*, 85s–98s.

Spivak, B. (1996). The shared feeling. In *Discovering the self through drama and movement.* London: Jessica Kingsley Publishers.

Stevens, A., & Price, J. (1996). *Evolutionary psychiatry.* London: Routledge.

Symons, D. (1987). *An evolutionary approach: Can Darwin's view of life shed light on human sexuality?* In J. H. Geer & W. T. O'Donohue (Eds.), *Theories of human sexuality* (pp. 91–125). New York: Plenum Press.

Winicott, D.W. (1958). *Collected papers.* London: Tavistock Publications.

Biography

Shinta Hermanns comes from an acting and directing background with a special interest in physical theatre. She holds a PG Dip and MA in Drama and Movement Therapy (Sesame). Since her qualification, she has been exploring the therapeutic use of drama and movement with a large variety of client groups, including young adults attending an eating disorder step–down–program, and working with adults in a closed eating disorders unit at a private hospital in London. In addition to working as a drama and movement therapist, she has worked as a lecturer and supervisor for dramatherapy student placements at the Central School of Speech and Drama, as well as lecturing on the MSc Counseling Psychology Course at London Metropolitan University. For more information please visit: www.dramaistherapy.com.

Chapter 15

THE USE OF SPIRITUALITY AS A CREATIVE THERAPEUTIC MODALITY IN THE TREATMENT OF EATING DISORDERS

AMY JERSLID

W omen struggling with eating disorders often use terms like "quest" and "journey" to describe their experience with starvation, purging, and weight loss (Garrett, 1989, p. 96). Their ritualistic behaviors, the devotion with which they pursue them, and their subsequent sense of being purified all seem to reference a spiritual calling (Lelwica, 1999). Many clinicians (Emmet, 1997; Jersild, 2002) liken the obedience that they show the diet industry to religious devotion.

Despite these spiritual undertones, the field of psychology has only recently begun to explore treatment approaches that incorporate clients' religion or spiritual world view. Until recently, traditional psychoanalytic theory has tended to pathologize religion, reducing and rejecting it as superstitious, neurotic, and even psychotic (Simmonds, 2006). Freud (1930) referred to religious devotion as "regressive" and "infantile" (p. 74), explaining that humanity's desire for a god figure arose out of oedipal needs for a protective father.

Although psychological literature reveals a warming attitude toward religion and spirituality by the 1960s, the field's desire to be seen as a hard science continued to hinder theoretical development regarding the spiritual elements of psychological wellbeing and pathology. By the 1970s and 1980s, psychologists began earnestly discussing spirituality as a healthy aspect of human consciousness and functioning (Rizzuto, 1981). Finally, the 1990s began to see work on the applicability of spirituality and religious faith to psychological treatment (Epstein, 1995; Johnston & Antares, 2005).

Several studies over the past decade have attempted to establish a correlation between eating disordered behaviors and adherence to particular religious faiths, with some (Crisp et al., 1992) yielding a positive correlation and others (Gordon, 1990) finding no such relationship. In their 2000 book, Richards and Bergin offer one of the most thorough discussions on this topic, detailing clinical issues that may arise from a broad spectrum of religious groups around topics relevant to eating disorders, such as sexuality, the body, and gender roles.

This chapter will focus specifically on treatment interventions which encompass spiritual concepts, practices, and relationships. After describing specific spiritual issues that may arise in eating disordered women, this chapter will detail several treatment interventions, including the assessment of spiritual world views, the reframing of spiritual concepts, and the use of spiritual structures already in place in the client's life. In doing so, this chapter hopes to increase practitioners' comfort with approaching their clients' spirituality, and well as increase practitioners' understanding of the spiritual and religious nature of eating disorders and recovery.

Definition of Terms

While no one definition can encompass each individual's experience of spirituality, faith, and religion, these terms will be described at the outset for the purposes of mutual understanding. Fowler (1981) stated that Western society has often confused faith with intellectual acceptance; in contrast, Fowler suggested that faith can refer to any relationship, belief system, environment, talent, or heritage that sustains us. Fowler's description of faith is primarily a relational one, and he used the Greek translation of the word ("to give one's heart to") to emphasize this (p. 76). In doing so, Fowler suggested that faith is an emotional investment in something that gives us meaning.

By extension, spirituality addresses *why* something gives us meaning. For example, what does an individual's investment in something say about her world view, her priorities, and her passions? In short, spirituality will be used to refer to the system of beliefs or the collection of values that orient someone in the world.

It is important to note that spirituality and faith may or may not refer to the transcendent or supernatural. In addition, they may or may not express themselves in a formally religious context. While faith and spirituality refer to a broad spectrum of experiences, religion refers more specifically to those "cumulative traditions" (Fowler, 1981, p. 9) that express a people's faith, including rituals, images, symbols, music, literature and architecture, among other elements.

Finally, the word "god" will be used throughout the chapter to refer to a belief in something greater than ourselves. Although many other terms exist to capture this, such as "higher power" or the "divine," the term "god" will be employed due to its applicability across many different cultures.

Spirituality and Eating Disorders

Although many women may experience their eating disorders as entirely secular, their symptoms and the cultural pressures that exacerbate them often parallel spiritual ideals. Regardless of a patient or clinician's spiritual orientation, understanding these associations can make it easier to help the patient identify the underlying meaning of her symptoms and combat the cultural messages that justify them.

Several authors (Emmett, 1985; Jersild, 2002; Lelwica, 1999) have noted that thinness has come to signify virtuousness much in the same way that chastity did up until the past century. Lelwica suggested that this shift happened as the Church's authority waned in the face of scientific progress, when the measurable and observable earned our faith. Virtue and piety were no longer abstract ideals but rather physical qualities; thin became morally right. How often does one hear a dieter exclaim, "I was very good today?"

The diet industry has exploited this spiritual association by framing their products and plans in terms of salvation. They invite consumers to escape their physical flaws and promise many versions of heaven on earth in return: eternal youth, the perfect partner, or boundless confidence. Not surprisingly, dieting women articulate their experience in strikingly spiritual language. Dieting and eating disordered women often describe feeling called to a higher standard and finding righteousness in their ability to forgo food; some even experience a natural high, a kind of altered state of consciousness when severely restricting their caloric intake (Lelwica, 1999, p. 105).

One of the reasons that the diet industry has been so successful in selling a spiritual dream is that women face a kind of role confusion in modern society that's left them craving a larger sense of purpose. Women's increasing economic, political, and educational options have left them with new relational dilemmas: surpassing their mothers, moving further away from their families of origin, delaying children for a career, and giving up hard-won careers for new families. And while the American dream involves consuming as much and as quickly as possible, women are encouraged to refrain, diet, and deny their way to a feminine ideal.

Because of these contradictory roles and messages, clinicians (Costin, 1996; Jersild, 2001) and writers (Pipher, 1994) are conceptualizing eating disorders as problems of the soul, suggesting that obsession with weight and appearance are symptoms of a frustrated "search for meaning" (Pipher, p. 71). That is, it may be easier for a woman to express displeasure with her tangible body than to articulate a vague feeling of disconnected malaise.

Assessing Spirituality

Although a discussion of standardized spiritual assessment measures are beyond the scope of this chapter, it is generally recommended that a therapist include questions about spirituality during the intake as part of a global assessment of the patient. These questions should assess for whether the patient identifies herself as spiritual, whether she identifies with a particular religious community and/or theology, how intensely her involvement in her faith life is, and whether she feels her faith life has bearing on those issues she brings to treatment.

Even if the patient does not immediately present with spiritual or religious conflicts, assessing for their spiritual and religious background can yield important diagnostic information and provide an opportunity to join with the client. Most importantly, assessing for spirituality as part of the global intake assessment signals to the client that the therapist is willing to adopt a multicultural perspective that values other worldviews.

Spiritual assessments offer information about a number of systems in the client's life. Because religion and spirituality are often ripe areas of boundary negotiation in families, knowing how intensively a patient adheres to her parents' religion may offer hints about adolescent individuation. In addition, research has documented that children and adults describe god in ways that reflect the quality of their relationship with their parents (Wulff, 1991). A child raised in a strict home may imagine god in authoritarian terms, whereas a child raised in a giving home may imagine god as a benevolent provider. Therefore, listening for the patient's language during an assessment is just as crucial as listening for content.

Spiritual assessments can also offer information about psychological and social strengths and weaknesses. For example, does she demonstrate cognitive flexibility or rigidity by describing her spiritual life in extreme or nuanced terms? Does she discuss friends she may worship with or pastoral counselors who may already be involved in her recovery? Attending to these kinds of variables allows the therapist to determine whether a patient's spiritual life is relevant to her presenting problem and potential recovery, and whether spiritual interventions are therefore warranted.

Contraindications

In addition to clients who specifically request not to engage in spiritual discussions or exercises, several other contraindications to the use of spiritual interventions should be considered. Because spiritual interventions can require clients to consider abstract concepts, the client's cognitive stability is of primary importance.

If a client's symptoms are severe enough to disrupt her ability to be oriented to time and place or distort her perception of reality, spiritual interventions should be avoided. These symptoms include psychosis (delusions, hallucinations, and paranoia), active and frequent flashbacks or dissociation. Clients whose nutritional status is severe enough to cause cognitive impairment should also be considered inappropriate.

While spiritual interventions may be crucial to their recovery, clients who have been traumatized in religious settings or by religious figures, including cultic abuse, should not be considered appropriate for spiritual interventions until a great deal of care has been used to assess the client's groundedness, evaluate her supports and resources, process her treatment expectations, and consider transference and counter–transference implications for the therapeutic relationship.

Ethical Issues

There are several ethical issues that require consideration when addressing patients' spirituality. In particular, therapists should avoid overlapping roles or functions with religious figures in the client's life (psychotherapy versus pastoral counseling), engaging in a dual relationship with the client (attending the same religious congregation) or undermining religious authority in the client's life (by failing to collaborate with religious figures in the client's life is she states that this would be helpful).

Although spirituality is a value–laden subject, it is possible to keep from imposing one's own beliefs on the patient by avoiding several boundary lapses. Examples of these include teaching clients about religious beliefs that are irrelevant to their clinical issues, using spiritual interventions without the client's consent, telling clients that they are spiritually wrong or bad because of their behavior or beliefs, giving clients religious literature that they have not requested or adding one's own "horror stories" (Richards & Bergin, 1997, p. 154) when a client expresses frustration with spiritual experiences or principles.

While it is clearly unethical to express judgment toward a client's religious beliefs through these means, helping eating disordered clients explore how their spiritual beliefs about the body, sexuality or pleasure, for example, may impact their symptoms and recovery is perfectly appropriate. In general, spiritual interventions should never be used to supplant a patient's ideology, but should instead seek to resolve clinical issues.

Interventions

Because of the complex needs of eating disordered patients, spiritual interventions should not be used as the primary treatment modality, but instead as a component of a cohesive treatment plan. While some interventions detailed below are specific to certain religions or denominations, most can be considered "ecumenical" (Richards & Bergin, p. 124, 1997). That is, they can be applied to a variety of clinical issues with clients who espouse a wide range of beliefs. Ecumenical interventions offer therapists a greater deal of flexibility in their application and do not require a deep knowledge of specific theologies. Despite their broad nature, therapists should still proceed responsibly by assessing the patient's interest in spiritual interventions, discussing any concerns about a spiritual approach, and getting written or verbal consent before commencing.

Writing

Writing exercises are a particularly effective way for patients to address complex emotional issues, and for this reason are ideal approaches to spirituality. The act of writing can often provide clarity, pace, and structure to a patient's exploration of complicated feelings, as the written words become a container for their emotional life (Greenspan, 1999). In addition, because writing exercises can be done outside of the session, it offers clients a way to carry their work from the session into their daily lives.

Spiritual Autobiographies

Spiritual autobiographies are a very flexible and open–ended way to approach spirituality in a clinical setting. They can range from an unstructured conversation about a patient's religious upbringing, or a formal series of questions meant to guide a patient in writing about her faith life development. Writing a spiritual autobiography can often stimulate insight about spiritual and non–spiritual issues for the client; sharing the autobiography with the therapist offers witness and validation. More importantly, providing an opportunity for clients to consider how their faith life has both fortified and challenged them models critical thinking; this is particularly relevant to women with eating disorders, who often encounter and absorb many social messages that count on their unquestioning acceptance.

Regardless of differences in spiritual orientation, many women in treatment for eating disorders identify several consistently recurring spiritual themes when discussing their symptoms (Jersild, 2001). These themes can often be natural starting points for spiritual autobiographies. Below are five such themes followed by sample questions to stimulate discussion or writing.

Anger

Because anger is often seen as incompatible with a feminine ideal, many women struggle with expressing this emotion. Eating disorders have therefore been conceptualized by many clinicians (Baker Miller, 1991; Larkin, Rice & Russell, 1996) as a way for women to turn their anger inward rather than risk expressing it. This difficulty with anger can be reinforced or mitigated by a number of spiritual belief systems. Many spiritual traditions contain icons of serenity, from the Virgin Mary to the Buddha, which are emulated as spiritual ideals and which may inhibit an individual's comfort with anger. On the other hand, many religious texts offer examples of positive anger, such as Jesus' political activism (Mathew, 21:12; Mark, 11:15, Revised Standard Version).

Questions regarding anger and spirituality: What are some examples of anger in the stories of your faith? Have any individuals modeled the expression of anger in your faith community? Are there opportunities in your faith life to express and feel anger?

Perfection

As mentioned above, the pursuit of bodily perfection often protects women from confronting complicated emotional and relational issues in their lives. Richards et al. (1997) suggest that women involved in certain religious traditions may also use the pursuit of perfection to compensate for feelings of spiritual unworthiness. In contrast, many religious traditions and spiritual belief systems establish broader parameters for what constitutes perfection, such as the Judeo–Christian ideal that we are all made in god's image (Genesis, 1:27; Genesis, 5:3, Revised Standard Version), and may provide an antidote to our current culture's stringent and narrow definition.

Questions regarding perfection and spirituality: Is there a concept of "perfect" in your faith tradition? Is perfection emphasized by your faith tradition?

Self–Care

Because they often play a nurturing role in individual relationships and social groups, many women fear that acknowledging their own needs and desires may lead to ruptures in their relationships. For this reason, clinicians conceptualize eating disordered symptoms as a means of detaching from one's physical and emotional hunger. Many images of sacrifice in different religious traditions, such as the Buddha's rejection of his princely wealth or Jesus' crucifixion, may exacerbate guilt about acknowledging one's own needs. However, it is important to note how and whether sacrifice has been framed by an individual's particular spiritual upbringing within a larger religion; some denominations emphasize that which was sacrificed for, such as peace or self knowledge, rather than the sacrifice itself.

Questions regarding self–care and spirituality: Are there examples of self–sacrifice and self–care in your spiritual tradition? Have any individuals in your faith community modeled sacrifice or self–care for you? Have you had any personal experiences with asking for you own needs to be met within your faith community?

Forgiveness and Guilt

In their 1989 study on religiosity and mental health, Kroll and Sheehan found eating disordered respondents to be among the two diagnostic groups "most absorbed with their own sinfulness" (p. 71). Because forgiveness and guilt are cardinal issues in many religious traditions, therapists should be aware of how a patient's faith life may affect their symptoms and recovery. Some patients, for example, have been able to use concepts or rituals in their faith life to forgive themselves for their perceived imperfections; others, however, have been told by religious figures that their eating disorders constituted a sin.

Questions regarding forgiveness, guilt, and spirituality: How have forgiveness and guilt been handled in your faith tradition? What have been your experiences with forgiveness and guilt in your spiritual upbringing?

Sexuality and Embodiment

Many clinicians (Hutchinson, 1994; McIntosh et al., 2000) conceptualize eating disorders as a means of starving off ones' sexual features or numbing the libido, thereby avoiding the interpersonal and physical risks that come with inhabiting a mature female body. These risks range from having one's sexual boundaries violated to having others confuse physical maturity for emotional readiness to make adult decisions. Conflicts around one's sexual desires or sexual features can be amplified in women who observe religious traditions that emphasize chastity. Some theologians (Gross, 1996; Heyward, 1982; Reuther, 1998) have even suggested that monotheistic traditions in general, which depict god as hovering above and outside of humanity, tend to polarize spirit and matter and see the body as working against spirituality. Many of those same traditions contain progressive voices (Harrison, 1989; Lorde, 1989; Plaskow, 1990) which honor the body as the center of spiritual morality, not its opposite, because of its capacity to register those emotions necessary for community and commitment, such as love, happiness, and desire.

Questions regarding sexuality, embodiment, and spirituality: How has the human body been discussed, treated, or portrayed in your faith tradition? Are there any rituals marking puberty or sexual maturity in your faith tradition? How have individuals in your faith community discussed sexuality?

Metaphor Work

Exploring spiritual metaphors is an effective way to discuss a patient's spirituality and the impact it may have on her body. Because metaphors provide a discreet word or image to convey complex issues or emotions, they can help patients approach feelings more comfortably. In addition, the abstract nature of metaphor work coupled with a discussion of their personal relevance to the patient offers a safe alternation between intimacy and objectivity (Greenspan, 1999).

Metaphor work can be especially powerful when addressing spirituality because of the rich volume of religious metaphor that exists even in the secular culture. A basic awareness of religious metaphor can help our clients become more culturally literate, fortifying them with an ability to identify the etiology of various cultural images and challenges those that feel harmful.

Theologians (Plaskow, 1990; Soelle, 1984) have written about the effect that metaphors for the divine have on larger social values, and argued that secular culture absorbs these metaphors, so that the metaphor itself becomes culturally idolized instead of that which it refers. Plaskow (1990) cited "God the Father" as a potent example, stating that all too often in Judeo–Christian societies, "maleness is what is worshiped, not God" (p. 128). Soelle (1984) asked us to consider how different Western values might be if the Judeo–Christian god were imagined more often with relational metaphors (healer, shepherd, mother) rather than metaphors based on power (king, lord, ruler).

These and other implicit values conveyed by spiritual metaphors and carried into secular society have a great impact on eating disordered women, who so often measure themselves against cultural standards. Consequently, the ability to explore, supplement, or replace these metaphors has tremendous relevance for women in treatment and recovery. Plaskow (1990) suggested creating more inclusive metaphors to capture the divine, such as Light

or Stream. Metaphors such as these, which are not anthropo[l]
far less likely to lead to assumptions about which group (or ge[n]
ple reflect the true image of god.

The following are questions that therapists can use to stimulate [l]
work with clients: What metaphors exist in your faith or religion to d[escribe]
god? What metaphors exist in your faith to describe those who beli[eve]
god? How do these metaphors invite you into relationship with god, oth[ers]
yourself, and your body? How might they exclude you from relationsh[ip]
with god, others, yourself, and your body? What new metaphors can yo[u]
create to better convey how you would like to feel valued in the universe?

Ritual and Worship

As discussed above, different teachings of various religious traditions (and
not necessarily the pure tradition itself) are more likely to portray the body
as something to overcome on one's way to spiritual awareness (Gross, 1996;
Reuther, 1998). This can unfortunately reinforce eating disordered efforts to
control the body's appetites and cut off emotional experiences from the
physical self.

Because of their sensual nature, G. K. Chesterton once compared Catholic
mass to a good stogie and a glass of port. Ritual and worship can be wonderful ways to decrease this split between body and spirit. Singing, moving
in unison, kneeling or even lifting an arm in praise can all evoke different
emotional experiences: catharsis, fear, serenity, or joy. In turn, these emotional experiences are felt in the body through tense or relaxed muscles, a
racing heart, or deepening breath. This joining of a physical and emotional
experience can reinforce the body as a necessary part of a spiritual life rather
than an impediment or burden (Harrison, 1989).

Many patients engage in formal or informal rituals of worship, from
attending temple to sitting yoga, on a weekly or monthly basis. Because of
these regular time intervals, worship practices provide an ongoing opportunity for patients to observe and attune to the reciprocity between her physical and emotional states, and can often compliment other, non–spiritual,
therapeutic endeavors.

Prayer

Prayer is, for many patients, an indigenous resource; that is, many have
been raised in religious traditions that practice some form of prayer and
therefore already have this as a coping skill at their disposal. In addition,
those patients who do not subscribe to a religious tradition but who see them-

odality
norphized, are
der) of peo-
netaphor
escribe
ve in
ers,

ιtual often engage in some type of prayer,
ηto their daily routine, yoga, or a regular
Because prayer can be as formal as recit-
ιeriod of silence, it is accessible to most

ρeutic functions. Asking a patient to
·r in her recovery and which prayer
. her own expert. In discussing and
ιne therapist, the prayer subsequently
..al object, something she can take from the ther-
...ιto her daily life. Because eating disordered clients
...nding adaptive ways to self–soothe and contain impulsivity,
.an offer the client an effective way to calm herself, as well as a delay
.ιtween an impulse (to binge, purge or exercise, for example) and an action.

Since prayer is often expressed as a petition (i.e., asking for something), it provides a natural opportunity for eating disordered women, who so often struggle with acknowledging their needs, to practice this. If a patient is currently praying, it can be helpful to point out the ways that her prayer life allows her to imagine, dream, hope, and want amidst an eating disorder that too often separates her from these desires. If she has not traditionally prayed but expresses a wish to do so, it can be helpful to offer very basic examples of the variations prayers might take, thereby increasing its accessibility. Although an exploration of prayer can provide rich therapeutic opportunities, it is not generally recommended that therapists pray with their clients in session, as this can create role confusion and blur relational boundaries.

Spiritual Imagery and Relaxation

Many patients come to therapy with images or symbols from their spiritual lives that can be incorporated into relaxation techniques, guided imagery, or other creative exercises. Because it is often difficult for eating disordered patients to surrender to therapeutic exercises that reduce their sense of physical or emotional control, using meaningful spiritual imagery may increase the exercise's resonance for patients and mitigate their resistance.

A number of elements common to many different faiths are ideal for experiential exercises and relaxation rituals. For example, the Judeo–Christian tradition uses water in rituals such as the mikvah and baptism to signify cleansing or rebirth. Native Americans use herbs and smoke in a practice called smudging, to cleanse and prepare for ritual, change or insight; the presence of fire (such as candles or incense) often accompanies both Christian and Hindu sacraments as well. Even basic spiritual postures carry meanings that are especially relevant to eating disordered women. Buddhists, for example, draw their hands together in meditation (reflecting a prayer stance common to most faiths) to signify the integration of mind and body (Smith, 1991).

These and other elements can be used in movement therapy, art therapy, psychodrama, and other modalities to add depth and sensuality to therapeutic exercises. In addition, offering a patient the opportunity to both inform the therapist about the personal significance of certain symbols and to integrate those symbols into treatment can increase the patient's sense of authorship and investment in her treatment.

It is also helpful to be mindful of various religious calendars. Many spiritual traditions observe days of atonement, such as Yom Kippur, days of feasting and fasting, such as Lent and Ramadan, and seasons of reflection or celebration, such as Advent and Easter. Because these spiritual themes often parallel stages and tasks in recovery, it is often possible to integrate them into a patient's therapy to reinforce positive change or to encourage movement from a point at which they may be stuck.

Conclusion

Processing faith–related experiences offers opportunities for insight for both therapist and patient, and models the critical thinking needed to challenge cultural pressures that too often justify eating disordered symptoms. Exploring spiritual resources currently in place in the patient's life allows her to recognize moments of embodiment she may already be enjoying. Because of its multifaceted nature, spirituality transcends simple intellectual exercise and bridges cognitive, emotional, physical, and relational experiences for the patient, ultimately inviting her to integrate those aspects from which her eating disorder has left her disconnected.

References

Baker Miller, J. (1991). Women and power. In J. V. Jordan, A. G. Kaplan, J. Baker Miller, I. P. Stiver & J. L. Surrey (Eds.), *Women's growth in connection* (pp. 197–205). New York: The Guilford Press.

Costin, C. (1996). *The eating disorder sourcebook.* Los Angeles: Lowell House.

Crisp, A., Joughin, N., Haleck, C., & Humphrey, H. (1992) Religious belief and anorexia nervosa. *International Journal of Eating Disorders, 12,* 397–406.

Emmet, S.W. (1985). Future trends. In S. W. Emmett (Ed.), *Theory and treatment of anorexia nervosa and bulimia: Biomedical, sociocultural and psychological perspectives* (pp. 304–319). New York: Brunner/Mazel Publishers.

Emmett, S. W. (1997) The last word. *Eating Disorders, 5,* 93–95.

Epstein, M. (1995). *Thoughts without a thinker: Psychotherapy from a Buddhist perspective.* New York: Basic Books.

Fowler, J. W. (1981). *Stages of faith: The psychology of human development and the quest for meaning.* San Francisco: Harper Collins.

Garrett, C. (1998). *Beyond anorexia: narrative, spirituality and recovery.* Cambridge, England: Cambridge University Press.

Gordon, R. (1990). *Anorexia and Bulimia.* United Kingdom: Basil Blackwell.

Greenspan, B. (1999, November). *Therapeutic writing.* Paper presented at the Ninth Annual Renfrew Center Foundation Conference: "Feminist Perspectives on the Process of Change: Exploring What Works and Why." Philadelphia, Pennsylvania.

Gross, R. M. (1996). *Feminism and religion.* Boston: Beacon Press.

Harrison, B. W. (1989). The power of anger in the work of love. In: J. Plaskow & C. Christ (Eds.), *Weaving the visions* (pp. 214–225). San Francisco: Harper.

Heyward, C. (1982). *The redemption of God: A theology of mutual relation.* Washington, D.C.: University Press of America.

Hutchinson, M.G. (1994). Imagining ourselves whole: a feminist approach to treating body image disorders. In P. Fallon, M. A. Katzman & S. C. Wooley (Eds.), *Feminist perspectives on eating disorders* (pp. 152–170). New York: The Guilford Press.

Jersild, A. (2002). Separation of church and weight: Fleshing out Christianity's contradictions. *Bitch: A Feminist Response to Pop Culture, 17,* 54–60.

Jersild, A. (2001). Field mice and mustard seeds: Approaching spirituality as a therapeutic tool. *Eating Disorders: The Journal of Treatment and Prevention, 9*(3), 267–274.

Johnston, A., & Antares, K. (2005) Eating disorders as messengers of the soul. In S. G. Mijares & G. S. Khalsa (Eds.), *The psychospiritual clinician's handbook* (pp. 97–112). New York: Haworth Reference Press.

Kroll, J. & Sheehan, W. (1989). Religious beliefs and practices among fifty–two psychiatric inpatients in Minnesota. *American Journal of Psychiatry, 146,* 67–72.

Larkin, J., Rice, C., & Russell, V. (1996). Slipping through the cracks: Sexual harassment, eating problems and the problem of embodiment. *Eating Disorders, 4,* 5–26.

Lelwica, M. M. (1999). *Starving for salvation.* Oxford, England: Oxford University Press.

Lorde, A. (1989). Uses of the erotic. In J. Plaskow & C. Christ (Eds.), *Weaving the visions* (pp. 208–213). San Francisco: Harper.

Pipher, M. (1994). *Reviving Ophelia.* New York: Ballantine Books.

Plaskow, J. (1990). *Standing again at Sinai.* NY: Harper Collins.

Reuther, R. (1998). *Women and redemption: A theological history.* Minneapolis, MN: Fortress Press.

Richards, P. S., & Bergin, A. E. (1997). *A spiritual strategy for counseling and psychotherapy.* Washington, D.C.: American Psychological Association.

Richards, P. S., & Bergin, A. E. (2000). *Handbook of psychotherapy and religious diversity.* Washington, D.C.: American Psychological Association.

Richards, P. S., Hardman, R. K, Frost, H. A., Berrett, M. E., Clark–Sly, J. B., & Anderson, D. K. (1997). Spiritual issues and interventions in the treatment of patients with eating disorders. *Eating Disorders, 5,* 261–279.

Rizzuto, A. (1981). *The birth of a living god: A psychoanalytic study.* Chicago: University of Chicago Press.

Simmonds, J. G. (2006). The oceanic feeling and a sea change: Historical challenges to reductionist attitudes to religion and spirit from within psychoanalysis. *Psychoanalytic Psychology, 23*(1), 128–142.

Smith, H. (1991). *The world's religions.* San Francisco: Harper Collins.

Soelle, D. (1984). *Strength of the weak.* Philadelphia: Westminster Press.

Wulff, D. M. (1991). *Psychology of religion: Classic and contemporary views.* New York: Wiley.

Biography

Amy Jersild is a licensed clinical social worker specializing in the treatment of eating disorders and sexual trauma at Temple University's Tuttleman Counseling Services. Amy received her BS from Northwestern University in 1994 and her M.S.W. from the University of Pennsylvania in 1999. Amy has worked with women and men suffering from eating disorders for the past decade, and received her training at The Renfrew Center, one of the country's first facilities dedicated to the treatment of anorexia, bulimia, compulsive over–eating, and body image disturbance. Amy has published articles on the role of spirituality and religion in the development of body image in both clinical and popular journals.

Chapter 16

NOURISHING THE YOUNG THERAPIST: ACTION SUPERVISION WITH EATING DISORDERED CLIENTS USING THE THERAPEUTIC SPIRAL MODEL

KATE HUDGINS

Introduction

Twenty years ago, I was an intern in clinical psychology at the University of Wisconsin Medical School, Department of Psychiatry. I arrived, already a Board–Certified Practitioner of Psychodrama, Sociometry, and Group Psychotherapy with a number of years of private practice as a psychodramatist on my resume. It was a good match for me as an experiential therapist and trainer as many of today's experiential therapies were researched there. The Eating Disorder Program was one of the most advanced in the United States at that time.

However, truly holistic, body–based, experiential psychotherapy treatment programs were fairly new to the healing of people with eating disorders (Hornyak & Baker, 1989). Today, experiential therapies are called the treatment of choice for many stress–related disorders (Elliott, Greenberg, & Lietaer, 2002). Van der Kolk (2003) specifically prescribes experiential treatment for men and women who have eating disorders. Given that disordered eating is at its core a body–based psychological illness, it makes sense that treatment must also include the recovery of the body–mind. Drama therapy, psychodrama, Gestalt therapy, and the creative arts bring together a rich history of theory and practice of experiential methods of change to help people heal from eating disorders.

Complex PTSD and Eating Disorders

In many cases, people with eating disorders are vulnerable clients, often with histories of physical and sexual abuse, family alcoholism, or other overwhelming stress in their childhood development. These clients may carry dual diagnoses, including complex post–traumatic stress disorder (PTSD), and personality, mood, addictive, and dissociative disorders. The eating disorder gets them into treatment, because in many cases it is life threatening and must be addressed immediately. At times, lifesaving interventions such as inpatient treatment or other medical intervention are indicated. At any rate, full recovery from an eating disorder is often a long–term psychological process that includes body, mind, heart, and soul healing. Clinical supervision is invaluable for therapists who are working with clients with eating disorders.

The Therapeutic Spiral Model

This chapter presents a treatment and supervision system of experiential psychotherapy called the Therapeutic Spiral Model (Hudgins, in press–a–c, 2002, 2000, 1998, 1989). TSM, as it is commonly called, is a clinical system of structured experiential interventions to treat PTSD, addictions, eating disorders, and other mental health problems. It has an integrated theoretical foundation in clinical psychology and the treatment of trauma using experiential methods of change. TSM is a clinical method of drama therapy that uses modified psychodrama, Gestalt therapy, and the creative arts to bring healing to clients with eating disorders.

This chapter describes Live Action Supervision by Doctor Kate Hudgins with a composite TSM therapist working with a client who has bulimia. Therapist concerns, skill development, and countertransference are all examined as we follow the TSM therapist and her client across six months of individual experiential psychotherapy using the Therapeutic Spiral Model for treatment and supervision.

TSM Action Supervision Model

TSM Action Supervision follows the same clinical map as does the experiential treatment of people with eating disorders. First, we build Prescriptive Roles of restoration, containment, and observation needed to directly address more difficult areas of the eating disordered behaviors. When safety is established, a history of trauma often emerges and must be contained so it can be expressed safely when using experiential methods. TSM Action

Supervision teaches the therapist new skills in a step by step model that includes a countertransference focus for the therapist.

There are three steps in TSM Live Action Supervision:

- Establishing a Cognitive Container
- Teaching structured Hands–On Skills
- Transference and Countertransference Intervention

This chapter follows the supervision of a TSM trained therapist with a client diagnosed with bulimia as they begin TSM therapy, following the disclosure of an eating disorder. Below you will see how TSM supervision provides the psychological container for the therapist who often feels inadequate, overwhelmed, and frustrated as she deals with the strong defenses and intense affect involved in work with people with eating disorders.

A TSM Clinician

Gina is a recently licensed clinical social worker in private practice in a Midwest state in America. She is a registered drama therapist. Gina is 31 years old and brings to her role of experiential therapist a true dedication to providing a healing environment for people she sees in her practice. She is talented, bright, and highly empathic. She recently started training in TSM to learn advanced methods of action change with people who have PTSD and eating disorders. She also brings a personal history of anorexia and childhood sexual abuse. She has been in recovery from her eating disorder for the past four years and has the support of a therapist as needed. She seeks TSM Action Supervision to help her deal with her own issues as a provider, as well as to bring better treatment to her clients.

A TSM Client

Gina's client is a 19–year–old college student named Alicia. She has been in therapy with Gina for six months. Initially, she sought treatment for low self–esteem and concentration difficulties in school. She recently disclosed to Gina that she has been bulimic since she was sixteen when her parents separated and the family fell apart. She had responded well to the use of the creative arts and drama therapy as support and ego–building therapy. Now, she was asking to deal with her "deeper issues" and her eating disorder. Gina wants to use TSM to facilitate this next state of experiential therapy with Alicia.

Stage 1: Prescriptive Roles for Therapist and Client Alike

Stage 1 in all TSM therapy and supervision focuses on three clinical goals: (1) Building the Witness Role; (2) Instillation of Strengths; and (3) Providing Psychological Containment. This is absolutely true for both TSM therapy and TSM Action Supervision. Before moving into Trauma–Based Roles with Alicia, Gina learns to build her own Prescriptive Roles in TSM Action Supervision. She learns intervention skills while working through her own trauma triggers as a woman in recovery from her own eating disorder.

Building the Witness Role

Often overlooked in experiential therapy, the Witness Role needs to be established first to create a cognitive container for any action interventions. In TSM, this is easily accomplished through the use of Inspirational Cards. Each TSM session begins by the client/s picking one or more cards out of a deck of inspirational cards on the floor, on the desk, or on a table as they come in the room. They are asked to imagine this role as one that can "neutrally observe you throughout your time in this session." They talk about the role and then physically place the card somewhere in the room to mark a physical space for the Witness Role.

Gina attended a supervision group one month and was greeted by the Louis Hay "Healthy Body" cards. People picked one or more cards that were true for them. The cards had pictures with statements like "I love my heart," "I love my hair," "I love my eyes," "I love my spine." They talked in groups of two to share why they picked the card they did to be the seed of a Witness Role. They put the cards up on the walls of the group room and gathered their papers and pen to present a case in action for the supervision group. Subsequently, many therapists in the supervision group used cards of Inspiration to start off their groups for women with eating disorders.

Instillation of Strengths

Gina comes into an individual supervision session feeling hopeless and in despair. Alicia has not been able to change her pattern of bingeing and purging up to 8000 calories a day more than one day in the past week, despite her best efforts. She feels like she is a total failure, that she can't do anything right. She is beating herself up with criticism and destructive self–blame. Gina is stuck in a parallel process, feeling incompetent and inadequate to "get" Alicia to change life–threatening behaviors. She brings her concerns into her individual TSM supervision session.

I ask her to pick two or three scarves to represent strengths she brings to her work with Alicia. We build a Circle of Safety (Cox, 2000) for her to provide containment and increase her experience of her own strengths as we begin the experiential component of our supervision session. Gina picks a bright Indonesian sarong to represent her own vitality. Next, she draws out a cool blue scarf to represent her calmness. Then she looks up at me and says, "I don't think I have any more strengths, Doctor Kate. I am so upset about not helping Alicia." I choose a pink scarf to add to her beginning circle and tell her it is my unconditional positive regard for her. I say: "I believe in you. You are very skilled and talented, just a little stuck right now. She just told you about her bulimia. That is a huge step. She will eventually be able to stop the bulimic eating patterns as well. You will help her. And I will help you."

She is then able to choose a multicolored cloth and name it as her determination to bring healing to others. I add a second strength of my own, that of a clear cognitive mind that can help her sort out what she needs to do next. I add a scarf that has many colours and patterns that still have an orderly pattern to it. She sighs and sits down in her chair with her Circle of Safety out in front of her in the room.

I ask Gina to imagine Alicia inside the circle. She is able to do this and describes her as curled up in a fetal ball, scared of the world, wanting to withdraw from college, her relationships, and actually life itself. She starts to get lost in the darkness and despair of Alicia's life, even from the witness role as client. I help her stop the seductive pull of the eating disorder. I ask her to look at her inspirational card that she picked as she sat down in the therapy chair. It says hope. I tell her, we have hope that Alicia can change. And this is just the beginning of the process.

To deepen her active experiencing of her own strengths, I ask Gina to take the role of one of her strengths in the Circle of Safety surrounding the client. She stands and picks up the scarf that represents her strength of Determination. I ask her to dress herself in this role. She adds a fur headband and picks up a rhinestone wand. She comes alive in the role. She takes the warrior pose from yoga and says she is "ready to fight." As you can see, this role reversal is done with full creativity so that it is anchored in at the somatic level of experiencing. We don't want strengths to just be words, but to have the actual experience of them in body, mind, heart, and soul. TSM experiential interventions allow this to happen.

GINA AS DETERMINATION: I am determined to help you heal. You are just scared. College is hard. There are so many pressures. Please know I am here for you and we can do this together. You are not alone.

SUPERVISOR: Use your body. Use your wand. Speak to Alicia and tell her how you two can do this together with others in her life.

GINA AS DETERMINATION: *(Her body sways. She uses her wand. She touches the pillow that is holding the role of Alicia.)* We don't have to do this alone. Come on. It's not that bad. We can do this. You've told me the secret. That is the important thing. Now, we can work with understanding and change your bulimic patterns. We can do this. OK?

Containment: The Body Double

Gina arrives at a later individual supervision session with a sense of depletion. She says "I don't' know what to do with Alicia. When I hear about her life, all I want to do is stop eating myself, never a good feeling for a recovering anorexic. I have actually lost three pounds in the last month and I am worried where we are both going with our issues. Please give me some guidance so I can stop my own emotional patterns that are connected to not eating for me. Help!"

We start supervision with a discussion of the parallel process she sees between herself and her client, Alicia. Whenever you think the supervision issue many contain an element of countertransference, it helps to set the cognitive container by naming the parallels between you and your client. Both the similarities and the differences, especially in terms of recovery. Simply putting words and narrative labels on the issues that are intersecting between therapist and client provides the first step in psychological containment. If you can admit what is in the way, you can change it. " No shame, no blame" is a core TSM mantra that allows therapists to bring up their personal issues without fear.

Next, I suggest that we set up an action scene where she talks to her client while I take the role of her Body Double (Hudgins, 2002). She knows that the Body Double (BD) is a role that speaks in the first person as a helpful inner voice that focuses on a positive experience of being in your body in the present moment, even under stress. As always, the BD focuses on increasing awareness of her own physical resources, helping her to calm and self–soothe. The BD also suggests psychological and social resources she can use. Because it is an inner voice, rather than the words of the supervisor per se, the teachings can often be more readily accepted. It also provides a container of nonverbal empathy and interpersonal support. as the BD sits beside the client rather than across from her.

Gina sets up two chairs across from each other. I suggest that it might be easier to talk to her client if they sit at a 45–degree angle rather than across from each other. She agrees to try this. She picks the black scarf to mark Alicia in the chair. She sits down in the therapist chair and I bring another chair in to her right and sit beside her as her Body Double. We begin our experiential TSM Action Supervision.

See the Appendix at the end of this chapter for session dialogue and supervisory interaction from the role of Body Double. As you will see, Gina experiences her own personal restoration at a body level, and also gains a powerful new action intervention, the Body Double, she can use directly with Alicia in their next session.

Stage 2: Working with the Eating Disorder

After building strengths and developing the capacity for self–observation and psychological containment, both therapist and client can move onto Stage 2 TSM therapy. Here we directly access the TSM trauma–based roles of victim, perpetrator, and abandoning authority through the use of a safe sociodramatic TSM experiential structure called "Walking the Trauma Triangle." This TSM clinical action structure teaches the therapist a frame to view the eating disorder as a set of internalized ego states or roles that maintain the downward spiral into eating disordered behaviors. It helps both therapist and client begin to contain, label, and express the self–hatred, rage, grief, and loss that fuel the eating disorder.

Stage 2 is often difficult work for therapists and clients as the intense feelings that the eating disorder had been holding at bay begin to surface into active experiencing of self and in the therapeutic relationship. This often, brings up counter transference and any unworked through trauma patterns for the new therapist working with eating disorders. When they can bring these issues to supervision, the therapists find their own healing and can then help the clients make further progress for themselves.

The clinical goals in Stage 2 of TSM therapy are: (1) identifying and labeling of internalized trauma based roles and patterns, (2) safe and conscious expression of feelings, and (3) integration of dissociated ego states. You will see here how we follow this template in working with therapists in supervision as they assist their clients in working directly with their own trauma material.

The Trauma Triangle

A couple of months later, Gina comes into the office telling me that Alicia is thinking of suicide because she feels so helpless. Three months into actively dealing with her eating disorder, Alicia can still only maintain normal eating for a few weeks at a time before she has a binge. Then she collapses in shame and overwhelming self–hatred. Gina asks for some tools to help Alicia see her trauma patterns, rather than just the eating disorder. I decide to teach her the Trauma Triangle, a TSM assessment tool to look at the internalization of victim, perpetrator and abandoning authority roles as they play out in an eating disorder.

While there are several others triangles that people use to look at addictions and other problems, what is unique to the TSM Trauma Triangle is the role of Abandoning Authority. The theory behind this role is that abuse cannot occur, in most cases, if there is someone holding the appropriate authority and intervening to stop the abuse. A father cannot sexually abuse his daughter if the mother takes her authority and throws him out or gets a divorce. Priests cannot molest young boys if the church does not cover up and abandon its authority for its congregation. Religions cannot oppress people if governments do not support their authoritarian beliefs and give them power.

When someone is victimized, not only do they internalize a sense of victimization and an image of the perpetrator, but they also internalize a sense of abandonment of authority for oneself. This is particularly true in people with eating disorders. We are talking basic self–care when one is struggling with disordered eating. Sometimes even life and death. The TSM Trauma Triangle can help people look at their own self–destructive patterns so they can identify them, where they came from, and how to use the Prescriptive roles to intervene in the trauma patterns.

Gina and I use the scarves to mark out a triangle in my office. We put down cards that label each point: victim, perpetrator and abandoning authority. I suggest that she role–play her client Alicia. I will be the therapist asking the client to walk the triangle so she can learn how to do this intervention in her next session.

CLIENT: I am seriously thinking about killing myself. I really really really don't want to be in this body anymore. I hate it so much!

THERAPIST: Yes, I can see and feel your self–hatred today and I'd like to help you release that and not turn it toward your body today. (*Establishes a clinical contract for the session.*) I don't want you to hurt yourself.

THERAPIST: OK, let's stand up. As you can see I have marked a triangle on the floor with the roles that are normally learned from trauma. You know what a victim is as you have lived that role in many relationships. From what you've told me, I think your mother's cold fury and out of control raging at you is where you internalized the self–blame that makes up your perpetrator role. And the third role in TSM is to look at how you abandon authority for making good self–care decisions for yourself today. . . . Do you understand those roles?

CLIENT: Mostly, I am not quite sure about how I do abandon my own authority. I try to be in control all of the time. So, what do you want me to do now?

THERAPIST: I'd like you to just start talking out loud about not wanting to live. If I hear you making statements from any of these roles, I will ask you to step onto the triangle at that point. If I hear you making statements where you are using your strengths, practicing good self–care, taking authority for yourself, I will ask you to step off the triangle. OK?

Let's put an empty chair in the center of the Trauma Triangle to represent your eating disorder. You can see how much of the dialogue inside your head is connected to your bulimia and how much too healthy self–care and recovery. No shame, no blame. Just listen to yourself as you walk through the thoughts in your head as you speak them out loud.

CLIENT: Sure sounds interesting.

THERAPIST: OK, step onto the triangle here at the victim role because you feel a sense of helplessness that you don't want to live anymore.

CLIENT: Oh . . . is that a victim statement? I didn't know that. It does feel like I have given up.

THERAPIST: Now, move to the abandoning authority role. You are saying you are actively giving up on yourself. That is an abandoning statement. Keep walking.

CLIENT: Well, shit . . . I just can't stop bingeing and purging? I just can't and it is driving me crazy. I mean, I'm just a stupid shit. I just can't do anything at all.

THERAPIST: Now, step over to the perpetrator role because you are calling yourself stupid and a shit. Where did you learn to call yourself those names? They aren't true you know? I have heard you express very smart ideas and certainly you are dedicated to doing it better, so I just don't see that view of yourself. I think you learned that from your mother or someone else.

CLIENT: When mom would rage, she would tell all of us that we were stupid, no good, and not wanted. I hated it, I just wanted to die. I couldn't get her to stop. There was nothing I could do.

THERAPIST: OK, come back to the abandoning authority role. Can you hear how you give up your ability to make different choices? Today, you are not little. Your mother cannot call you names anymore. Now, you have to stop calling yourself names. You've connected to a lot of your strengths. What do you think?

CLIENT: I can't do it any differently. I am lonely. I don't wanna do it all by myself anymore. I just wanna feel taken care of. That is what draws me to the food over and over again. That idiotic belief that food will make me feel better. It doesn't. It just makes me feel worse.

THERAPIST: Great. Let's step off the trauma triangle, because you are accurately labeling your distorted thinking, that food can make you feel better. The way you use food, it can only make you worse.

CLIENT: Oh, all it gives me is a fantasy. I know I am stronger than that now. I just wish it were easier for me. I wish I had a picture perfect recovery. But that's not how I am able to do it. So, today, right now, no shame, no blame. Only trying again.

THERAPIST: Great. Now, that kind of thinking gets you off the triangle. Say again what you just said. You are stronger now. You have more help. Step outside the trauma roles, and speak to your eating disorder, caught in the old patterns.

CLIENT: Ok, but ya know as soon as I stepped off the triangle, I could feel the pull to just stop eating for the next few days. It is just too hard to take care of myself. Sometimes, I just wanna give up too.

THERAPIST: OK, you just stepped back onto the triangle in the abandoning authority role. What do you think you are feeling now as you give up on yourself and think of turning to not eating to push your feelings down?

CLIENT: I think I am scared and angry and just want to get away from it all.

THERAPIST: Yes, let's step off the triangle again. Now let's sit down and you can tell me more about your feelings, your true feelings.

Working with Countertransference

Now nine months into TSM therapy with Alicia, Gina starts supervision off with the following statement:

"I am enraged at the eating disorder. Alicia's bulimia is still totally consuming her life. I remember that feeling. Getting on the scales 10x a day, trying to get the numbers to go down, down, down. Not dealing with my feelings. Not dealing with my family. I see her doing the same things. She is totally stuck again, and I just don't know what to do. I am so angry! I just want to hit something! I can't stand it! It totally reminds me of myself when I couldn't eat and just wouldn't do anything differently. I just wouldn't. What do I do now? I just can't stand it anymore!"

Wow, I say, "You are really angry today! I am glad you have brought these intense feelings into supervision today. Let's work with them together, OK? Gina continues to pace around the room.

I move in as her Body Double. I say, "Boy, I sure am angry. Far beyond what is just related to Alicia not eating. I'm guessing this is my own counter transference. Do I want to work on that today?" Gina sits down in the chair and starts crying. She says, "Yes, yes, I do. I just feel so out of control. And since I don't have my eating disorder anymore . . . sometimes it is just too hard. I just don't want to do it anymore. I am worn out. I am tired."

I sit down in my chair as supervisor. I get a contract with Gina to spend the session working on her countertransference. She is angry with herself, at Alicia, but most importantly she is angry at the eating disorder. I suggest an action structure to help her express her own feelings about having had an eating disorder and how it can cause so much damage in someone's life. I ask her to use the chairs, the scarves and anything else in the room she wants to create the role of the eating disorder, of anorexia, so she can have a conversation with it.

She takes one of the straight–backed chairs from the wall. Next she takes all the dark scarves . . . black, brown, dark blue . . . and she wraps the chair tightly, like a tourniquet, around and around the chair. Then she dresses it up with a vase of silk flowers that sit on my desk. She tells me, "That's it. That what anorexia looks like. It ties up the person. Controls them. And tries, all the time, to make you think it is so you can look prettier, be more in control on the outside, when inside everything is crazy."

I ask her to add the internal chaos to the sculpture. To concretize all of what anorexia is about, not just the outside, not just the control. She immediately gets up and takes the pad of colored paper that is always available for supervision. She tears up sheet after sheet after sheet as she starts to cry. She says these bits and pieces, brightly colored and dark alike are how it feels to have anorexia nervosa, little bits of self all torn and mixed up.

Once again, I step into the Body Double role and say, "Yes, I am crying for my self, for my own losses, the many pieces of myself I have struggled to put back together again. Today, it just feels like too much. I did it for me, but I'm not sure I can do it for Alicia. She has to decide to do it herself." She takes a deep breath and her tears begin to subside. She leans against my shoulder for a moment, taking in the physical support of her Body Double. I put words to this process: "It is good to lean against myself, to feel my solid and supportive body that is always there for me. I can just stop and take time for myself. This is good." She breathes in the support and says, "OK, I am ready to talk to the eating disorder. I know what I want to say now."

I move aside. I suggest that she feel her strength and says whatever she wants to say to the anorexia for herself and for Alicia. This is her statement:

"You don't have control of me anymore. You cannot hurt me. You cannot make me care about the numbers on the scale or the amount of calories that go into my mouth. I take

care of myself now. Food
nourishes me. Food is my friend. You are NOT my friend, nor are you Alicia's friend.
But ya know,
you aren't our enemy either. You are just a defense. Just a way to try to control feelings,
and
you know you aren't even very good at that. You can't scare me today. I know you. I
KNOW you."

We finish the supervision session by talking about how she could use this same action structure, a dialogue with the eating disorder with the support of the Body Double, to help Alicia express some of her feelings. Having released the intensity of her feelings that came from her counter transference, Gina is now ready to help Alicia begin to do the same.

Conclusion

As you can see in the above examples, TSM follows the same clinical map for supervision as it does in experiential psychotherapy to treat eating disorders. Prescriptive roles are firmly established before we move onto trauma–based roles in both therapy and supervision. When Gina came into her supervision sessions clearly distressed, supervision first focused on building up her own Prescriptive roles of restoration, containment, and observation. She learned how to use the inspirational cards to mark a Witness Role and then used the cards in her weekly Eating Disorder group. She role reversed with her Determination from her Circle of Safety to resource herself in the face of Alicia's own despair. She learned the Body Double in supervision when she was depleted and found it a clinical intervention she came back to time and time again with Alicia as her recovery continued. Together, they both learned to self–soothe and contain anxiety and defenses.

In Stage 2, Gina learned a TSM sociodrama structure called the Trauma Triangle that gave her a tool to help Alicia identify how she was repeating the Trauma–based roles of victim, perpetrator, and abandoning authority. She was able to clearly see how she was giving up on herself and to find ways to connect back to her strengths in order to decrease her suicidal ideation. Additionally, Gina was able to bring a strong countertransference reaction to supervision without shame or blame, Here she could work on the remnants of her own eating disorder and find release from her past once again.

While this is just a brief overview of TSM Action Supervision, I think you can see the safe psychological container it provides for therapists working with eating disorders. Live action supervision not only provides theories and ideas of how to treat clients, but also gives the therapist a chance to see the experiential interventions used. This promotes rapid learning of effective skills and thereby increases the therapist's view of self as competent even when the work gets difficult, as it will with people who have eating disorders. The no shame, no blame container of TSM allows the deepest of healing for therapist and client alike. It truly does nourish the soul.

To end this chapter, I want to discuss the research that is currently under-way testing the Therapeutic Spiral Model™ as an effective model of experiential psychotherapy to treat eating disorders and other stress related psychological problems.

Research on Experiential Psychotherapy: The Therapeutic Spiral Model

While TSM itself, is collecting on–going data of treatment effectiveness, the larger body of psychotherapy research already demonstrates the success of experiential methods of change. Proving itself equally effective as CBT and psychodynamic psychotherapy 10 years ago, experiential psychotherapy is now called for in treatment protocols for many psychiatric problems (Bergin & Garfield, 1994; Elliott, Greenberg & Lietaer, 2002; van der Kolk, McFarlane & Weisaeth, 1996). No less than Harvard neurobiologist, Besell van der Kolk (2003) stated that experiential methods are a must when treating eating disorders. Johnson (2000) demonstrated the use of drama therapy in the effective treatment of PTSD and called for a model that can be researched and tested. The Therapeutic Spiral Model (Hudgins 2002) is such a model of treatment and supervision.

A small body of clinical research shows TSM is a clinically significant model of experiential change for stress related disorders, including eating disorders. McVea and Gow (2006) did a process analysis of a TSM drama in Australia. They found the structured intervention of the Prescriptive Roles (Hudgins, 2002) were crucial in providing support and containment during the psychodramatic enactment of a mother talking to her daughter who is bulimic. A one–year pilot study conducted with Chinese clients, who had suffered from domestic violence in Taiwan, showed significant decreases in clinical levels of depression, anxiety, and general symptoms of PTSD using a three–day intervention module of TSM (Hudgins, Cho, Lai, Ou & Wen, 2005). Forst (2001) demonstrated the usefulness of TSM with drug addicts and alcoholics with PTSD. In 2000 (Hudgins, Drucker & Metcalf) demonstrated the use of the Body Double to significantly decrease dissociation across three individual therapy sessions with a woman who had a history of sexual abuse and suffered from anorexia (Hudgins & Drucker, 1998). Please see an earlier chapter (Hudgins, 1989) for a description of the three–stage model of experiential treatment that was the forerunner of the current TSM system with a client with anorexia. The specific intervention of the Body Double, which is demonstrated in this chapter, has particularly shown to be effective with people with eating disorders. In fact, it was developed to work with this clinical population. Ciotola (2006) mentions the usefulness of the Body Double as facilitating healing with clients with eating disorders. Other articles (Burden & Ciotola, 2003; Ciotola, 2004) discuss the usefulness of the Body Double for clients diagnosed with PTSD and an eating disorder.

My hope is that this chapter on TSM Action Supervision leaves your minds and hearts full of hope for your work with people with eating disorders. It is also my hope that it encourages you to seek out quality supervision for yourself so that you can stay nourished and contained as you contribute to the healing of these clients. Be well.

Appendix–Session Dialogue with a Body Double for TSM Action Supervision

BD (*sitting next to Gina, taking her same body posture*): I can take a deep breath as I see Alicia and sit with her again today. I can feel my feet on the floor. I can look around at my office and see the pretty colors and the books I love to read. I am OK today, just a bit overwhelmed.

Gina (*takes a deep breath and sighs*): Yes, I am OK today. I am OK even though I feel overwhelmed. I have help. I don't have to do it all alone.

BD: Yes, I forget that so easily, running around, still trying to do everything perfectly. Right now, I can just take a deep breath and relax, move my shoulders. Slooow down.

Gina: Yes, yes . . . that is right. When I sit with Alicia I feel helpless there is so much she is struggling with. Money, time, patience . . . having a hard time. She feels there is nothing she can do. I get caught in that (*sighs again*).

BD: Yes, I do feel helpless sometimes, but the reality is that I have support for myself. I have supervision. I have good women friends. I can take a deep breath and breathe in all the caring around me (*deep, slow, audible breath*).

Gina: (*sits back a bit in her chair and takes another deep breath*): Yes, I do have more support than Alicia does. But I still worry about her and what I should do. How can I help her? What can I do?

BD: Yes . . . as I breathe in the support of my friends and my supervisor, I also worry how to help my clients. Let me just take a moment to think of the resources I have that can help my clients (*another deep audible breath*). She is telling me she is bulimic. She wants me to help. She is asking for my help.

Gina: Alicia . . . I can help you. We have similar issues in some ways. We both struggle with our eating at times. We worry about everything. And . . . I have many resources to help you (*takes a deep breath*). Today, let's just take a breath together. Feel the support of Mother Earth under our feet. We can use this moment to gain the resources from the earth to be "good enough" today (*takes a deep breath*).

BD: Look, how I just brought in a very important transpersonal strength to Alicia. There is always the support of Mother Earth, an enduring mother who is always there to support us. That is good. I am good enough . . . as a therapist and as a woman (*deep breath*).

We end the role play and move to a brief discussion about what Gina learned in today's supervision. Mostly, she says she learned that she is different from her client. She ends truly feeling the support she has. She knows she can reach out and connect to the support she needs. It doesn't have to be all her responsibility. Freeing her up from her own parallel process gives Gina hope for her next few sessions.

We a discuss the experience of having a Body Double. Gina says it made all the difference in the world to her. It helped calm her down. To keep her anxiety at bay as she thought about what she could do differently with herself and her client. I suggest that in her next session, she begin to teach Alicia the Body Double, so she can internalize it quickly. Our research shows a client can internalize the Body Double n 3 sessions and begin to use it for her own self–soothing and to decrease dissociation (Hudgins, Drucker & Metcalf, 2000).

References

Bergin, A. E. and Garfield, S. L. (Eds.). (1994). *Handbook of psychotherapy and behavior change* (4th ed.). New York: John Wiley and Sons, Inc.

Burden, K., & Ciotola, L. (2003). *Report from a Body Double: An advanced clinical action intervention module in the therapeutic spiral model.* Workshop handout. Charlottesville, VA: Therapeutic Spiral International, LLC. www.therapeuticspiral.org

Ciotola, L. (2004). *The body dialogue.* Workshop handout. Charlottesville, VA: Therapeutic Spiral International, LLC. www.therapeuticspiral.org

Cox, M. A. (2000). The six safety structures in the Therapeutic Spiral Model™. Workshop handout. Charlottesville, VA: Therapeutic Spiral International, LLC. www.therpeuticspiral.org

Elliott, R., Greenberg, L. S., & Lietaer, G. (2002). Research on experiential therapies. In M. Lambert, A. Bergin, & S. Garfield (Eds.), *Handbook of psychotherapy and behavior change* (5th ed.). New York: John Wiley & Sons, Inc.

Hornyak, L., & Baker, E. (1998). (Eds). *Experiential therapy for eating disorders.* New York: Guilford Press.

Hudgins, M. K. (1989). Experiencing the self through psychodrama and gestalt therapy in anorexia nervosa. In L. Hornyak and E. Baker (Eds.), *Experiential therapy for eating disorders.* New York: Guilford Press.

Hudgins, M. K. (1998). Experiential psychodrama with sexual trauma. In L. S. Greenberg, J. C. Watson, & G. Lietaer (Eds.), *Handbook of experiential psychotherapy* (pp. 328–348). New York: Guilford Press.

Hudgins, M. K. (2000). The therapeutic spiral model: Treating PTSD in action. In P. F. Kellermann & M. K. Hudgins (Eds.), *Psychodrama with trauma survivors: Acting out your pain.* London: Jessica Kingsley Publishers.

Hudgins, M. K. (2002). *Experiential treatment of PTSD: The therapeutic spiral model.* New York: Springer Publishing Company.

Hudgins, M. K. (in press–a). *Action against trauma: A trainer's manual for community leaders following traumatic stress.* Charlottesville: University of Virginia, Virginia Foundation for the Humanities, Institute on Violence and Culture.

Hudgins, M. K. (in press–b). Clinical foundations of the therapeutic spiral model: Theoretical orientations and principles of change. In M. Marciano, J. Burgmesiter & C. Baim (Eds.), *Advanced theories of psychodrama.* New York: Routledge.

Hudgins, M. K. (in press–c). *Building a container with the creative arts: The Therapeutic Spiral Model™ to heal post–traumatic stress in the global community.* Springfield, IL: Charles C Thomas Publisher.

Hudgins, M.K., Cho, W. C., Lai, N. W, Ou, G. T., & Wen, J. (2005). *Therapeutic Spiral Model in Asia: 2001–2005,* International Association of Group Psychotherapy, Pacific Rim Conference on Trauma.

Hudgins, M. K, & Drucker, K. (1998). The containing double as part of the Therapeutic Spiral Model for treating trauma. *The International Journal of Action Methods, 51*(2), 63–74.

Hudgins, M. K., Drucker, K., & Metcalf, K. (2000). The containing double: A clinically effective psychodrama intervention for PTSD. *The British Journal of Psychodrama and Sociodrama, 15*(1), 58–77.

Johnson, D. R. (2000). Creative therapies. In E. B. Foa, T. M. Keane, & M. J. Friedman (Eds.), *Effective treatments for PTSD.* New York: Guilford Press.

McVea, C., & Gow, K. (2006). Healing a mother's emotional pain: Protagonist and director recall of a Therapeutic Spiral Model session. *Journal of Group Psychotherapy, Psychodrama and Sociometry, 59*(1), 3–22.

van der Kolk, B. (2003). In terror's grip. *Connections,* Feb/March. Washington, DC: International Association of Eating Disorders Professionals.

van der Kolk, B., McFarlane, A.C., & Weisaeth, L. (Eds.) (1996). *Traumatic stress: The effects of overwhelming experience on mind, body, and society.* New York: Guilford Press.

Biography

Doctor Kate Hudgins is a clinical psychologist; board–certified trainer, educator and practitioner of psychodrama, Sociometry, and group psychotherapy, international expert on experiential methods with PTSD, and an inspirational speaker in the global community. Doctor Kate is the developer of the Therapeutic Spiral Model and founder of Therapeutic Spiral International, LLC, and an international training institute to accredit practitioners and trainers in experiential methods. She is a widely published author with three books and several chapters and articles on the safe use of experiential therapy to treat PTSD and other stress–related disorders. She currently builds Action Trauma Teams in Asia, working in Mainland China, Taiwan, and Malaysia. The Therapeutic Spiral Model is the personal and professional weaving of her training as a psychologist and a psychodramatist and her personal experience as a survivor of childhood sexual abuse, an eating disorder, and family alcoholism. Please visit her website at www.therapeuticspiral.org for additional articles and information on the Therapeutic Spiral Model in your local area.

Chapter 17

A POSITIVE ETHICAL APPROACH TO USING CREATIVE ARTS THERAPIES WITH EATING DISORDERS

LISA D. HINZ

Introduction to Positive Ethics

Customary approaches to ethics often have a risk management focus. In this type of approach, practitioners are admonished to learn ethical standards and applicable state laws in order to prevent harm to clients (e.g., Dileo, 2000). While prevention of harm is a worthy goal, this chapter will focus on a positive approach to ethics in which practitioners actively strive to reach their highest potential as therapists (Knapp & VandeCreek, 2006). According to Knapp and VandeCreek (2006), a positive approach to ethics emphasizes how therapists can promote exemplary behavior in themselves, their colleagues, and their institutions. It promotes providing the highest possible standard of care. For example, a positive approach to ethics would not focus on avoiding illegal breaches of confidentiality; it would focus on striving to enhance trust in the therapeutic relationship. Each area of ethical thinking can be conceived in positive terms with practical methods suggested to help therapists achieve the highest standards.

In order to provide superlative care for eating disordered clients, practitioners should respect the power of creative arts therapies and be well trained in their use. Arts–based therapies are widespread weekly practices in treatment centers for eating disorders (Frisch, Franko & Herzog, 2006). Providing optimal care entails understanding specific characteristics of eating disorders and how these traits might interact with aspects of the therapeutic relationship, and the delivery and reception of creative arts therapies. This chapter will consider the positive ethical implications of using creative arts therapies

271

with eating disordered clients in the areas of achieving professional excellence, providing sensitive explanations, enhancing trust, and embracing cultural competence. Client resistances and transference issues will be viewed in a positive light. Creative arts therapies are vital and powerful treatments for eating disorders (Hinz, 2006) and their positive ethical implementation provides the best possible chance for their success.

Professional Excellence

Creative arts disciplines are overseen by credentialing bodies and guided by codes of ethics (American Dance Therapy Association, 2006; Dileo, 2000; Moon, 2006; National Association for Poetry Therapy, 2006; National Association of Drama Therapy, 2006). Each ethical code addresses professional competence, requiring therapists to be aware of the limitations of their competency and the restrictions of their techniques. It would be considered practicing outside ones area of professional competence to call oneself a creative arts therapist without meeting at least minimal educational and training standards. Therapists need to be aware of the scope and power of their remedies; creative arts interventions are not always benign. At the same time, the realities of agency staffing demands often require flexibility in providing services and leading therapy groups. Competent therapists *can* ethically incorporate the use of expressive techniques with thoughtful preparation and adequate supervision.

Wiener and Oxford (2003) stress the importance of obtaining appropriate training in the use of expressive therapeutic techniques. The authors state that without adequate training or supervision practitioners might find their first attempts at using creative arts techniques unproductive and dismiss them as ineffective. However, Wiener and Oxford argue that with appropriate training, creative arts techniques *can* work for most able practitioners. They add that because creative arts therapies are *action oriented*, words alone cannot adequately communicate their power. The authors emphasize that training should involve *practicing* techniques and ongoing supervision.

A positive ethical approach to competence means that therapists exceed minimal requirements for competence, strive for excellence, are self–aware, and regularly engage in self–care practices (Knapp & VandeCreek, 2006). In treating anorexia, bulimia, and binge eating disorders, therapists must be aware that the disorders are complex, sometimes resistant to improvement, and often require long–term care. Therapists can feel disheartened, pressured, and sometimes work excessively to change clients. The American Psychiatric Association in its *Practice Guidelines for the Treatment of Patients with Eating Disorders* (2000b) recognizes these potential emotional pitfalls and recommends therapists treating eating disorders participate in ongoing peer consultation.

Eating disorders can be associated with serious physical complications (American Psychiatric Association, 2000a). Therefore ethical treatment involves understanding the limits of one's professional training and abilities to deal with the complex physical realities that eating disorders present. Consultation with medical professionals is strongly advised (American Psychiatric Association, 2000b). Physical health status should be regularly monitored by a physician, and clients benefit from working with a dietitian who can supervise diet and exercise. With appropriate releases of information, treatment can be coordinated such that client frustration with repetition of eating disorder behaviors is reduced and effectiveness of treatment is increased (Thompson & Sherman, 1989). Coordinated treatment efforts help ensure that therapeutic gains are being made in all areas: physical, emotional, and spiritual.

Clients with eating disorders, particularly those with anorexia nervosa, may face death as a result of the considerable physical damage done by the disorder. Many treating professionals believe that they have an obligation to prevent self–harm including initiating life saving measures such as forced tube feeding (Werth, Wright, Archambault & Bardash, 2003). Others believe that clients have the right to refuse treatment for their life–threatening disorders unless they have been assessed and found incompetent to make treatment decisions (Giordano, 2005). Providing optimal treatment for life–threatening disorders will involve consultation among all treating professionals as well as clients and family members. Collaborative decisions must be made based on what is in the best interest of clients rather than focused on reducing therapists fears.

Sensitive Explanations

Ethics codes of creative arts therapies disciplines state that clients have a right to informed consent for treatment (American Dance Therapy Association, 2006; Dileo, 2000; Moon, 2006; National Association for Poetry Therapy, 2006; National Association of Drama Therapy, 2006). Sensitive explanations go beyond informed consent to incorporate knowledge of how client characteristics such as perfectionism and control might interact with the demands of creative arts therapies. Anticipating these interactions helps clients make better informed decisions about their participation. For example, expressive therapies quickly access deeply buried conflicts and emotions (Makin, 2002; Sloboda, 1995). Eating disordered clients might be especially vulnerable to rapid and profound exposure as they often enter therapy suffering from alexithymia, lacking conscious awareness of their feelings and needs (Bruch, 1973; Canetti, Bachar, & Berry, 2002). Without careful preparation about the power of the therapeutic endeavor they are beginning, clients might feel unmasked by creative arts therapies before they are prepared to verbally reveal the information contained in expressive sessions, especially when information is disclosed in a group context. Sometimes group members are able to respond to the content or process of another member's creative expression before they can attend to the same issues in their own work (Rust, 1995). Seeing or hearing conflicts raised by another person gives permission to one group member to discuss a conflict while another may still be avoiding it. Therapists must educate group members about how to respond sensitively to one another's creations, allowing that their own projections are likely in the forefront.

Not only do the creative arts therapies call for careful overall explanations, providing optimal treatment requires each sessions is structured to make it optimally beneficial. Both group and individual sessions can begin with a preparatory discussion of the proposed process and conclude with a detailed debriefing. Callahan (1989) explains that eating disordered clients require careful debriefing due to a tendency to dissociate in the presence of intense emotion. If strong emotions evoked during sessions are not fully processed, clients are left with unacknowledged or unresolved feelings which may lead to subsequent binge purge episodes or caloric restriction.

Sensitive explanations of creative arts therapies include information that clients often use their bodies and voices as tools in treatment (Totenbier, 1995; Young, 1995). Eating disordered clients will quickly be faced with body dissatisfaction and fears, and may require different treatment guidelines that those usually recommended. For example, Young (1995) writes that a developmental approach in drama therapy suggests that certain physical activities are used as warm up exercises and "icebreakers." Young emphasizes that due to deep seated body image conflicts typical warm up experiences would be a better ending point than starting point in the treatment of eating disorders.

Therapists must sensitively explain all expressive techniques, especially to clients in eating disorder treatment facilities where there might be limited choice about participation. Sensitive explanations imply an insightful understanding that many clients have not danced or used art materials since elementary school, and that their creative attempts at poetry might have been met with negative criticism by former teachers or parents. Many might not have been exposed to musical instruments in school or at home. Thus creative arts therapies might be considered foreign at best and threatening at worst, activating client fears and vulnerabilities.

Client Resistance in a New Light

Feelings of fear or vulnerability in new and unfamiliar situations might stir up perfectionist qualities that often characterize eating disordered clients and lead them to criticize and refuse creative arts therapies (e.g., Bruch, 1973; Rogers, 1995). Initial resistance can be decreased by understanding underlying perfectionism and performance fears and providing realistic reassurances *before* resistances occur (Rogers, 1995). For example, introducing creative arts therapies simply as unique ways of gathering and communicating information can help reduce performance fears. Further explaining how the right hemisphere of the brain processes information differently than the left, and that during creation clients will draw new and different information from their experiences, also can aid in reducing initial discomfort and resistance. In addition, reassurances of the therapist's nonevaluative stance are imperative.

Betensky (1973) points out that therapists must not be excessively invested in proving the effectiveness of their crafts. She adds that if practitioners are adamant about the helpfulness of creative arts therapies, they will inevitably make mistakes that can alienate clients who have had difficulty trusting people all their lives. Errors might include being overly eager to suggest interpretations, or insisting on therapist–determined meanings. With experience, expressive therapists will appreciate that participation in the creative process itself is healing and life enhancing; it does not always need language.

In fact, sometimes the overuse of language can be viewed as a form of resistance to creative arts therapies. Clients with eating disorders have been called super intellectualizers because they are most comfortable rationalizing, talking, and arguing about their eating disordered behavior (Matto, 1997). Resistance can take the form of defensively engaging in so much preparatory discussion that there is limited time for the creative process (Jacobse, 1995). According to Jacobse, therapists must gently curtail discussion and encourage creative action, because it is through active engagement in the therapeutic process, not talking about it, that emotion is experienced and expressed.

Resistance will not always take the form of outright refusal to participate in creative arts therapies. Some clients will unreservedly engage in therapy, but with stereotypical or rigid productions: Tuneless music with an unyielding beat, drama with stereotypical roles, and art with stereotypical images such as hearts and flowers (Henley, 1989; Jacobse, 1995; Sloboda, 1995). Therapists must accept clients' first creations and encourage further attempts, noticing any slight deviation in content or theme. When variation is noticed, clients can be asked to expand on that difference with new action (Henley,

1989). Thus, therapists allow clients' own comfort with divergence from the conventional guide them to freer expression. In addition, changing to a new creative modality also might help liberate clients from the stereotypical to authentic sharing of themselves and their emotions (McNiff, 2004).

Eating disorders often develop in part because the direct expression of emotions was disallowed in families of origin (Bruch, 1973; Reindl, 2001). When the direct expression of emotions and needs is discouraged clients develop issues with control, often replacing control over food for control over inner states. In the positive ethical treatment of eating disorders, clients actively participate in formulating treatment goals (Knapp & VandeCreek, 2006). Clients' active involvement reduces struggles for control that can plague the treatment relationship. For example, clients changing task instructions could be viewed as resistance stemming from a control issue. A positive ethical approach would encourage therapists to view the alteration of instructions as clients attending to their needs. Clients would not be chastised for deviating from provided instructions, but rather queried about how the new procedures better met their needs. Clients must be praised for paying attention to their needs, a particular problem for people with eating disorders.

Eating disordered clients often ignore their own needs and attempt to please therapists as they have attempted to please other people all their lives (Sloboda, 1995; Thompson & Sherman, 1989). Clients must be actively educated that they are not in therapy to please therapists. The use of creative arts therapies helps highlight that changes are made by and for clients, not for the therapists or anyone else. When clients create with movement, drama, music, art, or poetry they are not simply repeating what they think the therapist wants to hear. Powerful creative answers come from within clients and reflect their own internal wisdom. Creative arts therapists will help clients learn to honor this innate knowledge as well as apply it in original and innovative ways to change their lives.

Enhancing Trust

In a positive approach to ethics, confidentiality does not merely mean avoiding prohibited disclosures of information. It means providing a safe environment for therapy and doing everything possible to enhance trust (Knapp & VandeCreek, 2006). Attention to safety and trust are salient issues with eating disordered persons who consistently struggle with trust issues (Makin, 2002; Reindl, 2001). Promoting safety and trust in creative arts therapies involves many factors, among them are: Ensuring the physical space is respected and outside intrusions do not occur (Rust, 1995), providing high quality materials for client use (McNiff, 2004), informing clients of potential dangers inherent in materials (Moon, 2006), respecting time limits, and educating group members about appropriate behavior (Rust, 1995). Providing optimal creative arts therapy means delineating clear rules of engagement and at times participating side–by–side with clients in the creative process to provide immediate feedback, reassurance, and support (Moon, 2006; Stark, Aronow & McGeehan, 1989). These methods help define creative arts therapies and demonstrate their safe and effective use in an environment characterized by mutual trust.

Trust becomes an issue when therapists inquire about public displays of client art. Therapists must understand that they are not in equal relationships with clients. Due to their position of unequal power, clients may not feel able to decline participation in public demonstrations of their work. Creative products made in therapy are rarely appropriate for public viewing (Moon, 2006). Trust increases when therapists help clients think through their motivations and the possible consequences to everyone involved (e.g., nonclient family members) of public displays such as poetry readings and art exhibitions. Enhancing trust means that therapists value creative communication as highly as verbal communication and protect it in the same manner (Hammond & Gantt, 1998). Even within an agency care should be taken to share creative productions only when necessary to facilitate treatment. Creative arts therapies can involve potentially disturbing images (e.g., Makin, 2002; Sloboda, 1995; Totenbier, 1995). Hammond and Gantt (1998) write that inexperienced therapists are particularly vulnerable to becoming emotionally overwhelmed by the content of disturbing images and more likely to inappropriately disclose confidential information as they seek to process their feelings. Therapists need to be aware of the potential for compassion fatigue and take active steps to care for themselves physically, emotionally, and spiritually (Knapp & VandeCreek, 2006). Positive self–care efforts will help therapists maintain enthusiasm for their vital work.

The Gifts of Transference

Clients suffering from anorexia and bulimia demonstrate significant control issues which often are played out in the therapeutic relationship. Clients might project demanding, conflicting, or unrealistic parental expectations onto therapists and therefore must be actively involved in the formulation of realistic treatment goals (Giordano, 2005). They may project onto therapists qualities of controlling or ineffectual parents, ask therapists for behavioral suggestions, and then react with disdain to their advice (Rogers, 1995; Schaverien, 1995; Thompson & Sherman, 1989). Creative arts answers are more likely than verbal answers to be accepted because they come from within and stem from clients' own innate healing knowledge. When clients ask for suggestions therapists can guide them back to the gifts discovered in their own wise creative arts experiences.

Optimal ethical treatment means that therapists understand and anticipate the types of transference issues that might occur in the treatment of eating disorders (Knapp & VandeCreek, 2006). It has been my experience in a variety of situations that clients ask therapists about their own history of eating disorders. This question brings up two issues: First, what and how much personal information should therapists disclose; and, second, should therapists with a current or past history of an eating disorder treat eating disordered clients. In the first situation, therapist must carefully think through their motivation for self–disclosure and any impact that it might have on treatment outcome. In general, therapist self–disclosure should only take place if it will enhance clients' therapeutic outcomes (Moon, 2006). Client inquiries can be anticipated so that therapists are prepared with sensitive and therapeutic responses to them.

Understandable controversy surrounds the issue of whether therapists with current or past eating disorders should treat clients with similar disorders. In a survey of over 300 eating disorder patients and professionals, participants were asked to rate the quality of therapeutic relationships and advice from hypothetical therapists: Those with a history of eating disorder, a current eating disorder, or never having suffered from an eating disorder (Johnson, Smethurst & Gowers, 2005). Results showed that both professional and patient participants believed that therapists with a past history of an eating disorder might be more empathetic and demonstrate more clinical expertise than either therapists who never had suffered from an eating disorder, or those with current disorders. Little concern was shown for potential harm to clients being treated by therapists with an active eating disorder. But significant concern was demonstrated for the potential vulnerability of *therapists* with current eating disorders. It appears that clients with eating disordered therapists would find themselves worried about or placing therapists' needs before their own. As mentioned above, clients must learn to put their needs first, especially in therapy. Having a worrisome therapist is not optimally therapeutic and thus therapists with current eating disorders probably should not treat clients with similar disorders.

Andersen and Corson (2001) delineate the characteristics of an ideal psychotherapist for eating disordered clients and list nonpossessive warmth as an optimal personality trait. It has been my experience and that of other authors (e.g., Winn, 1995) that therapists with *current* eating disorders have difficulty expressing warmth and can be too directive and overly controlling. I also have worked with therapists who had recovered from eating disorders.

I believe that the *past history* of an eating disorder might have helped them become highly perceptive and effective therapists. Regardless of personal history, *all* therapists who work with eating disorders must be very comfortable with their own bodies (Totenbier, 1995). Even if the body is not used directly as an instrument in therapy, transference issues regarding weight and body image will arise. Therapists must be comfortable having their bodies scrutinized, evaluated, and discussed. Modeling comfort with ones body is a gift to young men and women who often loathe their own.

Transference can be a valuable asset in creative arts therapies because counselors offer their clients the gifts of real and challenging materials and tasks (Betensky, 1973). The gift also includes therapists' faith in clients' abilities to create. Betensky mentions that therapists indicate through regularly offering materials and instructions that they are available to help, but have faith in clients' abilities to create independently. The fundamental message of these gifts is that clients have something unique and important to convey, and their productions are healing.

Embracing Cultural Competence

Ethics codes sometimes contain a section on non discrimination with wording to the effect that therapists shall respect diversity and not discriminate against clients on the basis of gender, religious beliefs, ethnicity, and other factors (Dileo, 2000; Moon, 2006). Some ethical codes do not specifically address the issues of diversity (e.g., American Dance Therapy Association, 2006; National Association for Poetry Therapy, 2006). The positive ethical treatment approach would encourage understanding and appreciation of how eating disorders are expressed differently in various cultures and require cultural competence in their treatment.

In the past, eating disorders were thought of as disorders impacting only upper class white women. Ethnic minority status was seen as a "protective factor" against the development of eating disorders (Smolak & Striegel–Moore, 2001). However, membership in an ethnic minority group only seems to be a protective factor if an ethnic beauty standard is embraced and the Eurocentric beauty standard is eschewed (Presnell, Bearman, & Stice, 2004). For example, ethnically identified Black and Latina women demonstrate concern about the physical nurturance of their bodies *not* the typical concerns about how their bodies look (Rubin et al., 2003). However, as increasing numbers of men and women from diverse ethnic backgrounds have internalized the Eurocentric beauty standard idealizing thinness, eating disorders have become more common in many cultures (Presnell et al., 2004; Smolak & Striegel–Moore, 2001).

Direct communication and open discussion of personal and emotional issues are not valued or allowed in many non–Western cultures (Sudarsky–Gleiser, 2004). Therefore the metaphorical communication characterizing creative arts may facilitate therapy where verbal therapy might be intimidating. Eurocentric counseling professionals value individual therapy. However, people raised in communal societies such as the native Hawaiian culture would most likely benefit from group counseling and experience individual counseling as uncomfortable (Sudarsky–Gleiser, 2004). Further, individuation of young adults is a value based in certain western cultures and often described as a goal in eating disorder therapy. However, independence would be an inappropriate goal in cultures where separation from parents is viewed as disrespectful. Younger members of immigrant families can feel divided between their two cultures and uncertain of how to respect both, while maintaining a personal identity. I have witnessed clients using art to express elements of both cultures and begin to experiment with of integration.

A positive ethical approach requires that therapists are competent to deal with the cultural issues mentioned here and many others. Creative arts therapies can bridge cultural gaps because they do not depend on language for their full effect. Not speaking the dominant language could possibly cause inhibition and reservation in clients. Writing about the use of visual art in therapy, but equally applicable to all expressive therapies, Henderson and Gladding (1998) argue that art can draw clients out of self–consciousness into self–awareness by using symbolic expression. In addition, art can call attention to the universal nature of creative expression, and at the same time highlight the distinctive nature of creativity in various cultures. Creative arts therapies can help clients integrate their unique experiences into meaningful accounts of their past, present, and future.

Again, it is not enough for therapists to be *aware of* cultural struggles and how they impact the use of creative arts therapies with eating disordered clients. Therapists must be able to use creative arts therapies to their full effect when treating diverse clients. They must be knowledgeable about and capable of handling issues of culture, ethnicity, minority status, and privilege and their impact on the therapeutic relationship (George, Greene, & Blackwell, 2005; Smolak and Striegel–Moore, 2001).

Conclusion

The positive ethical approach to the treatment of eating disorders ensures that creative arts therapists strive to reach their utmost potential as therapists and provide the highest standard of care to their clients. A positive ethical orientation does not focus on the avoidance of harm, but rather on the promotion of excellence in individuals and institutions. This viewpoint keeps creative arts therapists aware of the unique power of their modalities and helps them actively strive to use these compelling methods in considered ways to ensure their effectiveness. Attaining the highest standards of knowledge and competence is essential when dealing with eating disordered clients and mindful self care is necessary in order to maintain enthusiasm for the work. Enhancing trust and providing sensitive explanations of creative arts therapies can reduce client resistances and enhance the quality of treatment.

Positive ethics encourages collaboration among professional colleagues and the inclusion of clients in treatment planning and decision making. These two factors reduce client repetition of eating disordered symptoms and thus increase a positive focus in therapy. In addition, collaboration and inclusion reduce conflicts about control and enhance client motivation for recovery. Finally, in striving to reach the highest level of competence, creative arts therapists become knowledgeable about other cultures, how eating disorders are expressed in various cultures, and how creative arts therapies can help bridge cultural gaps.

References

American Dance Therapy Association. (2006). *Code of ethical practice of the American Dance Therapy Association* (On-line). Available: http://www.adta.org/ethics.cfm

American Psychiatric Association. (2000a). *Diagnostic and statistical manual of mental disorders* (4th ed., text rev.). Washington, DC: Author.

American Psychiatric Association. (2000b). *Practice guidelines for the treatment of clients with eating disorders* (2nd ed.). Washington, DC: Author.

Andersen, A. E., & Corson, P. W. (2001). Characteristics of an ideal psychotherapist for' eating–disordered patients. *Psychiatric Clinics of North America, 24*(2), 351–358.

Betensky, M. G. (1973). *Self-discovery through self-expression: Use of art psychotherapy with children and adolescents.* Springfield, IL: Charles C Thomas.

Bruch, H. (1973). *Eating disorders: Obesity, anorexia, and the person within.* New York: Basic Books.

Callahan, M. L. (1989). Psychodrama and the treatment of bulimia. In L. M. Hornyak & E. K. Baker (Eds.), *Experiential therapies for eating disorders* (pp. 101–120). New York: Guilford Press.

Canetti, L., Bachar, E., & Berry E. M. (2002). Food and emotion. *Behavioural Processes, 60*(2), 157–164.

Dileo, C. (2000). *Ethical thinking in music therapy.* Cherry Hill, NJ: Jeffrey Books.

Frisch, M. J., Franko, D. L., & Herzog, D. B. (2006). Arts–based therapies in the treatment of eating disorders. *Eating Disorders, 14*(2), 131–142.

Giordano, S. (2005). *Understanding eating disorders: Conceptual and ethical issues in the treatment of anorexia and bulimia nervosa.* Oxford: Clarendon.

Hammond, L. D., & Gantt, L. (1998). Using art in counseling: Ethical considerations. *Journal of Counseling and Development, 76,* 271–276.

Henderson, D. A., & Gladding, S. T. (1998). The creative arts in counseling: A multicultural perspective. *The Arts in Psychotherapy, 25,* 183–187.

Henley, D. R. (1989). Stereotypes in children's art. *The American Journal of Art Therapy, 27,* 116–125.

Hinz, L. D. (2006). *Drawing from within: Using art to treat eating disorders.* London: Jessica Kingsley Publishers.

Jacobse, A. (1995). The use of dramatherapy in the treatment of eating disorders. In D. Doktor (Ed.), *Arts therapies and clients with eating disorders* (pp. 124–143). London: Jessica Kingsley Publishers.

Johnson, C., Smethurst, N., and Gowers, S. (2005). Should people with a history of an eating disorder work as eating disorder therapists? *European Eating Disorders Review, 13,* 301–310.

Knapp, S. J., & VandeCreek, L. D. (2006). *Practical ethics for psychologists: A positive approach.* Washington, DC: American Psychological Association.

Makin, S. (2002). *More than just a meal: The art of eating disorders.* London: Jessica Kingsley Publishers.

Matto, H. C. (1997). An integrative approach to the treatment of women with eating disorders. *The Arts in Psychotherapy, 24,* 347–354.

McNiff, S. (2004). *Art heals: How creativity cures the soul.* Boston: Shambhala.

Moon, B. L. (2006). *Ethical issues in art therapy* (2nd ed.). Springfield, IL: Charles C Thomas Publisher.

National Association for Poetry Therapy. (2006). *Poetry therapy code of ethics* (On-line). Available: http://poetrytherapy.org/codeofethics.html

National Association of Drama Therapy. (2006). National association of drama therapists code of ethical principles (On-line). Available: http://www.nadt.org/codeofethics.html

Presnell, K., Bearman, S. K., & Stice, E. (2004). Risk factors for body dissatisfaction in adolescent boys and girls: A prospective study. *International Journal of Eating Disorders, 36,* 389–401.

Reindl, S. M. (2001). *Sensing the self: Women's recovery from bulimia.* Cambridge, MA: Harvard University Press.

Rust, M-J. (1995). Bringing "the man" into the room: Art therapy groupwork with women with compulsive eating problems. In D. Doktor (Ed.), *Arts therapies and clients with eating disorders* (pp. 48–59). London: Jessica Kingsley Publishers.

Rogers, P. J. (1995). Sexual abuse and eating disorders: A possible connection indicated through music therapy? In D. Doktor (Ed.), *Arts therapies and clients with eating disorders* (pp. 262–278). London: Jessica Kingsley Publishers.

Rubin, L. R., Fitts, M. L., & Becker, A. E. (2003). "Whatever feels good in my soul": Body ethics and aesthetics among African American and Latina woman. *Culture, Medicine, and Psychiatry, 27,* 49–75.

Schaverien, J. (1995). The picture as transactional object in the treatment of anorexia. In D. Doktor (Ed.), *Arts therapies and clients with eating disorders* (pp. 31–47). London: Jessica Kingsley Publishers.

nothing   nothing

Sloboda, A. (1995). Individual music therapy with anorexic and bulimic patients. In D. Doktor (Ed.), *Arts therapies and clients with eating disorders* (pp. 247–267). London: Jessica Kingsley Publishers.

Smolak, L., & Striegel–Moore, R. H. (2001). Challenging the myth of the golden girl: Ethnicity and eating disorders. In R. H. Striegel–Moore and L. Smolak (Eds.), *Eating disorders: Innovative directions in research and practice.* Washington, DC: American Psychological Association.

Stark, A., Aronow, S., & McGeehan, T. (1989). Dance/movement therapy with bulimic patients. In L. M. Hornyak and E. K. Baker (Eds.), *Experiential therapies for eating disorders* (pp. 121–143). New York: Guilford Press.

Sudarsky–Gleiser, C. (2004). The voice of the eating disorder is loud among us too: Challenging the Euro–centric bias of our profession. *The Renfrew Perspective, Winter,* 22–24.

Thompson, R. A., & Sherman, R. T. (1989). Therapist errors in treating eating disorders: Relationship and process. *Psychotherapy, 26,* 62–68.

Totenbier, S. L. (1995). A new way of working with body image in therapy, incorporating dance/movement therapy methodology. In D. Doktor (Ed.), *Arts therapies and clients with eating disorders* (pp. 193–207). London: Jessica Kingsley Publishers.

Werth, J. L., Jr., Wright, K. S., Archambault, R. J., & Bardash, R. (2003). When does the "duty to protect" apply with a client who has anorexia nervosa? *Counseling Psychologist, 31*(4), 427–450.

Wiener, D. J., and Oxford, L. K. (Eds.). (2003). *Action therapy with families and groups: Using creative arts improvisation in clinical practice.* Washington, DC: American Psychological Association.

Winn, L. (1995). Experiential training for staff working with eating disorders. In D. Doktor (Ed.), *Arts therapies and clients with eating disorders* (pp. 144–158). London: Jessica Kingsley Publishers.

Young, M. (1995). Dramatherapy in short–term groupwork with women with bulimia. In D. Doktor (Ed.), *Arts therapies and clients with eating disorders* (pp. 105–123). London: Jessica Kingsley Publishers.

Biography

Lisa D. Hinz, Ph.D., ATR is a clinical psychologist and registered art therapist. She is an adjunct faculty member in the Saint Mary–of–the–Woods College masters degree program in art therapy. Dr. Hinz is a consultant to the St. Helena Hospital Transformations Weight and Lifestyle Management Program in St. Helena, California.

AUTHOR INDEX

SUBJECT INDEX

A

ANAD, 57, 59, 78, 79

APA, 60, 63, 84, 92, 111, 124, 170, 172

Abuse, 9, 28, 38, 42–43, 49, 59–60, 62, 69, 73, 76, 78–81, 83–86, 89–90, 92–95, 97, 106–107, 113, 117, 119–120, 123, 138–139, 141, 160–161, 244, 255–256, 261, 267, 270, 282

Acculturation, 4–6, 9, 11, 161–162, 164, 170

Addiction, 14, 74, 101, 239, 255, 261

Alcohol, 59, 73, 78, 255, 266, 270

Alexithymia, 63, 74, 98, 215, 216, 273

Anger, 35, 59, 62, 75, 106, 151–152, 178, 190, 193, 229, 246, 252

Anorexia nervosa, 8, 9, 12, 14–16, 18, 26–27, 29, 32, 46, 48, 52–55, 57, 59, 62–63, 78–79, 84–85, 91, 93–97, 107–115, 119–125, 128–129, 131, 138–141, 146, 150, 156–158, 170, 176, 192, 195–196, 199, 202, 207, 210, 225–226, 228–230, 232–233, 238–239, 251–253, 256, 264, 267, 269, 272–273, 277, 281–283

Art therapy, 12–94

Attachment, 57, 60, 61, 78, 85, 86, 151, 193, 227, 234,

Binge, 7, 9, 12, 60, 73, 84, 87, 91, 95–96, 111, 138–140, 144, 146, 159–161, 163, 174, 176–177, 179, 182–185, 187–189, 192–193, 196, 199, 203–204, 226, 230, 250, 257, 260, 262, 272, 274

Bipolar, 73, 124,

Body Image, 4–5, 7, 9, 11, 13–17, 19, 22–23, 27–31, 34–36, 38, 43–44, 46, 49, 51–53, 55, 79, 83–88, 90–94, 116–117, 124, 126, 127, 129, 134, 162, 165, 171–172, 178–179, 184, 190, 193, 197, 208, 211, 216, 231, 252–253, 274, 279

Borderline Personality Disorder, 59, 60–61, 67–69, 80–81, 123, 139, 140, 175, 190

Bulimia, Bulimia nervosa, 4–6, 8–10, 12, 15, 27, 29, 46, 48, 52, 54–56, 59, 84, 94–96, 107–108, 122–123, 128, 138, 139–140, 150, 157, 161, 176, 195–196, 199, 202, 210, 225–226, 228, 230–233, 239, 251, 252–253, 255–256, 258, 262–263, 272, 277, 281–283

C

Cognitive Behavioral, 8, 10, 39, 64, 93, 117, 126, 139–141, 144, 175, 192–193

Collage, 37–38, 42–45, 49–51, 175, 179, 181, 188, 190

Collectivism, 9

Compartmentalization, 67–71, 76, 197

Compulsion(s), 59, 173, 175, 194–195, 200–206

Counter–transference, 38, 46, 244, 260, 264–265

Culture, 4–11

Cultural relativism, 9

D

Depersonalization, 67, 70, 74–75

Depression, 7, 41, 124, 126–127, 131, 138, 145, 176, 207, 226, 228, 239, 266

Diagnostic Drawing Series, 21, 27

Denial, 29, 67, 144, 164, 205, 288

Dissociation, 41, 59, 81, 87, 94, 149, 244, 266, 268

Drama therapy, 194–224